Immunosorption Techniques
Fundamentals and Applications

Immunosorption Techniques Fundamentals and Applications

by

Peter Mohr, Martin Holtzhauer
and Günter Kaiser

Akademie Verlag

Authors:

Prof. Dr. sc. nat. P. Mohr
Märkische Allee 62
O-1140 Berlin

Dr. rer. nat. Günter Kaiser
Erich-Kuttner-Str. 30
O-1156 Berlin

Dr. sc. nat. M. Holtzhauer
Max Delbrück Zentrum für
Molekulare Medizin
Robert-Rössle-Str. 10
O-1115 Berlin

1st edition 1992
Editorial Director: Christiane Grunow
Production Manager: Christian P. Biastoch
Composition: DARGE Fotosatz GmbH, Berlin
Printing and Bookbinding: Druckerei „G. W. Leibniz“, Gräfenhainichen
Cover design: Ralf Michaelis

with 54 Figures and 32 Tables

Die Deutsche Bibliothek – CIP-Einheitsaufnahme

Mohr, Peter:
Immunosorption techniques : fundamentals and applications ;
with 32 tables / by Peter Mohr ; Martin Holtzhauer ;
Günter Kaiser. – 1. ed. – Berlin : Akad.-Verl., 1992
ISBN 3-05-501350-6
NE: Holtzhauer, Martin:; Kaiser, Günter:

Printed of acid-free paper

Printed in the Federal Republic of Germany

Preface

The increasing interest in the application of immunoaffinity methods both for analytical and preparative purposes and for research as well as for commercial exploitation results primarily from the specificity and universality of the antigen-antibody reaction. Accordingly, it is possible today to obtain antibodies with high selectivity to nearly all organic and bioorganic molecules or parts of them.

Increasing knowledge of immunological structures and processes at the molecular and cellular level as well as better understanding of protein chemistry and biochemistry in the last few years were essential prerequisites for the present state-of-the-art in this field named 'immunosorption techniques'.

Though the development of the hybridoma techniques for generation and propagation of monoclonal antibodies has contributed substantially to the rapid progress of immunsorption techniques, the use of polyclonal antibodies is also still far from reaching its limits.

Whereas the first area of extended application of immunoaffinity techniques has been medical analysis (RIA, EIA), numerous immunosorption procedures are now increasingly introduced into other fields of analysis in both research and for commercial purposes. Moreover, many substances of biological origin have been identified, separated and purified in a preparative scale by using immunosorption methods. Immunoaffinity chromatography has also opened new possibilities for the separation of both subcellular particles and cells from biological material. Certainly, this trend will continue, and immunosorption techniques will gain increasing importance in the years to come.

The aim of the authors was to review the present knowledge of the application of immunosorption techniques with emphasis on separation processes. Other topics are immunoassays, immunoblotting and immunodot techniques, as well as immunosorption methods for therapeutic purposes and immunosensors. Immunoaffinity methods in clinical analysis have already been reviewed extensively elsewhere, and are therefore omited.

To facilitate the understanding of the matter fundamentals of immunology and affinity chromatography are dealt with in a condensed form. To present the practical approach too, some experimental protocols are also enclosed. An extensive literature index should facilitate a deeper penetration into special topics.

With this review, the autors address themselves above all to interested biochemists, physicians, pharmacists etc. in research and development as well as to students.

Many colleagues have supported our project. In particular, we should like to express our great appreciation for helpful critical discussions to Prof. Dr. F. Noll (Chapter 4.1.), Dr. H.-D. Hunger (Chapter 4.2.) and Prof. Dr. F. Scheller (Chapter 4.4.), which we hope have enabled us to provide a comprehensive, up-to-date coverage of these topics.

Thanks are also given to Prof.Dr. J. Lasch (Martin Luther University, Halle/Saale) and Drs. M. Gloger and K. Hallermayer (Boehringer Mannheim GmbH, Tutzing) for their helpful criticism of the manuscript.

Finally, we are indebted to Dr. R. Schön and Mr. H. Marquardt for linguistic help, Mrs. Ch. Meusel for the artwork, and Mrs. K. Haase for typing large parts of the manuscript. Moreover, we wish to express our gratitude to Mrs. Ch. Grunow and the staff of the Akademie Verlag for all their efforts.

Peter Mohr, Martin Holtzhauer, Günter Kaiser

Content

List of Abbreviations

ab = antibody
ABTS = 2,2'-azinobis(3-ethylbenzthiazoline-6-sulfonate)
Abx = mixed mode ion exchanger (BAKER CHEMICALS)
ACD = acid citrate dextrose blood
AET = 2-aminoethylisothiouronium bromide hydro-bromide
AFP = α-fetoprotein
AP = alkaline phosphatase
BLV = bovine leukemia virus
BMNC = bone marrow mononuclear cells
BSA = bovine serum albumin
CEA = carcinoembryonic antigen
ClCOONB = N-(chlorocarbonyloxy)-5-norbornene-2,3-dicarboximide
CM = carboxymethyl
CNBr = cyanogen bromide
ConA = Concanavalin A
D = Dalton (unit of molecular mass, 1 kD = 1,000 D)
DPBS = Dulbecco's PBS
DEAE = diethylaminoethyl
DMSO = dimethyl sulfoxide
DTT = dithiothreitol
EDTA = ethylenediaminetetraacetic acid
EGTA = ethylene glycol bis(2-aminoethylether)-N,N,N',N'-tetraacetic acid
FACS = fluorescence activated cell sorter
FCFD = fluorescence capillary fill device
FCS = fetal calf serum
FITC = fluorescein isothiocyanate
FL = fluorescein-labeled
FPLC = fast protein liquid chromatography (trade mark of PHARMACIA-LKB)
GOD = glucose oxidase
GPC = gel permeation chromatography
HAT = hypoxanthine/aminopterine/thymidine
Hb = hemoglobin
HBsAg = hepatitis B surface antigen
HBSS = Hank's balanced salt solution
HCG = human choriogonadotropin
HEPES = N-(2-hydroxyethyl)piperazine-N'-ethanesulfonic acid
HGG = horse gamma-globulin
hGH = human growth hormone
HIC = hydrophobic interaction chromatography
HLA = human leukocyte locus A-system
HPAC = high performance affinity chromatography
HPIAC = high performance immunoaffinity chromatography
HPIEC = high performance ion exchange chromatography
HPLC = high performance liquid chromatography
HRP = horseradish peroxidase
HSA = human serum albumin
IEF = isoelectric focusing
Ig = immunoglobulin (e.g. IgG, IgA, IgE, IgM, IgD)
IL = interleukin
IM = immunomagnetic
K = equilibrium constant
K_D = dissociation constant
KLH = keyhole limpet hemocyanin
lac = β-lactoside
mab = monoclonal antibody
MPC = magnetic particle concentrator (e.g. a cobalt-samarium magnet)
OA = ovalbumin
PAGE = polyacrylamide gel electrophoresis
PAN = PHARMACIA Application Note
PAP = prostatic alkaline phosphatase
PBMC = peripheral blood mononuclear cells
PBS = phosphate buffered saline
PEG = polyethylene glycol
PEM = PEM buffer = 100 mM PIPES, 1 mM EGTA, pH 6.75
pI = isoelectric point
PIPES = piperazine-N,N'-bis(2-ethane sulfonic acid)
PNP = p-nitrophenyl
POL = polymerized flagellin
PVP = polyvinylpyrrolidone
QAE = quarternary aminoethyl
QMA = quarternary methylamino
RP = reversed phase
SAW = surface acoustic wave
SC = secretory component
SDS = sodium dodecylsulfate
SGG = sheep gamma-globulin
SP = sulfopropyl
SPR = surface plasmon resonance
SRBC = sheep red blood cells
T-gel = $HO-C_2H_4-S-C_2H_4-SO_2-C_2H_4-$MATRIX
TBS = Tris buffered saline
TNP = trinitrophenyl
TSH = thyroid stimulating hormone

1. Introduction

Immunoaffinity chromatography combines both the advantages of solid phase liquid chromatography procedures and the highly specific reversible immunocomplex formation, thus resulting in one of the most powerful and almost universally applicable separation techniques so far developed. The other immunoaffinity applications also rest on antigen-antibody interactions. Generally, however, the reversibility of the complex formation does not play an essential role in these techniques. Although the principle of immunoaffinity methods is rather simple, a fundamental knowledge in immunology at molecular level is useful for a more profound understanding of these methods.

In the first chapters following, this monograph will deal briefly with some of the problems of antibody production as well as with antigen-antibody interaction. For more detailed information the reader should consult a textbook (e.g. Bier, 1986; Roitt et al., 1989).

1.1. Fundamental Remarks on the Immune System

The fundamental principle of immunology is that the organism of humans and almost all animals is more or less able to distinguish between "self" and "nonself" and to eliminate "substances" (e.g. microorganisms, viruses, soluble and insoluble biomacromolecules) recognized as "nonself". In autoimmune diseases this capability is disturbed, and antibodies as well as cellular reactions against "self" tissues are induced.

During evolution, protection systems have developed from simple immunocytes (amoebocytes) in azoelomates to a very sophisticated immune system in vertebrates (deuterostomiata), consisting of several organs and a network of specific, nonspecific and regulatory mechanisms.

Skin and mucous membranes normally are a first efficient barrier to prevent "substances" from entering the body. Fig. 1.1. shows in a very simplified manner what happens if this first barrier is surmounted (fat arrows in Fig. 1.1. - 1.4. indicate special relevance for antibody production). Substances recognized as "self" are tolerated (e.g. autotransplantates). "Nonself substances", especially particles such as viruses and cells can be attacked by phagocytes (micro- and macrophages) or by natural killer cells. These mechanisms are nonspecific and do not have any relevance to immunoaffinity techniques. "Nonself substances", either not or not completely eliminated by phagocytosis cause a specific immunoresponse and are designated as antigens.

Strictly speaking, a definite distinction between specific and nonspecific mechanisms is impossible since there are several important interactions (not shown in Fig. 1.1.). On the one hand, the specific response can be triggered by a nonspecific mechanism. In this case special nonspecific cells pick up the antigen and "present" it (antigen-presenting cells) to other immunocompetent cells (lymphocytes), thus improving or even allowing antigen recognition and activation of these cells. On the other hand, phagocytosis and killer cell activities can be improved or mediated by specific antibodies reacting with the antigen or by specifically activated complement factors (immunophagocytosis, antibody dependent cellular

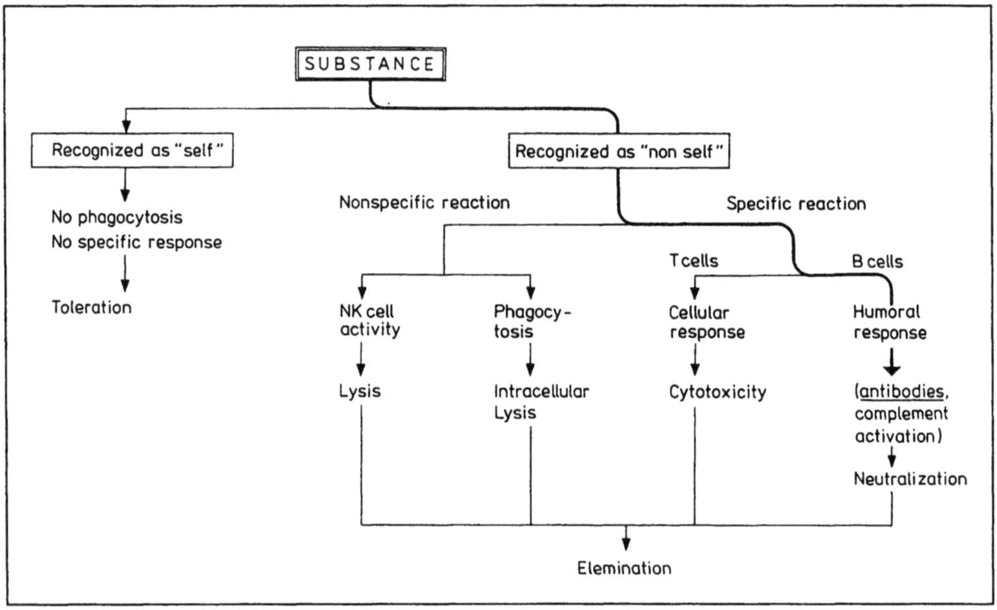

Fig. 1.1. Main effects of the immune system in vivo.

cytotoxicity) or by products of antigen specific T cells.

Thus because of the essential interactions and cell cooperation both (a) the humoral immunity which is very important in acute bacterial infections and (b) the cellular immunity which plays the dominant role in response to viral, fungal and chronical bacterial infections, in autoimmune diseases and in transplantate rejection, cannot be strictly separated from each other.

1.1.1. Differentiation of B and T Lymphocytes

All important processes of specific response are regulated or even performed by B and T lymphocytes. All the lymphocytes and other blood cells originate from pluripotent stem cells permanently produced in bone marrow, the most important organ of hematopoesis and immune system. Already, in this organ, first differentiation of these cells occurs. A scheme of immune and blood cell differentiation is presented in Fig. 1.2. All cells resulting from the myeloic stem (polymorph cells, mast cells, monocytes etc.) are not of direct interest in respect of antibody production, despite antigen presentation. Differentiation of lymphoid cells is markedly determined by the primary lymphatic organs (Fig. 1.3.). Lymphocytes developing in the thymus become T cells (T from thymus), whereas B cells were named according to a special organ in birds - the bursa fabricii - where they are developed. An equivalent organ was not found in mammals, but the function of B cell formation is fulfiled by other organs: mature bone marrow, fetal liver and spleen. Further proliferation and differentiation of both B and T lymphocytes mainly occurs in the secondary lymphatic organs (spleen, lymph nodes and lymphoepithelial system; see Fig. 1.3.) and not in circulation. Although receptors and mechanisms of antigen recognition are quite different for B and T cells, the subsequent processes of proliferation and differentiation occur in a very similar manner for both (Fig. 1.4.). Antigen specific cells of a pool of resting B and T lymphocytes are sensitized by antigen contact. After a period of latency they start to proliferate (B and T blasts) and differentiate to

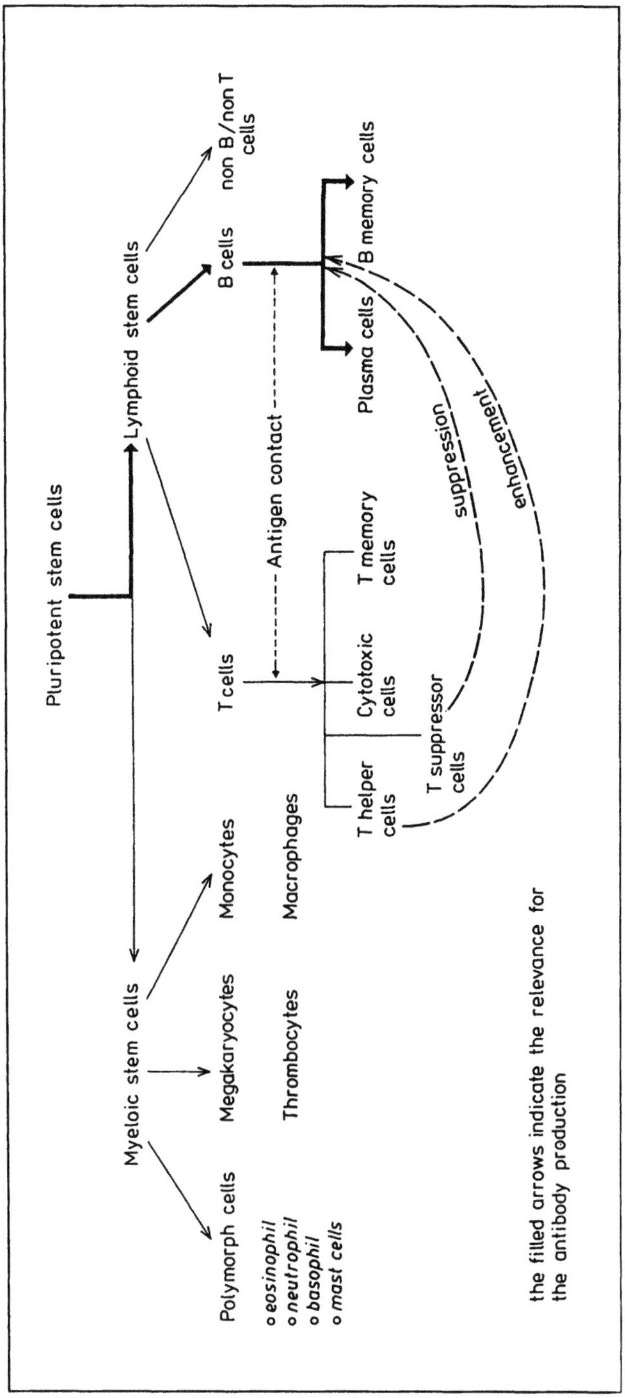

Fig. 1.2. Differentiation of cells of the immune system.

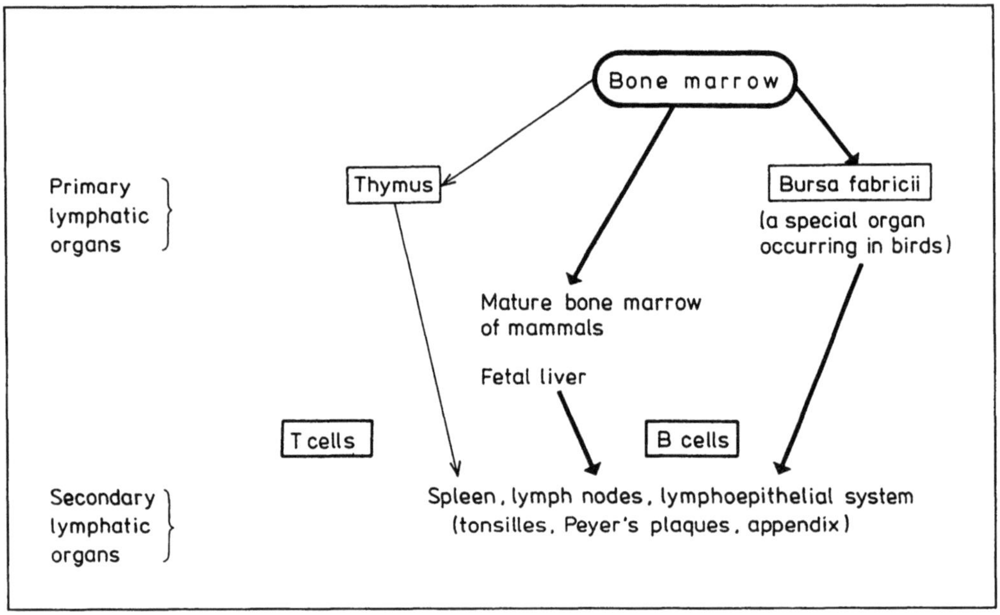

Fig. 1.3. Organs of the immune system.

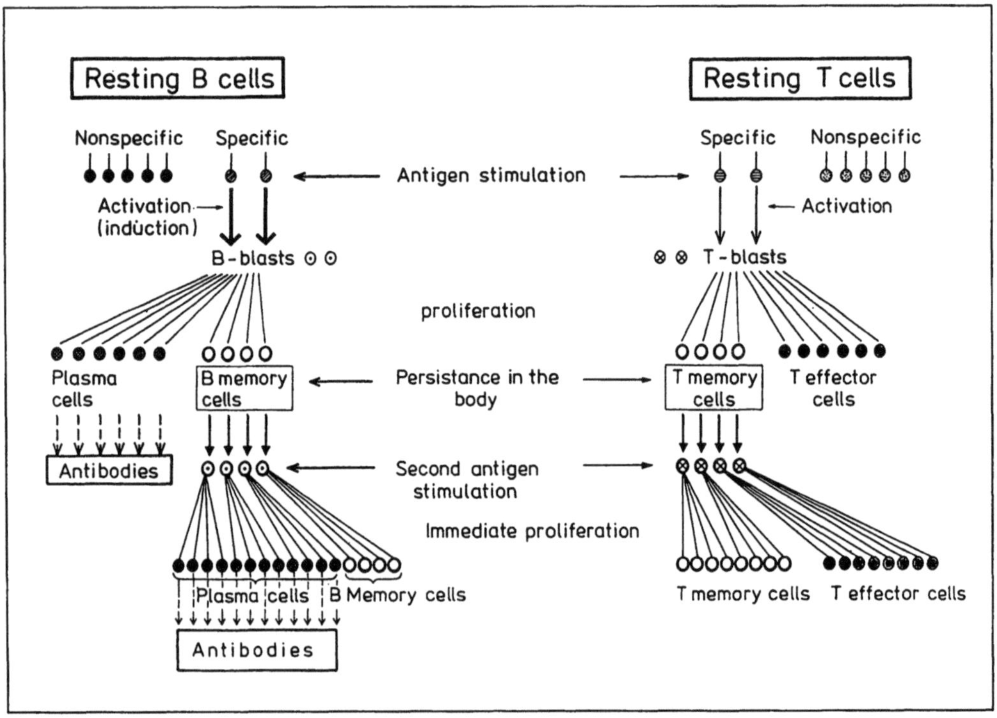

Fig. 1.4. Primary and secondary B and T cell response.

effector cells (plasma cells and cytotoxic or regulatory T cells, respectively) and to memory cells which do not continue to proliferate. Whereas effector cells fulfil their specific functions (as will be described later on) and die, this is not the case with memory cells. They persist in the body for a long period of time (often for the whole life) as resting, but antigen sensitized lymphocytes (designated as immunological memory). In the case of repeated contacts with this antigen, they "remember" the first antigen stimulation, start immediately to proliferate and produce an increased number of new effector and memory cells, thus ensuring a markedly accelerated and increased second immunoresponse in comparison to that after the first antigen contact. The early period of the first B cell response results mainly in IgM antibodies, whereas later on and in a second or following response, IgG antibodies dominate. These facts have to be taken into account when developing immunization strategies for specific antibody production.

1.1.2. Antigen Recognition and Immunoresponse

Resting B and T lymphocytes carry receptors on their surface that are capable of recognizing and binding the antigen specifically (Fig. 1.5.). The capability of binding the antigen is a prerequisite for specific activation of these cells, e.g. for the processes described above. Antigen receptors of B and T cells recognize, like antibodies, only a small part of the antigen (see Chapter 1.2.3.), designated as the antigenic determinant or **epitope**. It is important to know that all receptors expressed by a single lymphocyte normally are specific only for a given epitope (polyfunctional antigen-binding sites covering more than one epitope can occur), i.e. a cell can be activated only by antigens possessing its specific epitope. Different lymphocytes carry different receptors. The large diversity of immunoresponse is guaranteed by the large number of lymphocytes and the large diversity of receptors. An efficient co-operation between T cells and B cells is possible, since B cells and T cells recognize *different* epitopes of the antigen, e.g.

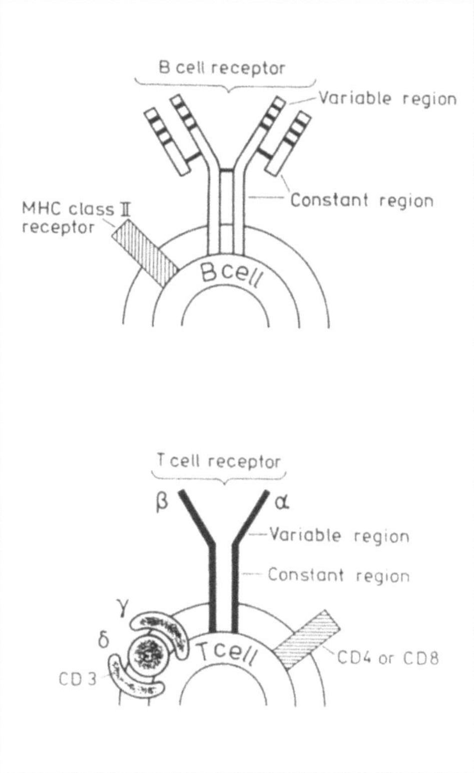

Fig. 1.5. Comparison of B and T cell receptors.

haptens (cf. Chapter 1.2.3.) are recognized by B cells, whereas T cells recognize the immunogenic carrier.

B cells and most T cells are not able to recognize free antigens. For an efficient recognition, the antigen has to be brought into close association with molecules of the "self" MHC (**m**ajor **h**istocompatibility **c**omplex). Antigen presenting cells that carry MHC molecules on their surface meet these conditions. Whereas antigen receptors of B cells are known to be immunoglobulins in neighbourhood to a MHC class II receptor, the T cell receptor is a more integrated system, consisting of an antigen recognizing part and a MHC recognizing part, which can function only together (Fig. 1.5.).

Cytotoxic T cells recognize antigens in connection with MHC class I molecules, whereas T helper cells need MHC class II molecules for antigen recognition. T suppressor cells are MHC independent and capable of binding free antigen. T helper cells promote and T suppressor cells decrease immunoresponse. The regulatory T cells can affect either T cells or B cells.

Strictly speaking, T cells and T cell products are not relevant to immunoaffinity techniques since T cells themselves do not produce antibodies. But T cells merely affect B cell activation (T inducer cells) or proliferation (T suppressor and T helper cells), thus being an important regulatory factor of antibody production and of humoral response in general. Most antigens even essentially need T cells to be capable of B cell induction (thymus dependent antigens).

Antibodies, the specifically reacting molecules used in all affinity techniques, are produced by B lymphocytes. However, most steps of B cell development are antigen independent.

Differentiation of B cells in mammals is markedly influenced by fetal liver and after birth by mature bone marrow. The most important B cell markers are surface immunoglobulins (sIg) functioning as antigen receptors. During differentiation from lymphoid stem cells to B cell precursors, the many different genes coding for the immunoglobulins are accidentally rearranged, thus resulting in the large diversity of immunoglobulins. B cell precursors still do not express sIg, but free μ chains are found in their cytoplasm. During further differentiation other heavy chains are expressed (α, γ, δ, ε). With the synthesis of light chains (κ or λ) and the arrangement to Ig molecules the specificity of a cell is permanently fixed. Imature B cells express only sIgM and are capable of only IgM response, whereas on mature B cells different classes of sIg (cf. Chapter 1.2.1.) can be found even on one cell. This is the case since B cells can switch to other sIg classes without loosing sIgM, but only the new receptor can be activated thereafter.

All receptors on a single B cell have the same specificity, and all plasma cells originating from this cell (B cell clone) produce antibodies of this specificity and of only one class or subclass. Since most antigens carry many different epitopes, they can activate different B cells with receptors also specific for different epitopes. Fig. 1.6. shows the principle of clonal selection in B cell activation.

Mature plasma cells (Fig. 1.7.) - the "factories" of antibody production - are widely differentiated cells which do not continue to proliferate. Normally they do not carry sIg since its receptor function is no longer necessary. Plasma cells contain a large amount of basophil (high RNA content) cytoplasm and a large endoplasmatic reticulum responsible for antibody synthesis. Glycosylation of the antibody molecules is performed by the Golgi apparatus. The antibodies produced fill the whole cytoplasm and are secreted into the body fluid.

The main physiological function of the antibodies is to bind the antigen forming an immunocomplex. This reaction alone normally does not result in an elimination of "nonself" substances. Only several bacterial toxins and viruses can be directly eliminated by neutralizing antibodies. But antibodies perform several effector functions which are important for antigen elimination. Most important among these functions is the activation of the complement system which represents a group of serum proteins. The activated complement components can either themselves eliminate the antigen, activate phagocytes or "label" antigens (e.g. bacteria) for an improved phagocytosis (opsonization). Furthermore, antibodies can interact with several types of cells via Fc receptors. When bound to macrophages, IgG can improve and specify phagocytosis (immunophagocytosis) and IgE can activate mast cells (histamin production) and basophil cells. Interactions with lymphocytes are also possible (e.g. feedback regulation of the antibody production). These examples demonstrate that antibodies play a central role in the complex immune system of vertebrates.

1.2. Antibodies and Antigens

1.2.1. Structure of Immunoglobulins

On account of their physicochemical properties (the globular structure) and immunological

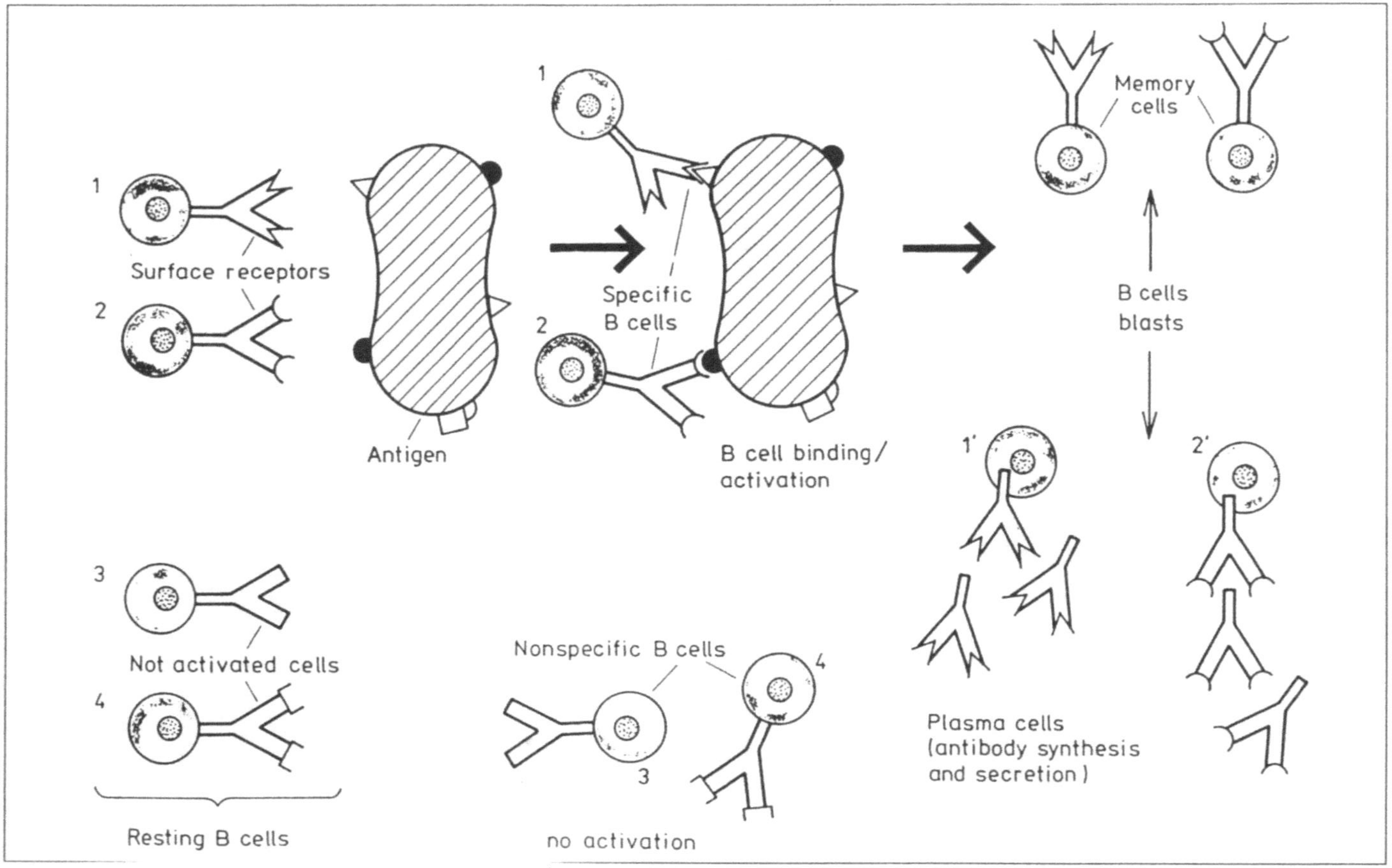

Fig. 1.6. Principle of clonal selection in antibody production.
The B cells 1 and 2 carry receptors (surface immunoglobulins) fitting epitopes of the antigen. They are bound to the antigen and activated. Subsequently, they proliferate and differentiate to plasma cells (1' and 2') which produce and secrete two different antigen specific antibodies. The receptors of the B cells 3 and 4 do not fit the antigen and, therefore they are not activated.

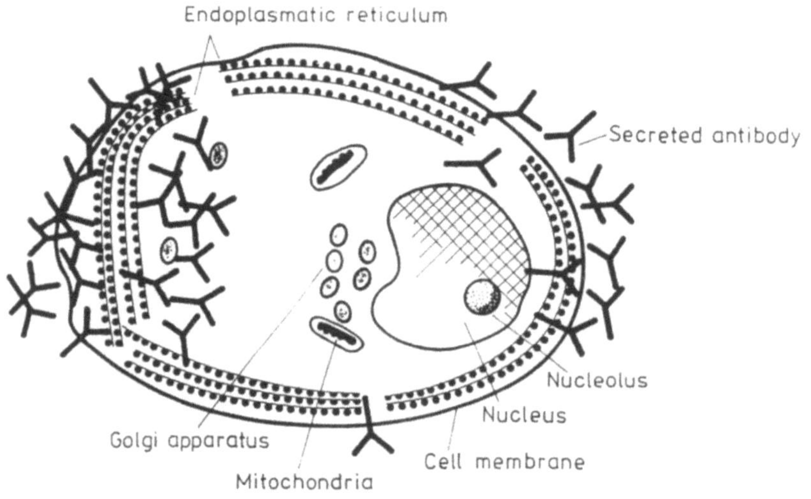

Fig. 1.7. Mature plasma cell with antibodies both even secreted and still contained in the cytoplasma. The rough endoplasmatic reticulum is arranged in parallel rows. The Golgi apparatus is responsible for glycosylation of the antibodies. All cytoplasma spaces are filled with antibodies which permeate through the cell membrane and leave the cell. Sometimes, antibodies are located in Russel's bodies.

activities, the whole group of antibodies and the antigen receptors of B cells were named immunoglobulins. The only difference between secretory (antibodies) and surface immunoglobulins (receptors) is in the C terminal sequence of amino acids of heavy chains. The surface immunoglobulins are prolonged by several additional amino acids, these being anchored in the B cell membrane, thus fixing the receptor to the cell surface.

The basic structure consisting of four polypeptide chains is practically the same in all immunoglobulins (Fig. 1.8.). Two identical heavy chains (H) and two identical light chains (L) are connected jointly by disulfide bonds and non-covalent interactions. In all immunoglobulins the H chains are associated with carbohydrate residues. Therefore, immunoglobulins are glycoproteins. The L chains do not carry carbohydrates. The C terminal regions of the H and L chains show a high degree of homology in their amino acid sequence and structure (constant regions: C_L and

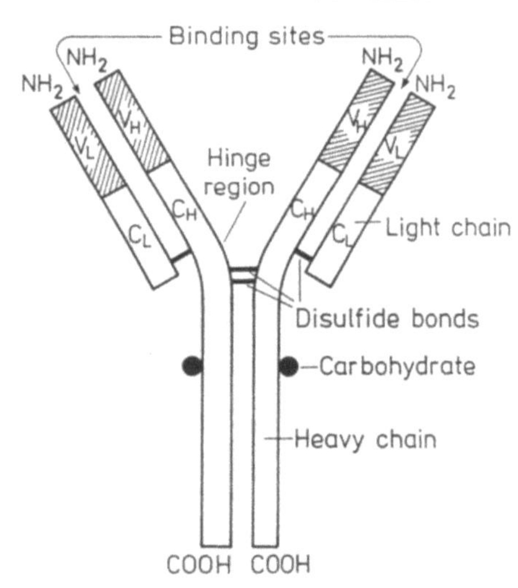

Fig. 1.8. Y model of immunoglobulins.
V_H and V_L, variable regions of heavy and light chains, respectively. —, disulfide bonds.

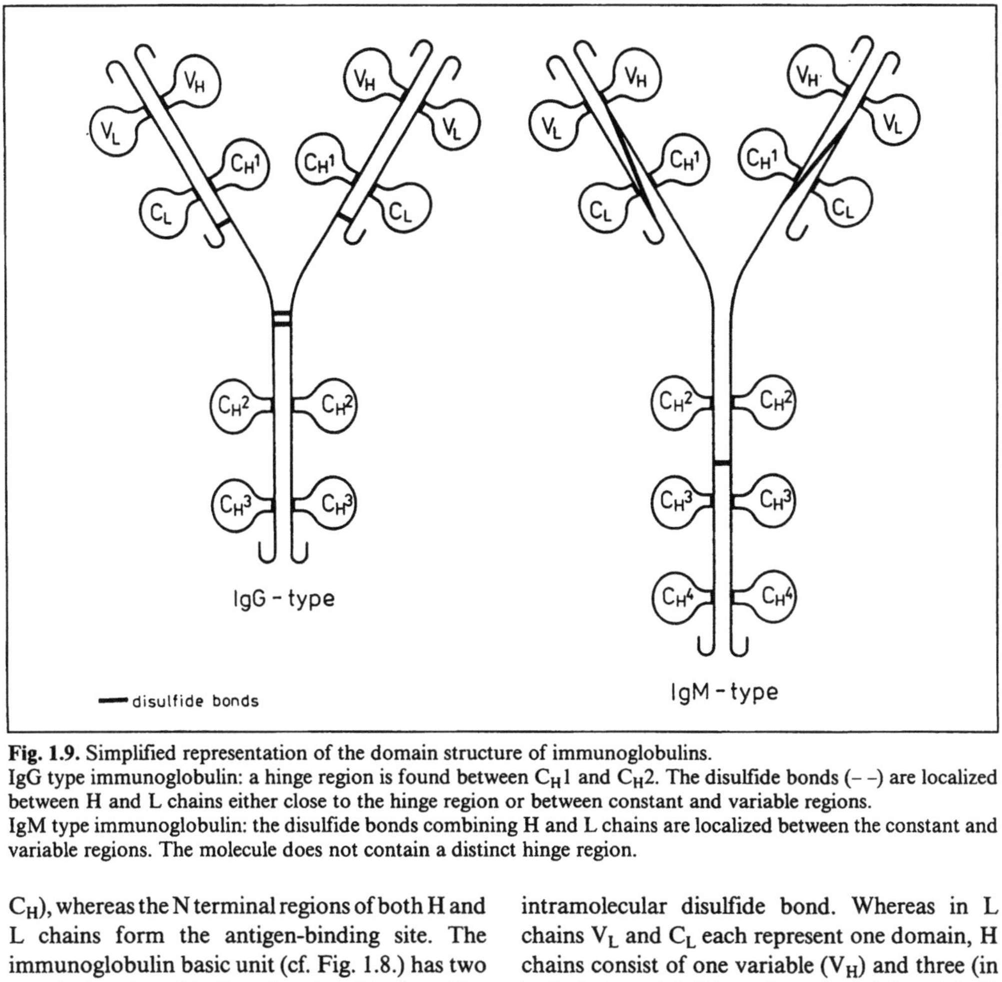

Fig. 1.9. Simplified representation of the domain structure of immunoglobulins.
IgG type immunoglobulin: a hinge region is found between C_H1 and C_H2. The disulfide bonds (– –) are localized between H and L chains either close to the hinge region or between constant and variable regions.
IgM type immunoglobulin: the disulfide bonds combining H and L chains are localized between the constant and variable regions. The molecule does not contain a distinct hinge region.

C_H), whereas the N terminal regions of both H and L chains form the antigen-binding site. The immunoglobulin basic unit (cf. Fig. 1.8.) has two identical antigen-binding sites; it is **bivalent**. The hinge region is a part, not exactly defined, of the constant regions of H chains between the domains C_H1 and C_H2 (see below), which is very flexible in the tertiary structure. This flexibility makes it possible to alter the distance between the two antigen binding sites, so that sterical hindrance can be overcome. The constant regions are not involved in the binding of antigens, but they stabilize the structure of the antibody molecule, and the C_H regions are responsible for the effector functions of antibodies.

Both H and L chains consist of globular domains, each of these being stabilized by an intramolecular disulfide bond. Whereas in L chains V_L and C_L each represent one domain, H chains consist of one variable (V_H) and three (in IgG, IgA and IgD) or four (in IgM and IgE) constant domains (C_H1, C_H2, C_H3 and C_H4). The additional domain in IgM and IgE is placed between C_H1 and C_H2 and a hinge region has not been found there. Fig. 1.9. shows the domain structure in a very simple manner. In reality the polypeptide chain within each domain is folded several times to form the globular structure.

Immunoglobulin Classes and Subclasses

In most mammals there occur five different classes of immunoglobulins: IgG, IgM, IgA, IgD and IgE.

Table 1.1. Most Important Physiological and Chemical Parameters of Human Immunoglobulins

Immunoglobulin	IgG1	IgG2	IgG3	IgG4	IgM	IgA1	IgA2	sIgA	IgD	IgE
Middle of serum concentration [mg/ml]	9	3	1	0.5	1.5	3.0	0.5	0.05	0.03	0.00005
Molecular mass [D]	146.000	146.000	170.000	146.000	970.000	160.000	160.000	385.000	184.000	188.000
Chain structure	$2\gamma_1$; 2L	$2\gamma_2$; 2L	$2\gamma_3$; 2L	$2\gamma_4$; 2L	$10\,\mu$; 10L; 1J	$2\alpha_1$; 2L	$2\alpha_2$; 2L	$4\alpha_1$; or α_2; 4L; 1J; 1SC	2δ; 2L	2ε; 2L
Molecular mass of heavy chain [D]	51.000	51.000	60.000	51.000	65.000	56.000	52.000	52.000-56.000	69.700	72.500
Number of heavy chain domains	4	4	4	4	5	4	4	4	4	5
Carbohydrate content [%]	2-3	2-3	2-3	2-3	12	7-11	7-11	7-11	9-14	12
Localization of carbohydrates	C_H2	C_H2	C_H2	C_H2	C_H1-4	C_H1-3	C_H1-3	C_H1-3	C_H1-3	C_H1-3
Disulfide bonds between heavy chains	2	4	15	2	1	1	1	1	1	2

Light chain (L) can be κ or λ in each case SC secretory component J joining chain

The class of an antibody is determined by the type of the H chain it contains ($\gamma, \mu, \alpha, \delta$ or ε). L chains occur in two different types (κ or λ). Each type of L chain can combine with each type of H chain, but within one molecule the L chains are of the same type, thus each class of immunoglobulins can occur in κ or λ form.

Furthermore, the immunoglobulin classes differ in their carbohydrate content and localization as well as in the degree of polymerization. For instance, the carbohydrate content of human immunoglobulins varies between 2 - 3 % in IgG and 12 - 14 % in IgM, IgD and IgE. Whereas in IgG carbohydrates are localized only in the C_H2 domain in other classes carbohydrates are found in several C_H domains. In IgA, IgD and IgE the C_H1 domain is particularly rich in carbohydrates, and in IgA even the V_H domain can carry carbohydrate residues. IgA in human serum is mainly monomeric, whereas in sera of most mammals IgA polymers (mainly dimers) dominate. Dimeric secretory IgA, found in all seromucous secretes, is a very important factor in the infection barrier. IgM normally occurs as pentamer. The γ and α chains occur in different subtypes, e.g. in humans the γ_1, γ_2, γ_3, γ_4 chains and α_1 and α_2 chains respectively, thus forming the immunoglobulin subclasses: IgG1, IgG2, IgG3, IgG4 and IgA1, IgA2, respectively. The subclasses of any class show a higher degree of homology among one another than do immunoglobulins of different classes. The immunoglobulin classes and subclasses and the types of L chain can be discriminated by specific antibodies, thus an exact classification of immunoglobulins is possible. As an example Table 1.1. lists the most important physiological and chemical parameters of human immunoglobulins. Immunoglobulins of other species are similar in their properties.

Although IgG subclass variations are found in most mammals, these subclasses are not comparable from species to species, because obviously the

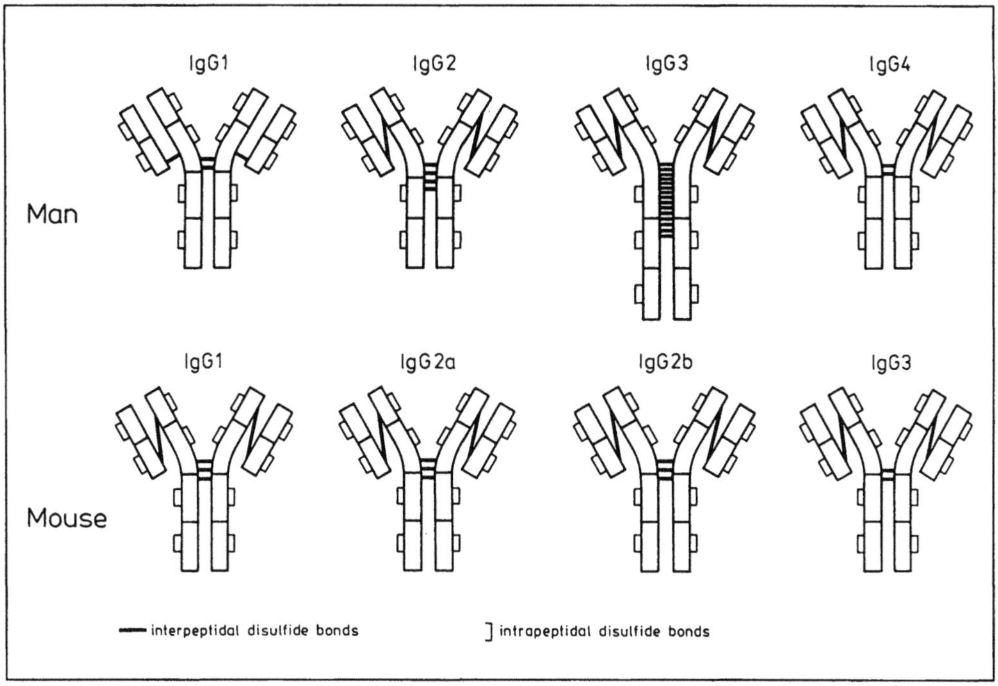

Fig. 1.10. Arrangement of polypeptide chains in IgG subclasses of man and mouse.
The C_H2 domain of human IgG3 is markedly prolonged (cf. the molecular weight of heavy chains in Table 1.1.). In mouse IgG2a and IgG2b the number of disulfide bonds is the same and their position is very similar, but there are differences in the chain structure.

subclass variations have developed phylogenetically very late. Fig. 1.10. illustrates the differences between IgG subclasses of man and mouse. The differences are clearly visible concerning the number and the position of interpeptidal disulfide bonds, but there are also clear differences in the molecular structure of the chains. In these properties even rat and mouse subclasses differ markedly from each other.

In polymeric immunoglobulins (IgA and IgM) an additional polypeptide chain is found, the joining chain (**J**), which together with disulfide bonds between the single units stabilizes the structure of the whole molecule. Secretory IgA, furthermore, contains a secretory component (SC), which is synthesized not in B cells, but in epithelial cells and which is bound to the dimeric IgA molecule during passage through the epithelial tissue. SC improves the transport of sIgA and prevents it from proteolytic degradation. The structure of IgM is similar to a star, whereas sIgA looks like a doubled Y (Fig. 1.11.).

The immunoglobulin classes most frequently used in immunoaffinity techniques are IgG and IgM, with IgG by far dominating. But IgA is also used, and tests for specific IgE are important in diagnosis of allergies. IgD is not relevant for *in vitro* methods.

Variations and Diversity of Immunoglobulins

Three important types of variations determine the variability of antibodies:

The genes for **isotypical** variants are present in all healthy individuals of a species. These variations mainly concern the C_H region, e.g. the immunoglobulin classes and subclasses), but also

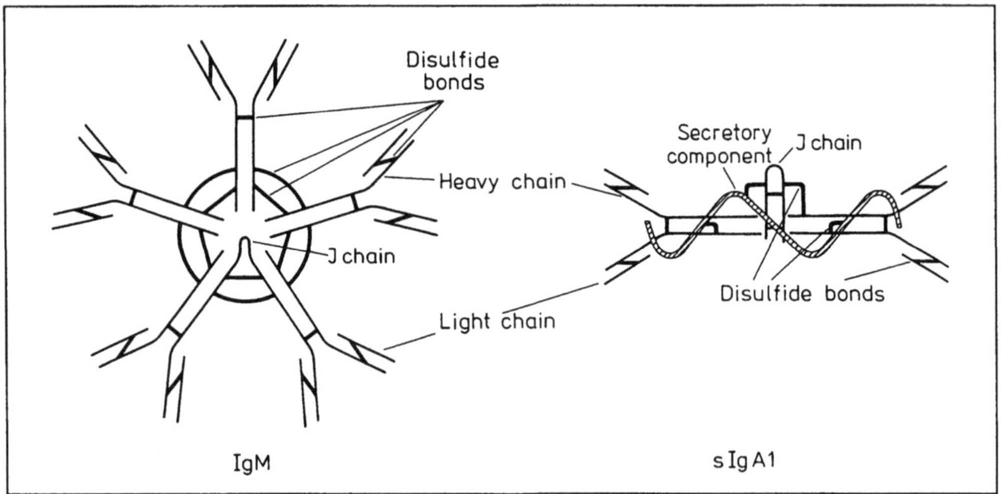

Fig. 1.11. Simplified representation of the structure of IgM and secretory IgA1.
IgM. The subunits are connected by disulfide bonds between C_H3 domains. The localization of the J chain is not exactly known.
Secretory IgA1. The J chain is connected via disulfide bonds with the C_H3 domains, and the secretory component with the C_H2 domains of each IgA1 subunit.

the C_L region (type of L chain) and the framework (relatively constant) parts of V_L and V_H (subgroups) contribute to the isotype. The **allotypical** variations are such within one species concerning different allels of special gene loci in C_L and C_H. The special allotypes are not expressed by all individuals of the species. Neither isotypical nor allotypical variations concern the antigen-binding site. The **idiotypical** variations concern the diversity of V_H and V_L, i.e., the *antigen-binding site* or regions close to it, which means that idiotypical variations determine the specificity of the antibody. The idiotype is the complete set of determinants of the variable regions. Idiotypes are normally specific for individual antibody clones but can also be common to several clones. The single determinants recognizable by anti-idiotypical antibodies are **idiotopes**, these being localized inside and outside the antigen binding site (the paratope) of the antibody molecule. Anti-idiotypical antibodies against an idiotope inside the paratope inhibit antigen binding, whereas those recognizing an idiotype outside the pararatope do not. The idiotypical variations are independent of class, subclass, type and allotype of the antibody.

The genetic origin of the large diversity of immunoglobulins cannot be explained here in detail. The NOBEL Prize of 1986 was awarded to S. TONEGAWA for his outstanding results concerning generation of antibody diversity (see TONEGAWA, 1983). During B cell development there occurs an extensive rearrangment of DNA which is briefly explained here for mouse immunoglobulins. The L chains are coded by a VJ system. For κ chains this means that during rearrangement, one of several hundred different V genes coding for the main part of the V region can combine with one of four J genes (a fifth one is never translated) coding for that part of the V region which is joined to the C region, and with the C gene for the C domain. Thus a large number of different combinations is possible. The λ chains are less variable (two different V genes and four different J genes). The V region of heavy chains is coded by three gene segments, VJ and an additional D (diversity) segment. Here, one of several hundred different V genes can combine with one of 12 different D

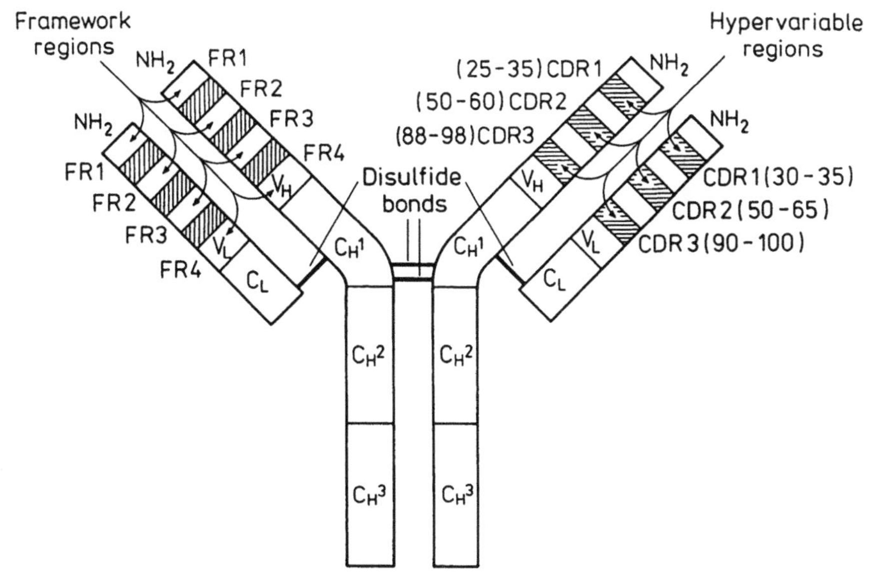

Fig. 1.12. Hypervariable and framework regions of V_H and V_L.
The hypervariable regions (hatched) of V_H and V_L named CDR1 - CDR3 (complementarity determining regions) starting from the N terminus.
The framework regions (FR1 - FR4) which are relatively homologous in different antibodies are responsible for folding of the polypeptide chains. In the drawing the polypeptide chains are unfolded. The numbers in brackets indicate the approximate amino acid positions of CDRs.

segments and one of four different J segments, and each of the possible VDJ combinations can combine with each of the different C gene combinations coding for the constant region, i.e. the immunoglobulin classes and subclasses. This guarantees an enormous diversity. Additionally, diversities are generated by variable recombinations and by somatic mutations. Thus, one can assume that the B cells are capable of synthesizing antibodies against any possible antigen.

The Antigen-binding Site

The antigen-binding site is formed only by the V domains of both heavy and light chains. The variability is not distributed homogeneously over the whole V domain: there exist three parts with a very high variability (hypervariable regions) and four parts with a relatively high degree of homology (framework regions) in both V_H and V_L (Fig. 1.12.). The hypervariable regions are numbered CDR1 - CDR3 (complementarity determining regions) starting from the N terminus of the chains. The six CDRs of V_H and V_L together form the antigen-binding site, whereas the eight framework regions (FR1 - FR4 of each chain) together with the intrapeptidal disulfide bonds fold the polypeptide chain in a manner arranging the CDRs of both chains spatially close together, so that they can form a "bag" similar to that known from the active center of enzymes (Fig. 1.13.). Several amino acids of the single CDRs are directly involved in the antigen binding, but the exchange of only one of them in one of the CDRs would alter the shape of the "bag" sufficiently so as

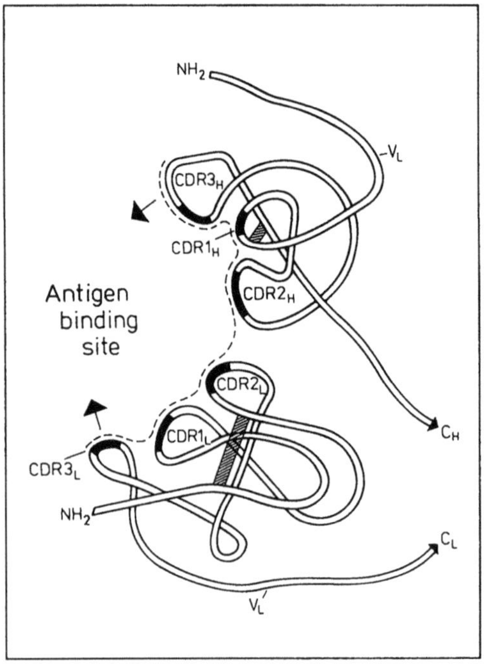

Fig. 1.13. Simplified representation of the antigen-binding site.
CDRs (filled) of V_H and V_L are arranged close together to form the antigen-binding site. The structure is stabilized by the framework regions (blank) and the intrapeptidal disulfide bonds (hatched).

to result in a different specificity of the binding site. The three-dimensional structure of the "bag" is the most important factor of the antigen recognition.

Taking into consideration that there are six CDRs, each consisting of 10 - 15 amino acid positions, and that each of these positions can be occupied by one of 20 different amino acids, the variability of binding sites is immense. By altering the folding of polypeptide chains the framework regions can also influence the antigen-binding site, although they are never directly involved in the binding of antigen.

1.2.2. Antibody Fragments

For some applications (e.g. for therapeutical use) it can be useful to separate antigen binding from other functions of antibodies, such as complement activation or binding to monocytes. Since these functions are localized in the constant regions of the heavy chains far away from the antigen-binding site, fragmentation of antibodies can solve this problem. Two enzymes are mainly used in the fragmentation of IgG molecules (Fig. 1.14.):

(a) The plant proteinase **papain** cleaves the chains in the hinge region of the IgG molecule resulting in two identical Fab fragments (**a**ntigen **b**inding **f**ragment antibodies; molecular weight 50,000 D) and one Fc fragment (**f**ragment **c**rystalline; molecular weight 60,000 D). The Fab fragments are monovalent antigen binding units. The disulfide bonds between the γ chains stabilize the Fc fragment. It is possible to cleave the Fab fragment by mild reduction into the free L chain and the Fd fragment (N terminal half of the H chain), which usually do not bind antigen.

(b) **Pepsin** digestion results in a $F(ab')_2$ fragment (molecular weight 100,000 D), and a pFc' fragment (mainly the C_H3 domain). The C_H2 domain is split into small peptides. $F(ab')_2$ is a bivalent antigen binding fragment which contains the complete hinge region, i.e. concerning the antigen binding it has the same properties as a complete antibody, but it does not bind to complement or monocytes.

Mild reduction of IgG results in two monovalent half molecules, i.e. only the disulfide bonds between the H chains are cleaved, whereas by strong reduction the four single chains are obtained. Half molecules can be recombined to complete antibodies. Even combination of two different half molecules (NISONOFF and PALMER, 1964) or Fab' fragments (NISONOFF and RIVERS, 1961) is possible, resulting in a bivalent hybrid antibody with two different antigen-binding sites within one molecule. Such bispecific antibodies are produced today more efficiently by the hybrid-hybridoma technique (cf. Chapter 1.3.3.).

1.2.3. Antigens and Haptens

In this section in the main we are concerned with defining terms:

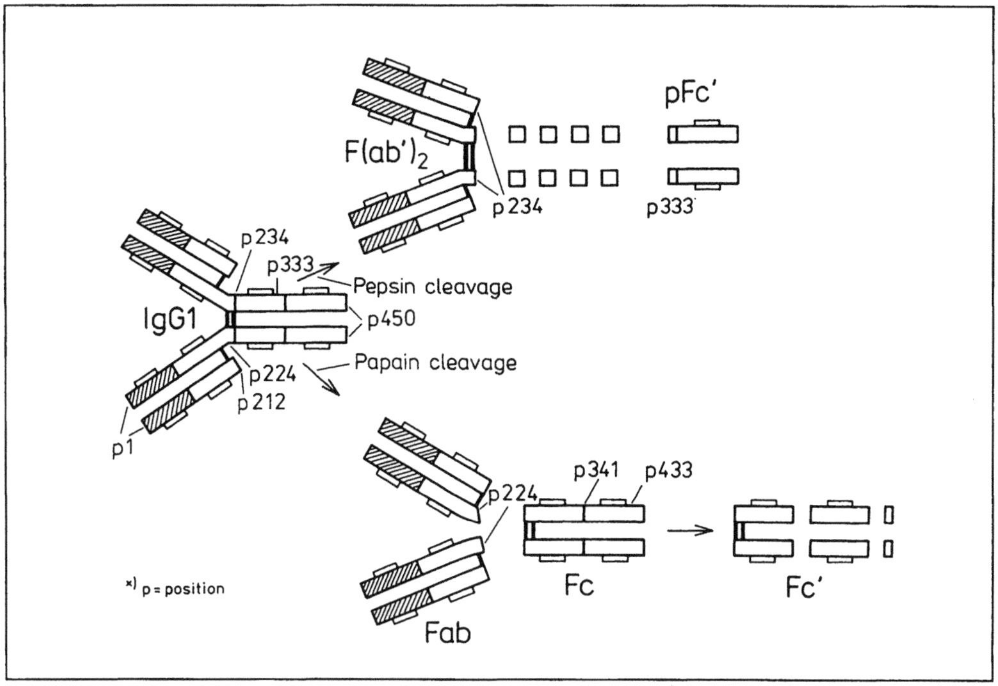

Fig. 1.14. Enzymatic cleavage of IgG (human IgG1).

Antigens are substances which are able to elicit an immunoresponse. A prerequisite is that they are "nonself", because "self" substances are tolerated. Against "self" substances an immunoresponse is induced only in exceptional cases (autoantigens, tumor antigens = altered "self", idiotypes of antibodies). Most antigens are very complex compounds (e.g. biomacromolecules like proteins, glycoproteins, polysaccharides, bacterial toxins, surface antigens of viruses or microorganisms, allergens). Antigens can be classified from several points of view (chemical structure, origin, marker antigens etc.). Concerning immunoaffinity chromatography for example the chemical classification is of special interest for the choice of appropriate running conditions.

Antigenicity is the ability of a substance to induce an immunoresponse and to react specifically with the products of this response (antibodies or sensitized lymphocytes); this means that an antigen is characterized by two important properties: Specificity and immunogenicity.

Specificity of an antigen means that the antigen induces antibodies which react selectively with the inducing antigen or with compounds very similar to it (cf. Specificity of antibodies). The specificity is markedly determined by the spatial structure and charge distribution within the antigen. Charged structures normally induce antibodies with opposite charge in the antigen-binding site. But only small parts of the antigen molecule (e.g. 7-8 amino acids in proteins; 3 - 7 sugar residues in polysaccharides) designated as antigenic **determinants** or **epitopes** (both terms are used almost equivalently in the literature) are directly concerned. Normally an antigen has many different epitopes, which can overlap. In this case it is polyvalent (Fig. 1.15.) and the sum of epitopes is the valency of the antigen. This means that one antigen can induce many different antibodies, each of them specific to a single epitope, but all of them are able to bind the whole antigen molecule. Such antibodies can be produced as monoclonal antibodies, and these can be used for analyzing the epitope pattern of the

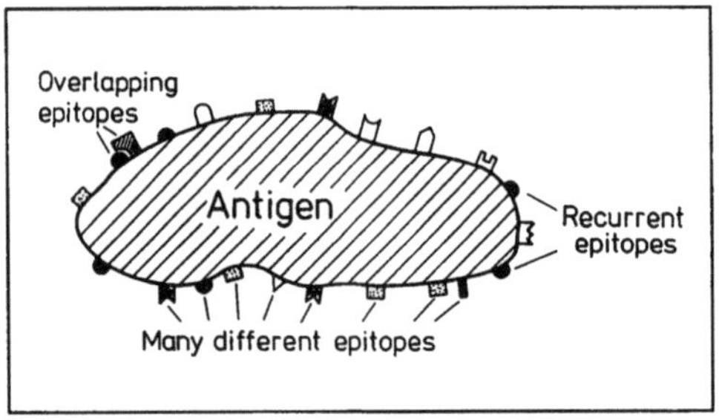

Fig. 1.15. Simplified representation of the polyvalency of an antigen.
The antigen carries numerous different epitopes; overlapping and recurrent epitopes occur.

antigen (epitope mapping). This has been done for many proteins, e.g. for human α-fetoprotein (MICHEEL et al., 1984).

Epitopes can occur several times on an antigen (recurrent antigens), but single epitopes can also occur on different antigens. Antibodies specific to those epitopes would react with all of these antigens (cross-reactivity). In proteins one can distinguish between sequence epitopes and conformational epitopes. Sequence epitopes enclose a distinct amino acid sequence within a polypeptide chain. Antibodies against sequence epitopes also react with denatured protein or with peptides containing the appropriate sequence. Conformational epitopes dominate by far in most native proteins. These epitopes are formed by groups of amino acids arranged closely together in the **spatial** structure of the proteins. Conformational epitopes are demolished by protein denaturation, whereas other epitopes can be found in denatured proteins which do not occur in the native molecules, i.e. preferably the complementary three-dimensional structures of epitope and paratope are responsible for antigen-antibody reaction. This has to be taken into consideration when immunization is performed using denatured proteins or peptides.

Immunogenicity is the ability of a substance to induce an immunoresponse. This depends on many factors (e.g. species and constitution of the immunized animal, dosage, application mode, degree of aggregation, molecular weight). Normally, corpuscular substances (microorganisms, viruses, cells) are more immunogenic than molecular substances. High molecular and aggregated compounds (e.g. aggregated immunoglobulins) are very immunogenic. As a rule immunogenicity decreases with a decrease of the molecular weight; however, the chemical nature of a compound markedly determines its immunogenicity. Proteins are strong immunogens, thus polypeptides of 4,000 - 5,000 D (in exceptional cases even smaller) can induce an immunoresponse. A high content of aromatic amino acids and a large heterogeneity further improve immunogenicity of polypeptides. Polysaccharides are less immunogenic than proteins and, indeed, a much higher minimal molecular weight is necessary (e.g. in humans, dextrans of more than 500,000 D). In rabbits pure polysaccharides do not induce an immunoresponse. Pure nucleic acids and lipids normally are not immunogenic.

Haptens are compounds which in pure form are not able to induce an immunoresponse but which can react with specific antibodies (nucleic acids, lipids, different low molecular weight compounds). An immunoresponse against haptens can be obtained by coupling them covalently to strong immunogens (e.g. proteins). Immunization then results in formation of antibodies against both the hapten and the carrier protein. Thus the possibility to generate antibodies against low molecular weight compounds has rendered immunological methods to become useful tools in drug research, drug monitoring, several diagnostics and even plant hormone investigations.

1.2.4. Antigen-antibody Reaction

An antigen-antibody reaction is the specific binding of an antigen to an antibody, thus forming an antigen-antibody complex. The reaction is reversible. As already described in Chapter 1.2.1., only a small number of amino acids of the hypervariable regions V_L and V_H are directly involved in the binding of an antigen - or better in the binding to a distinct epitope of the antigen. This means that most parts of the two molecules

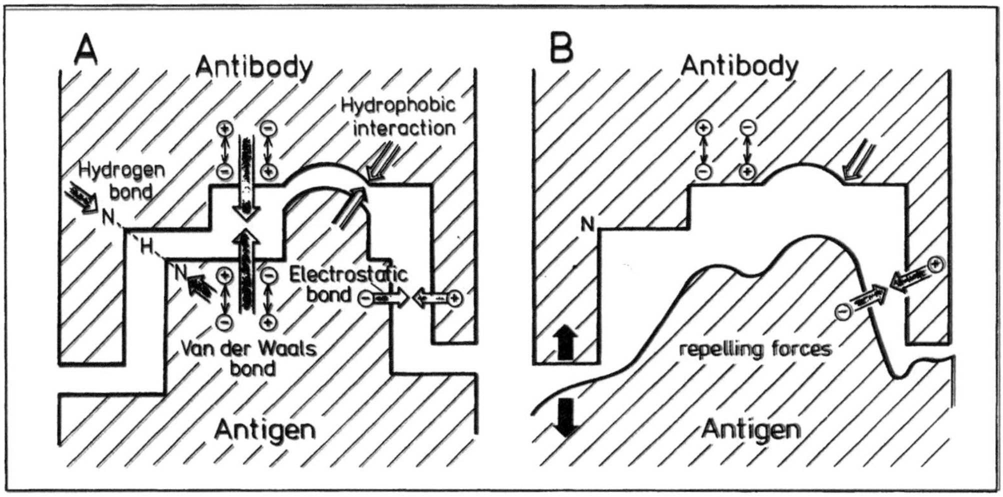

Fig. 1.16. Fitting of antigen and antibody.
A. The shape is ideally complementary, i.e. formation of many noncovalent bonds and no repelling forces.
B. No or poor complementarity in shape, i.e. few noncovalent interactions and strong repelling forces.

only influence the antigen- antibody reaction by stabilizing the spatial structure of the molecules.

The binding of an antigen to an antibody is performed exclusively by **noncovalent** bonds between several amino acids of the antigen-binding site and complementary chemical structures of the epitope. Several types of non-covalent bonds contribute to the total binding energy:

Hydrophobic interactions, the most important ones are based on a displacement of water molecules contacting apolar groups (e.g. hydrophobic amino acid residues) or molecules.

Electrostatic bonds arise from the attractive power of contrarily charged groups (e.g. $-NH_3^+$, $-COO^-$).

Van der Waals bonds which originate from non-covalent interactions between the electron clouds of different molecules (e.g. oscillating dipols).

Hydrogen bonds which form bridges between certain atoms (e.g. =NH ··· NH= or -OH ··· OH-) of different molecules.

The optimal distance between the interacting groups is different for the single binding types, but in all cases a relatively close contact is necessary because the binding energy decreases rapidly with an increase of the distance, e.g. the binding energy is proportional $1/d^2$ for electrostatic bonds and $1/d^7$ for van der Waals bonds (d is the distance between the interacting molecules, groups or atoms, respectively). The binding energy of a single non-covalent bond is very low compared to that of covalent bonds, but the formation and cooperation of many single bonds result in an enormous total binding energy. Therefore two important prerequisites are essential for an optimal antigen-antibody reaction:

(a) Appropriate atom groups of the antigen-binding region and an epitope must be arranged close together to form the above mentioned bonds.

(b) The antigen-binding site and the epitope must have the best possible complementary three-dimensional shape.

A little steric hindrance (interference of the electron clouds) already induces repelling forces and results in a significant decrease in the total binding energy. Therefore, these forces are probably responsible for the specificity of an antibody to a distinct epitope. Fig. 1.16. demonstrates both good and inadequate fitting of antigen and antibody. A partial fitting still with a dominance of attractive forces would correspond to an antibody of lower affinity (see below).

Specificity of Antibodies

Specificity of an antibody is the ability to bind selectively to complementary structures (epitopes of the antigen). Antibodies in most cases recognize the whole antigen better than isolated parts of it, i.e. the three-dimensional shape seems to play the most important role. In several cases antibodies can distinguish between native and recombinant proteins (ASTON et al., 1985) or between small conformational differences (COLLAWN et al., 1988), but antibodies can also detect single amino acid exchanges in proteins (STANKER et al., 1986) and even differences in the chemical configuration. Sometimes the antigen-binding site of an antibody can cover two (or more) independent or overlapping subsites specific to different epitopes. These antibodies are induced by one of these epitopes, but they can also react (in most cases competitively) with other(s) (Fig. 1.17.). Taking all these facts into consideration, an absolute specificity of an antibody to a given antigen is possible only if:

(a) The recognized epitope does not occur on different antigens,
(b) Different antigens do not carry epitopes similar to this epitope,
(c) In the case of polyfunctional binding sites neither the recognizable epitopes nor similar epitopes occur on different antigens.

If only one of these conditions is not met, then the antibody will **cross-react** with one or more different antigens. Nevertheless, for single antibody molecules, and in an adequate manner for monoclonal antibodies (see Chapter 1.3.3.), an absolute specificity is imaginable, and indeed monoclonal antibodies of a very high specificty could be obtained, i.e. these antibodies react with one antigen and do not cross-react with any of the molecules known to be related to this antigen. Proof of absolute specificity is practically impossible and not necessary.

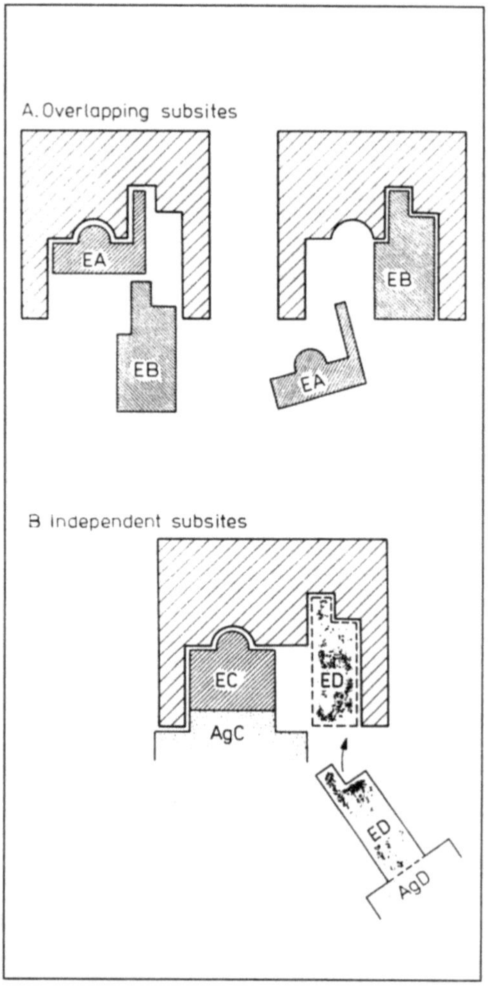

Fig. 1.17. Polyfunctional antigen-binding sites (here: bifunctional).
A. A bifunctional antigen-binding site with overlapping subsites can bind either of the recognized epitopes.
B. A bifunctional antigen binding site with independent subsites can bind both epitopes at the same time. In practice this is imaginable only for very small haptens. In most cases steric hindrance by the rest of the antigen molecule will result in competetive reaction like in A.

Antisera (polyclonal antibodies) consist of a lot of antibodies directed against many different epitopes of the inducing antigen. Therefore, an antiserum generated against a distinct antigen will cross-react with all molecules expressing one or more of the epitopes found on the inducing antigen. For this reason, the probability of obtaining absolutely specific antisera is very low. Indeed, highly specific antisera in most cases could be obtained only by immunoaffinity chromatography using either the desired antigen or cross-reacting antigens in immobilized form (Swaab and Pool, 1975), often in several steps. In this way cross-reacting antibodies can be removed from the serum, thus improving specificity for the target antigen (Köves and Arimura, 1989).

Qualitative and Quantitative Determination of Antibodies

Antigen specific antibodies can be detected by *in vitro* methods. For many years these methods have been based on either of the two classical *in vitro* reactions of antibodies: **Immunoprecipitation** and **agglutination**. Both reactions function only with polyclonal antibodies and polyvalent antigens.

Precipitation is the formation of higher molecular, insoluble (precipitating) network immunocomplexes of molecular (soluble) antigens and at least bivalent polyclonal antibodies at equivalent concentrations. Haptens are not precipitated.

Agglutination is the same reaction with corpuscular antigens (e.g. cells, viruses or antigen-loaded synthetic particles).

Methods based on precipitation are immunodiffusion techniques according to Ouchterlony (1962) (double diffusion of antigen and antibody in agar gel) or according to Mancini et al. (1965) (single radial diffusion of an antigen in antiserum containing agar), electroimmunodiffusion or immunoelectrophoretic techniques. These methods together allow both quantitative and qualitative estimation of antibodies and antigens, but they are not very sensitive. Passive hemagglutination can improve the sensitivity 100 - 1,000 times. In this method, soluble antigens are coupled covalently to the surface of erythrocytes, and these are then agglutinated by antiserum in test dilutions. The complement of the antisera has to be inactivated for this method.

Independent of specificity, immunoglobulins in sera and other body fluids can be conveniently quantified by laser nephelometric methods (Bergmann et al., 1978), these having been continuously improved. Automatic laser nephelometers now available make nephelometry a valuable tool for differential determination of serum proteins, including differential quantitation of IgA, IgG and IgM in clinical practice (Mencke et al., 1986).

Today precipitation and agglutination in antibody screening are widely replaced by radio- or enzyme-immune tests. These are more sensitive and can also detect monoclonal antibodies and even Fab fragments and may be performed with haptens too. Most convenient of them are solid phase antibody screening tests. Fig. 1.18. shows a convenient test principle for the detection of antigen specific mouse monoclonal antibodies. Cross-reactivity can be tested in the same manner. Labeling of antigen with ^{125}I or selected enzymes can sometimes be complicated, but protein and peptide antigens can easily be labeled with biotin or fluorescein isothiocyanate (FITC). In these cases, labeled avidin or labeled anti-FITC antibody can be used as universally applicable detectors. In large scale screening of different antibodies this can simplify the labeling expense enormously.

Screening methods for antibody specificity are an essential prerequisite for any kind of antibody production, because the specificity determines the practical value of antibodies.

Affinity and Avidity of Antibodies

Affinity is the binding energy of a single antigen-binding site of an antibody to the antigen. It is determined by the attractive and repelling forces discussed at the beginning of the chapter.

Thus, strictly speaking, an exact measurement of the affinity is possible only for the reaction of a monovalent antibody (e.g. a Fab fragment) with an antigen or hapten. In practice, antibodies are bi-

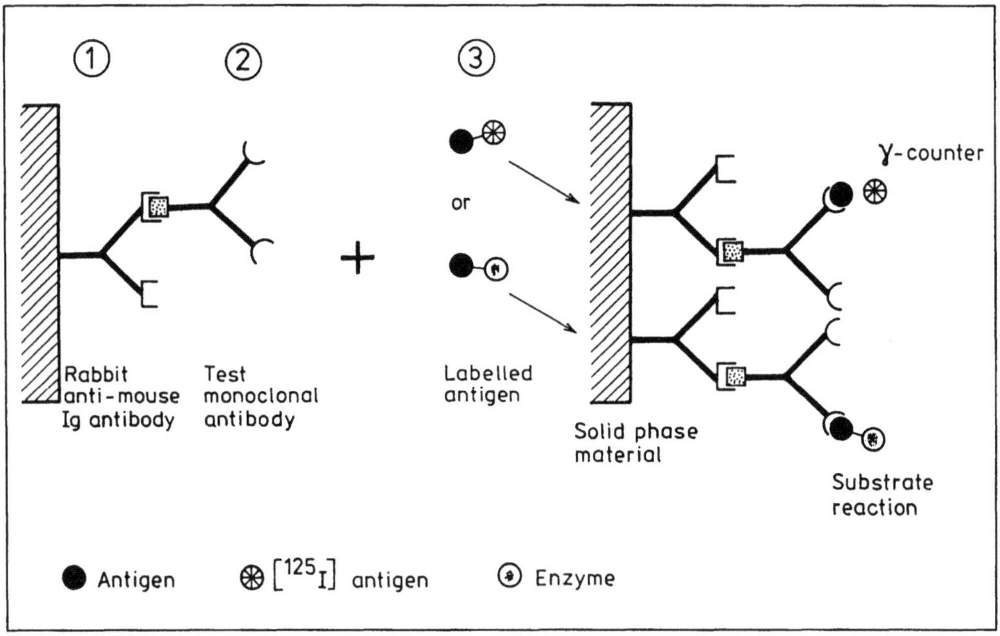

Fig. 1.18. Screening for antigen-specific mouse monoclonal antibodies.
(1). A purified helper antibody (e.g. rabbit anti-mouse immunoglobulin antibody) is bound to a solid phase (e.g. adsorbed to wells of flexible micro test plates or plastic foils). This step is necessary, since a direct adsorption of the test antibody would be inhibited by the serum proteins contained in the culture medium. Unbound material is extensively washed away with PBS or tap water.
(2). The plate is incubated with the test solution (e.g. culture supernatants from a clonation experiment). In this step the monoclonal antibodies are bound by the helper antibody. It is extensively washed once more.
(3). The plate is incubated with ^{125}I- or enzyme-labeled antigen. If the test solution contains antigen-specific antibodies, the labeled antigen is bound to form the solid phase complexes shown in the figure.
After washing, the bound ^{125}I-antigen can be measured in a gamma-counter. Bound enzyme-labeled antigen is incubated with an appropriate chromogenic substrate and then determined by a photometer or visually. The same test system can be used to titrate antibody solutions for the estimation of antibody concentration (sequential dilutions of the test solutions).

or polyvalent, and most antigens are polyvalent too. This means that the antigen can bind to more than one binding site of the antibody. In this case, the resulting binding energy is by orders of magnitude higher than the sum of the binding energies of the single contacts (bonus effect), since for dissociation of the antigen-antibody complex all bindings have to be split at the same time. The overall binding energy of a polyvalent antibody to a polyvalent antigen is termed **functional affinity** or **avidity**. Under physiological conditions, avidity plays a much more dominating role since naturally occurring antigens are polyvalent, and natural antibodies at least bivalent. In contrast, the affinity of bi- or polyvalent antibodies to a monovalent antigen or hapten is not higher than that of a Fab fragment, since in this case the dissociation of a single binding always results in the dissociation of an antigen molecule from the complex.

In polyclonal antibodies (antisera) even affinity to a single epitope is heterogeneous. This heterogeneity is a disadvantage in several immunoaffinity techniques (e.g. immunoaffinity chromatography).

In monoclonal antibodies all binding sites have the same affinity (exclusive affinity). For monovalent antigens, i.e. molecules that carry the recognized epitope only once, and ideally for haptens which normally represent a single epitope, the affinity can be measured.

Determination of the affinity constant

Since the antigen-antibody reaction is reversible, an equilibrium is established which can be described as:

$$Ag + Ab \rightleftharpoons AgAb \qquad (1)$$

According to the law of mass action it follows:

$$K = \frac{[AgAb]}{[Ag] * [Ab]} \qquad (2)$$

In this equation [AgAb] is the equilibrium concentration of the bound antigen. [Ag] and [Ab] are the equilibrium concentrations of the free antigen and antibody, respectively. The equilibrium constant K is a measure for the affinity and is termed the affinity constant. Since all concentrations are given in mol/l, K has the units l/mol and is the reciprocal of the concentration of the free antigen, when one half of the binding sites of the antibody are occupied, because from [AgAb] = [Ab] it follows K = 1/[Ag]. The higher the numerical value of K, the greater the affinity. In analogy to the K_m value in enzyme kinetics, the reciprocal affinity constant 1/K is used in some methods of affinity determination. In this case, the relation is the smaller the numerical value, the higher the affinity.

Determination of the affinity constant can be performed by different methods. In most cases, the antigen and the antibody are incubated together and are allowed to establish the equilibrium. Usually, the initial concentration of one of the components (mostly the antibody) is kept constant, whereas the other is varied. At the equilibrium the free and bound antigen are separated from each other by an appropriate method, so that the bound antigen can be measured. A separation can be achieved by different methods. FRIGUET et al. (1985) compared immunoprecipitation, fluorescence transfer and solid phase ELISA methods for two different monoclonal antibodies and obtained comparable K values in all three tests. Separation can be further achieved by precipitation of immunocomplexes using ammonium sulfate (GRISWOLD and NELSON, 1984) or 13% polyethylene glycol 6000 (CHARD, 1980) by equilibrium filtration (STONE and METZGER, 1968) or by use of solid phase-bound catcher antibodies (VAN HEYNINGEN et al., 1983). In the case of antibodies reacting with the active site of an enzyme, the separation can even be omited, since the inhibition of enzyme activity is a direct measure of the bound antigen in equilibrium (EHLE et al., 1989). The affinity constant K can also be calculated from elution data in immunoaffinity chromatography (BRUERA et al., 1983).

The determination of the value of K is often performed according to STEWARD and PETTY (1972):

Substituting [Ab] = [Ab_o] - [AgAb], where [Ab_o] is the total antibody concentration, equilibrium (2) can be written:

$$[AgAb] = K * [Ag] * ([Abo] - [AgAb]) \qquad (3)$$

Considering the valency of the antibody (n) and the heterogeneity exponent (a) by simple transformations of (3) the general binding equation (4) is obtained:

$$[AgAb] = \frac{n * K * [Ab_o] * [Ag]^a}{1 + K * [Ag]^a} \qquad (4)$$

For Fab fragments n and a are 1. In the case of monoclonal IgG antibodies is n = 2, and one can ideally assume a = 1. Using [Ab_+] = 2[Ab_o], where [Ab_+] is the initial concentration of the antigen-binding sites of bivalent antibodies, and [Ab_o] = [Ab_+] for Fab fragments equilibrium equation (4) can be transformed to:

$$\frac{1}{[AgAb]} = \frac{1}{K} * \frac{1}{[Ab_+]} * \frac{1}{[Ag]} + \frac{1}{[Ab_+]} \qquad (5)$$

From this term [Ab_+] can be determined, which is important for crude antibody preparations. If

$1/[Ag] = 0$, then $1/[AgAb] = 1/[Ab_+]$. Thus a plot of $1/[AgAb]$ against $1/[Ag]$ allows the determination of $[Ab_+]$ extrapolating the curve to $1/[Ag] = 0$, and the determination of $1/K$ from the slope of the curve after determination of $[Ab_+]$. The transformation of (3) or (4) according to SCATCHARD (1949) results in:

$$\frac{[AgAb]}{[Ag] * [Ab_+]} = -K * \frac{[AgAb]}{[Ab_+]} + K \qquad (6)$$

K can be calculated from the slope of $[AgAb]/[Ab_+][Ag]$ against $[AgAb]/[Ab_+]$ (SCATCHARD plot). The logarithmic transformation of (4) according to SIPS (1948) resulting in:

$$\log \frac{r}{n-r} = \log K + a * \log [Ag] \qquad (7)$$

with $r = [AgAb]/[Ab_0]$ and $n = 2$ for IgG, allows the determination of K from a plot: $\log r/(2-r)$ against $\log [Ag]$. Using (6) or (7) $[Ab_+]$ must be known.

All three methods were shown to give similar results in the determination of K for six monoclonal antibodies by JACOBSEN et al. (1982), considering that they had to be corrected for a bivalent antigen (human IgG). STEVENS et al. (1987) demonstrated that even for monovalent antigens a correction procedure is necessary to determine the true affinity constants of bivalent antibodies.

As an alternative to these methods, WAGENER et al. (1983) calculated affinity constants of monoclonal anti-CEA antibodies from inhibitor curves of ^{125}I-CEA binding at a constant concentration of antibody by "cold" CEA as an inhibitor in different concentrations. Using the equation of MÜLLER (1980):

$$K = \frac{1}{(I_t - T_t) * (1 - 1.5b + 0.5b^2)} \qquad (8)$$

where I_t is the total inhibitor concentration at 50 % inhibition of the tracer binding, T_t is the total concentration of the tracer and b is the fraction of the tracer bound in absence of the inhibitor.

A simple method based on a solid phase radioimmunoassay allows ranking of affinities of different monoclonal antibodies against one antigen directly from the antibody dilution curves at half maximal antigen binding (VAN HEYNINGEN et al., 1983). By this method the order of affinities can even be ranked more or less correctly by performing dilution rows of culture supernatants of unknown antibody concentration. Thus, the method is an ideal tool for selecting high and low affinity antibodies in screening tests after clonation in monoclonal antibody production.

A method for calculation of affinity constants directly from antibody dilution curves has been described by GRISWOLD et al. (1985).

Determination of affinities plays an important role concerning further use of antibodies. Most monoclonal antibodies have affinity constants in the range of 10^6 to 10^{12} l/mol. For use in antigen determination assays (RIA, ELISA), antibodies of high affinity (10^8 to 10^{12} l/mol) should be selected to ensure a very stable binding of the antigen, whereas in immunoaffinity chromatography antibodies of moderate affinity (10^6 to 10^7 l/mol) should be used to allow a sufficient binding of antigen as well as a mild elution.

1.3. Antibody Generation and Propagation

Antibodies, because of their outstanding specificity to the corresponding antigen, are widely applied in medical diagnostics and therapy, drug research, biological investigations and in the study and purification of proteins and other substances. Today, antibodies can be raised against almost any desired chemical compound and any corpuscular antigen, even if only a small amount of antigen (or hapten) is available. Worldwide there is a great need for specific antibodies. Before KÖHLER and MILSTEIN (1975) introduced the hybridoma technique for the production of **monoclonal** antibodies in vitro, antibody production had been limited to immunizing animals and collecting the immune serum. Antibodies from immune sera are **polyclonal.** Monoclonal antibodies have some notable advantages over polyclonal antibodies; they are homogeneous in class (subclass), type of light chain, allotype and what is most important, in antigen binding properties, e.g. specificity and affinity. Since hybridoma cell lines are immortal, monoclonal antibodies can be produced, furthermore, in almost any desired amount in a standardizable quality. Even today commercial production of monoclonal antibodies is performed in kilogram quantities. An advantage of polyclonal antibodies is their ability to precipitate or to agglutinate antigens, which today is still used in many test systems. In their favour too is that they do not require cell culture equipment for their production and, therefore, can be raised in any laboratory, animal supply provided.

1.3.1. Immunization

A lot of factors have to be taken into consideration, when developing an immunization strategy for a distinct antigen. Low molecular compounds, lipids and nucleotides are not immunogenic. They have to be coupled to suitable strong immunogens to become immunogenic (haptens, see Chapter 1.2.2.). Keyhole limpet (*Megathura crenulata*) hemocyanin, *Helix pomatia* hemocyanin, bovine serum albumin and ovalbumin are often used for this purpose. In order to improve the antibody response, the antigen for primary immunization is mixed normally with an **adjuvant**. For this purpose bacteria, cellulose, mineral oils, detergents, aluminium compounds and other materials have been applied. The best results were obtained using a water-in-oil emulsion containing heat-killed mycobacteria (FREUND'S complete adjuvant = FCA). The bacteria stimulate the immune system and the emulsion guarantees a slow release of antigen into the circulation of animals. Booster (secondary) injections of antigens are necessary in most cases to achieve high antibody levels because secondary immunoresponse is markedly increased (memory). These injections are performed without adjuvant or using FREUND'S incomplete adjuvant (FIA, without bacteria).

The success of an immunization depends decisively on:

- the immunized animal (immunological constitution, genetic relation to antigen donor; and immunogenicity of an antigen is different in different species),
- antigen dose (too low and too high doses cause tolerance, whereas **low immunogenic** doses induce high affinity antibodies, and high immunogenic doses induce low affinity antibodies),
- mode of application (i.v., i.p., i.m., s.c., i.d.; number of application sites; adjuvant),
- antigenicity of antigen (molecular weight, chemical structure, resorption, degradation),
- number and time of booster immunizations.

The choice of an animal for immunization further depends on the amount of antiserum required, the amount of antigen available, animal supply and, in the case of monoclonal antibody production, it has to be compatible to the available fusion partner. Anti-idiotypical antibodies should be raised in the same species or even in the same strain as is the "antigen" donor, so as to exclude response against other parts of the antibody molecule, whereas in most cases it is advisable to immunize animals of a species phylogenetically distant from the antigen donor.

If enough antigen is available, it is always advisable to immunize several animals by the same or slightly different methods. Although the immunization procedure has to be optimized for each particular antigen, Table 1.2. provides some guidelines which are useful in polyclonal antibody production. However, very different methods can also be successful and other animals can be immunized (for procedures in detail including serum preparations see JOHNSTONE and THORPE, 1982).

Primary immunization of rats and mice can also be performed in a similar manner for generation of monoclonal antibodies but normally only one or two booster injections at intervals of 1 - 4 months are necessary then. Occasionally, different injection sites are chosen, e.g. into foot pads or directly

Table 1.2. Immunization Procedures for Protein Antigens [a)]

Species	Dose [μg]	Primary immunization [b)] Mode	Sites	Alternative	Minimal interval [days]	Booster immunization(s) [c)] Dose [μg]	Mode	Sites
Mouse	5-50	**i.p.**	1	i.v., s.c.	7-8	5-50 or more	i.v., i.p.	1
Rat	10-100	**i.d.**	4-6 in back	i.m., s.c.	7-8	10-50	i.m., s.c., i.v., i.p.	2-4
Guinea pig	10-100	**i.d.**	4-6 in back	i.m., s.c.	7-8	10-50	i.m., s.c.	2-4
Rabbit	50-200	**i.d.**	6-8 in back	i.m., s.c.	10	50-200	i.m., s.c., i.v.	several
Goat/sheep	500-2000	**i.d., i.m., s.c.**	several in back	-	21	500-2000	i.m., s.c., (i.v.)	several
Chicken	50-200	**i.m.**	2-4	-	10	50-200	i.m.	2-4

[a)] especially for mice there exist many different immunization procedures; [b)] adjuvant: FCA; [c)] adjuvant: none or FIA
i.d., intradermal; i.m., intramuscular; i.p., intraperitoneal; i.v., intravenous; s.c., subcutanous; FIA, incomplete Freund's adjuvant

into lymph nodes (Raymond and Suh, 1986). Spleen is "harvested" 3 - 4 days after the last booster injection, when the number of actively dividing B lymphocytes (blast cells) reaches its maximum. At the time of the highest serum antibody level (7 - 8 days after booster injection, i.e. the time for bleeding), the yield of hybridomas is low, i.e. mature plasma cells are not suitable for cell fusion, whereas a larger number of freshly stimulated large B lymphocytes (blast cells) is a prerequisite for good fusion results (Stähli et al., 1980). Multi-dose injection can be disadvantageous to hybridoma production (Oi et al., 1978), but an enormous increase in antibody-forming cells can be achieved by transfer of spleen cells from a freshly boostered mouse together with antigen to an irradiated syngeneic recipient and restimulation after four days (Kenny et al., 1981). A single injection can often be sufficient for production of monoclonal antibodies (Trucco et al., 1978). Single dose immunization directly into the spleen (Spitz et al., 1984) can improve efficiency and minimize the amount of antigen necessary for immunization. Furthermore, it lasts a few days only and has been shown to be particularly efficient for large or aggregated molecules (Thorpe et al., 1984). Taking into consideration that IgM antibodies dominate only in the first stage of primary immunoresponse and play a subordinate role later on when IgG antibodies reach the highest levels, single shot methods are particularly useful for generation of monoclonal IgM antibodies.

Last but not least it should be mentioned that immunization of B cells for monoclonal antibody production under special conditions can be performed *in vitro* (in cell culture). Experience with this method has been reviewed by Reading (1982). There are several advantages over *in vivo* immunization: very small amounts of antigens are necessary, immunized cells for fusion are available within a few days and immunization is also successful with poor immunogens (e.g. autoantigens). Furthermore, *in vitro* immunization enormously improves the possibility of producing human monoclonal antibodies, since *in vivo* immunization of humans must not be performed in most cases. Because monoclonal antibodies can be generated from *in vitro* immunized peripheral blood lymphocytes (Borrebaeck, 1988), the provision of sensitizable human cells is not a problem either.

Antigen can be used for *in vitro* immunization (for in vivo too), even bound to nitrocellulose (GRATECOS et al., 1987). Thus, antigens purified by electrophoretic methods can be used directly from Western blot.

1.3.2. Polyclonal Antibodies

Polyclonal antibodies are normally obtained from the serum of immunized animals. Test bleedings to monitor the antibody level are always advisable, also prior to fusion experiments. For this purpose small amounts of blood are removed in an appropriate manner (e.g. from the tail of mice or from ear vein of rabbits), and animals are allowed to recover. When the specific serum antibody level is high enough (high titer), smaller animals (mice, rats, guinea pigs, hamsters) are sacrificed and bled exhaustively by heart puncture, to obtain a larger volume of blood. Rabbits, goats, sheep and other large animals can be bled weakly over 1 - 2 months and will deliver large volumes of blood. Blood is normally taken from the jugular vein.

For serum preparation blood is preferably collected in glass containers, allowed to clot (1h at room temperature, then overnight at 4 °C) and clots are removed by centrifugation. Serum is stored at 4 °C (a preservative should be added) or in aliquotes frozen at -20 °C or -70 °C. Chicken serum should not be frozen. Immune plasma prepared from blood after addition of coagulants (e.g. heparin) should be defribrinated prior to antibody purification because clotting factors can disturb in purification.

1.3.3. Monoclonal Antibodies

The hybridoma technique introduced by KÖHLER and MILSTEIN (1975) is based on the fusion of spleen cells (or lymph node cells; cf. MIZRA et al., 1987) of an immunized animal with neoplastic B cells of a myeloma cell line of the same animal strain. The resulting hybrid cells exhibit the most important properties of both parent cells; they produce and secrete antibodies such as sensitized B lymphocytes, and they are immortal, a characteristic of the myeloma cell line.

Most of the monoclonal antibodies are of the IgG or IgM classes, but monoclonal IgA antibodies could also be obtained in rare cases. Incidence of IgA mab's is markedly higher when using gut-associated lymphoid tissues instead of spleen cells for fusion (KOMISAR et al., 1982). Allergen specific monoclonal antibodies have been described by BÖTTCHER et al. (1978). The magnitude of monoclonal antibodies is derived from rodents (mice, rats), but mouse-human and human-human hybridomas play an increasing role (see LARRICK and BUCK, 1984).

A schedule for hybridoma generation and propagation is presented in Fig. 1.19.

Cell fusion

Cell fusion can be induced by different agents. Usually cells are incubated at high density in the presence of 30 - 50 % polyethylene glycol (PEG) 1500 or 4000, with spleen cells being 3 - 12 fold in excess. Fusion rate normally is not more than 1 of 1,000 spleen cells. Results of PEG- mediated fusion can be improved by addition of 5 - 10 % dimethylsulfoxide, which protects cells (NORWOOD, 1976).

Under certain conditions PEG can contain toxic aldehydes (KADISH and WENC, 1983). Suitability of PEG differs from batch to batch, thus making PEG an uncertain parameter in cell fusion. Some viruses can also induce cell fusion. Cell fusion mediated by an electric field, originally developed for plant protoplasts by ZIMMERMANN and SCHEURICH (1981) is applicable to mamalian cells. In comparative experiments it has even been shown to result in higher fusion rates and better hybridoma growth than PEG fusion (KARSTEN et al., 1988).

Cell fusion can further be laser-induced (SCHIERENBURG, 1987). Binding of antigen to the surface of myeloma cells can improve hybridoma yield in chemically induced fusions (KRANZ et al.,

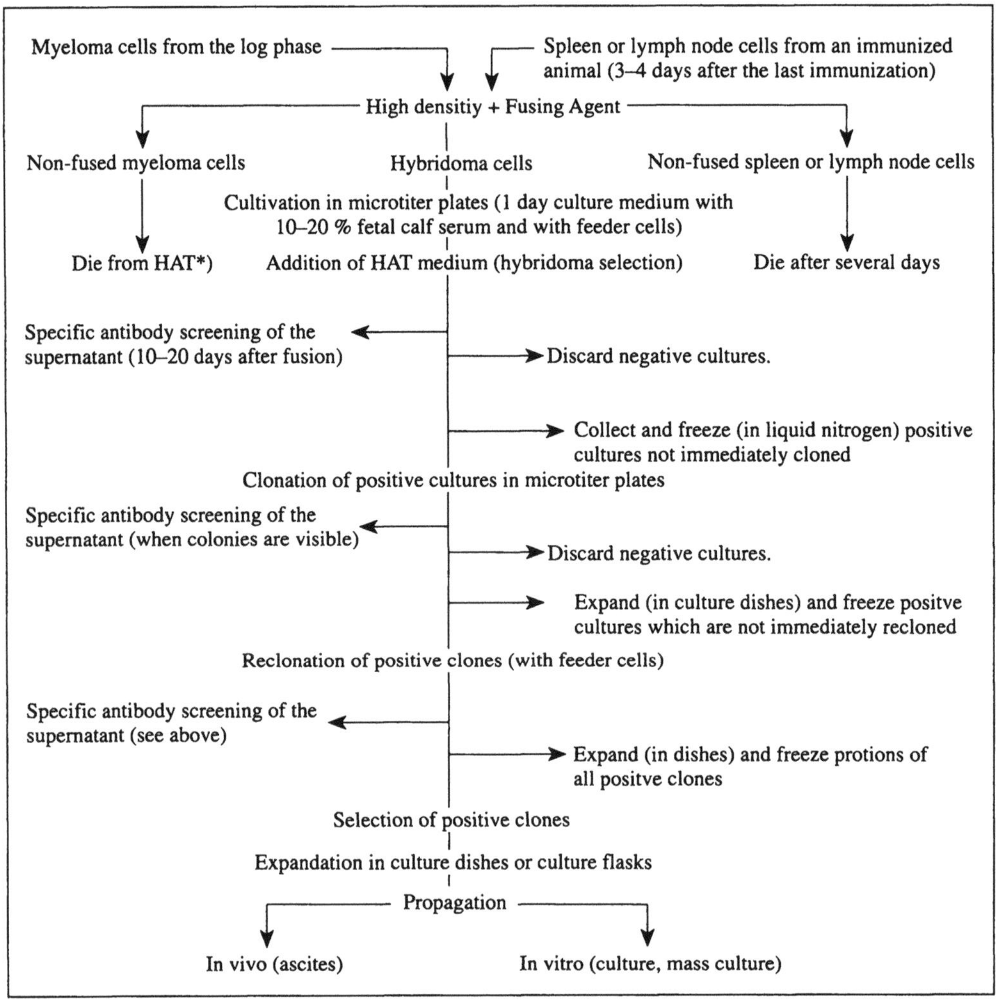

Fig. 1.19. Generation and propagation of hybridoma cell lines (*in vivo* immunization).
*) Hypoxanthine/aminopterine/thymidine (instead of aminopterine also azaserine can be userd)

1980) or can even result in spontaneous fusion of antigen-labeled myeloma cells selectively with antigen-reactive spleen cells (Bankert et al., 1980).

Hybridoma Selection and Clonation

Myeloma cells used for cell fusion should meet two important requirements: (1) they should themselves not produce immunoglobulins or single immunoglobulin light chains because these would contaminate the antibodies produced by the hybridomas. (2) They should die in a selective culture medium in which hybridomas survive. Usually hypoxanthine-guanine phosphoribosyl transferase (HGPRTase) deficient cell lines are used, which die in a culture medium containing hypoxanthine, aminopterine (or azaserine) and thymidine (HAT medium). Aminopterine or azaserine inhibit de novo synthesis of nucleic acid, and the salvage pathway is impossible without HGPRTase. Other possible methods of hybrid cell selection were reviewed by CLEMENTS (1975).

Suitable cell lines include amongst others NSO, P_3X63-Ag8.653, SP_2OAg14 (no immunoglobulin at all) from mice, Y3 and 210RC43.Ag1 (κ chains) from rats or the human cell line SKO-007 (although producing IgE). Under these conditions, after fusing and HAT selection only hybridoma cells survive since non-fused spleen cells die after a period in culture and non-fused myeloma cells die from HAT.

Selection is usually performed in cell culture plates (24 or 96 wells). After selection, the growing hybridoma colonies are screened for specific antibody production and antibody-producing colonies of interest are cloned. Normally this is done by diluting the cells in culture medium and placing them into microtiter plates (96 wells) in a manner whereby not more than one cell is transferred to each well. Growth of these single cells is supposed to be accomplished by feeder cells (spleen cells, peritoneal macrophages). In most cases a repeated clonation (reclonation) is necessary to obtain stable clones. Cells now growing in one well have all derived from one hybridoma cell. Thus the antibody molecules produced and secreted by them are all identical. The hybridoma cell lines, and the produced antibodies, are **monoclonal**. Although such cell lines are relatively stable after prolonged cultivation or after freezing, reclonation is advisable. While investigators have long believed that plate cultivation and clonation could not be automated because of the many different processes to be considered, recently an automated system (robotic sample processor RSP 5052) was developed by TECAN, which can fulfil all feeding and cloning operations (WILTON-SMITH, 1987).

Bispecific and Engineered Antibodies

It is even possible to fuse cells of two hybridoma lines, or hybridoma cells with spleen cells to form hybrid hybridomas (tetradomas or triomas, respectively), which produce a mixture of both "parent" antibodies and a hybrid antibody with antigen binding sites for two different antigens (bispecific monoclonal antibodies). In the case of triomas, the hybridoma line (MILSTEIN and CUELLO, 1983) and in the case of tetradomas one of the hybridoma lines, has to be sensitive to a selection medium (STAERZ and BEVAN, 1986) or the "parent" cells are labeled by different fluorescent dyes (e.g. FITC or TRITC), and hybridomas showing double fluorescence are selected using a fluorescence activated cell sorter (FACS) (KARAWAJEW et al., 1987, 1988). Bispecific antibodies provide an opportunity to improve application of antibodies in biological and medical test systems or in medical therapy. The production of chimeric antibodies consisting of mouse V regions and human C regions (humanized antibodies) by recombinant cell lines is also possible (WHITTLE et al., 1987), being more useful in therapeutic application than murine antibodies. Single chain antigen-binding proteins can be produced as recombinant polypeptides in *E. coli*, consisting of V_H and V_L sequence of a monoclonal antibody connected by a linker polypeptide. BIRD et al. (1988) have constructed three different proteins of this type: one against human growth hormone and two against fluorescein. Advantages from single chain antibodies are anticipated for *in vivo* use (small size, low immunogenicity and less nonspecific reactions because of the lacking Fc portion).

Hybridoma propagation

Once established, important clones have to be propagated to obtain larger amounts of antibodies. This can be performed *in vivo* and *in vitro*.

In vivo propagation

For this pupose hybridoma cells are injected into the peritoneal cavity of syngeneic animals. Usually, animals (Balb/c mice or LOU rats) are primed with 0.1 - 0.5 ml/animal tetramethylpentadecane (pristane) at least 1 day (better 5 - 14 days) prior to inoculation of 10^6 - 10^7 hybridoma cells per animal. Ascitic fluid can be collected within 5 -

30 days after inoculation of cells. In most cases, repeated collections are possible. The efficiency of antibody production in vivo depends on the productivity of the cell clone itself, on the number of inoculated cells, the amount and time of pristane priming, age and sex of animals. These parameters have been optimized for Balb/c mice by Brodeur et al. (1984) and for rats by Kints et al. (1989). Furthermore, hybrid mice can yield 3-4 times more ascites than Balb/c (Brodeur and Tsang, 1986). Antibody concentration in ascites may vary between 1 and 10 (rarely 15) mg/ml depending on the hybridoma clone. For instance, Chandler (1987) has described the ascites production of 37 different cell lines, requiring between 9 to 15 mice to produce 1 g of antibody. Because of the high specific antibody content, *in vivo* propagation has been preferred in laboratory practice. It is possible to produce considerable amounts of monoclonal antibodies without a sophisticated equipment in a relatively short period of time. Nevertheless, there are some disadvantages which call this method in question when considering large-scale production:

1. Ethical points of view ("mass murder" of animals),
2. Impracticability of handling large numbers of animals (manual labour),
3. Host immunoglobulins render the purification process more difficult,
4. Difficulties in "standardizing" animals for reducing lot-to-lot variations (Chandler, 1987),
5. Lipids and pristane residues in ascitic fluid,
6. Difficulties in meeting regulatory demands for *in vivo* use of the products in humans.

Therefore, in the eighties the trend in large-scale production of monoclonal antibodies has been in favour of *in vitro* propagation.

In vitro propagation

Since the low antibody content of only 10-100 μg/ml, the low productivity of only millilitre amounts of culture supernatant per day and the large portion of manual labour required do not allow an efficient scale-up of hybridoma culture in plates or flasks, the aim was to develop in vitro systems allowing the production of large amounts of antibody containing fluid in a short period of time, to increase the antibody content in this fluid and to find methods for automation and continuous culturing. Different strategies were chosen to solve the problem. The most important methods are covered here briefly (for detailed information see Seaver, 1987). Airlift bioreactors have been driven at 10, 100 and 1,000 liter scale and can be used for many mammalian cell lines, with hybridomas giving better results in batch or fed-batch culture than in continuous culture (Rhodes and Birch, 1988). High hydrostatic pressure in large airlift fermentors does not negatively affect growth and productivity of hybridoma cells (Lambert et al., 1987). Reuveny et al. (1986) compared different cell propagation methods in stirred reactors using very low serum concentrations. The production rate based on one liter culture per day allows consideration of scaling-up and demonstrates that the perfusion method gives by far the best results (Table 1.3.).

Backer et al. (1987) used retrofitted 150 and 1300 liter computer-controlled stirred fermentors for automated hybridoma culture and could demonstrate that there is no noticable cell damage at cell densities of more than 5 x 10^6 cells/ml and agitation rates up to 150 rpm. Antibody concentrations of more than 100 μg/ml could be obtained. Although cell density and concentration of product are relatively low, suspension culture reactors are a viable technology for large-scale production of monoclonal antibodies because these reactors are flexible in use and can achieve full production rates within a few days (an advantage too in cases of contamination or technical failure).

Good results were also obtained using bioreactors where cells are encapsulated or immobilized in or on matrices, e.g. ceramics (Putnam, 1987) or semipermeable membranes (Posillico et al., 1987). Hollow-fiber reactors have been used and optimized by many authors (Andersen and Gruenberg, 1987; von Wedel, 1987). In this technique, cells grow entrapped in membrane fibers of defined porosity. Already in 1986 Altshuler et al. reported that porosity of hollow

Table 1.3. Results of Monoclonal Antibody Production in Stirred Fermentors Using Different Propagation Modes [a)]

Propagation mode	**Antibody concentration** [μg/ml]	**Production rate** [mg/l culture per day]
Batch	100-200	15
Fed-batch (daily addition of fresh medium)	> 200	27
Semi-continuous (partical medium replacement twice a day 200 ml)	170	34
Semi-continuous (periodical feeding with glucose and glutamine)	310	62
Perfusion culture (5 μm filter); continuous feeding and product "harvest"	390	660

[a)] according to REUVENY et al., 1986

fibers plays an important role in the productivity of hybridomas. Best results (260 μg/ml) were obtained using a pore size of 100,000 Daltons cut-off, because serum constituents are widely removed from the product, but the best yield was only 4 mg/day. Recently HEIFETZ et al. (1989) reported results obtained with a VITAFIBER V bioreactor (AMICON) using serum-free medium. Within 40 days of run they could produce 15 g of antibody, with a per day production of 579 mg of IgG during the productive phase. More than 95 % of total protein in "harvest" was IgG. In general, cell densities are higher in encapsulation and hollow-fiber techniques (10^7 - 10^8 cells/ml) than in suspension cultures (10^4 - 10^7 cells/ml), and in addition antibody concentration in supernatant may reach 0.1 - 10 g/l as compared to 0.01 - 0.5 g/l for suspension cultures. Using roller flasks SJÖGREN-JANSSON and JEANSSON (1985) grew cells in different types of dialysis tubing in a low protein medium, whereas feed medium outside the tubing was supplemented with 10 - 30 % fetal calf serum. Antibody concentrations between 1.2 and 5.4 mg/ml in the tubing could be obtained, depending on the given cell line. A disadvantage is the low volume of tubing, despite high concentration resulting in the production of only a few milligrams per bottle per day. However, purification is simplified and, furthermore, different hybridomas can be processed at the same time without using sophisticated equipment.

For many years, mammalian cell cultures could be grown only in culture media supplemented with fetal calf serum or other suitable serum. In hybridoma culture, FCS is most frequently used (6 - 30 %) because it contains only negligible amounts of immunoglobulins. Nevertheless, it is expensive and can complicate large-scale purification processes because of lot-to-lot differences. Already in 1976 GUILBERT and ISCOVE could demonstrate that hemopoietic cells are able to grow in a medium in which serum was replaced by selenite, transferrin, albumin and lecithin.

In a series of studies, KOVAR et al. (1985, 1986a, 1986b, 1987) have developed serum free culture media for hybridoma cultivation. Starting with the growth supporting media supplemented with transferrin, insulin and other growth factors including ethanolamin, vitamins and other low molecular weight substances, they were able in 1987 to grow hybridomas in protein-free media supplemented with iron compounds in high concentration. GLASSY et al. (1988) reported the following advantages:

- Chemically defined composition,
- Better reproducibility of growth and product yield,
- Lower cost,

- Reduced difficulties and cost of antibody purification,

and as disadvantages:

- Optimization is necessary for each cell line,
- Not all cell lines grow in serum-free media,
- Often longer lag periods occur,
- Growth rate, cell density and viability are sometimes reduced.

Furthermore, they listed albumin and lipids, insulin, transferrin, ethanolamine, selenium, and β-mercaptoethanol as the most frequently used supplements. For several hybridomas, a slightly prolonged doubling time was observed, whereas a few hybridomas grow even faster in serum-free media, and in optimized serum-free media many hybridomas produced larger amounts of antibody (expressed in $\mu g/10^6$ cells per day). Also, MURAKAMI (1984) found insulin, transferrin, ethanolamine and selenite (ITES) to be essential for hybridoma growth, with ethanolamine being most important. For an excellent review on basal media, medium supplementation, productivity and use of serum-free media in suspension and membrane bioreactors, including a cost comparison to serum-supplemented media under identical conditions see MURAKAMI (1989).

Since antibody productivity in serum-free media is similar to that in serum-supplemented media, or even better for several hybridomas, and as costs are lower, the trend will be towards these media, regardless of the reported disadvantages, because of the great advantage of simpler purification of products.

During all stages of the hybridoma cultivation process - hygiene is by far the most important factor for successful antibody production. This starts with a strictly aseptical handling of spleen and myeloma cells and continues in clonation. Cells free of any infection are a prerequisite for mass culture. Mycoplasma contamination is one of the major and most serious problems. If possible, contaminated cultures should be discarded to prevent other cultures from being infected (OSTERHAUS and UYTDEHAAG, 1985). Valuable cell lines can be cured by animal passage (ascites cells) and recultivation, by short heat treatment (42°C) or by chemicals and antibiotics, but success is not guaranteed.

In large-scale cultivation, once established, cultures can be quite easily prevented from contamination by sterile application of feeding and "harvest" of product, and by use of efficient filter and sealing systems.

A completely new way of monoclonal antibody production has been opened by HIATT et al. (1989), who were able to transform tobacco leaf segments by complementary DNA derived from a mouse hybridoma messenger RNA, and to regenerate mature plants from these. Crossing of plants, that produce γ or κ chains respectively, resulted in plants which contained the functional antibody in concentrations of up to 1.3 % of total leaf protein, thus providing a real alternative to mass culture of mammalian cells.

2. General Problems

2.1. Solid Supports

Steps in planning (immuno)affinity separations are (i) selection of a suitable matrix, (ii) choice of an appropriate activation method, (iii) pick of the ligand which should be fixed, (iv) selection of immobilization method (coupling) of the ligand, and (v) choice of the conditions for adsorption/desorption steps.

Mostly solid supports are used for separations, but also soluble macromolecular materials (e.g. dextran, poly(ethylene glycol) = poly(ethylene oxide)) are applied for two-phase aqueous affinity partition processes (cf. reviews by CHASE, 1984, JANSON, 1984, BASKIR et al. 1989).

A support (matrix) for affinity chromatography or another kind of separation of biomolecules should have some properties which are sometimes contradictory. An ideal matrix should be:

- chemically inert (no reactions with solvents or constituents of the buffers used)
- easy to activate for covalent fixation of ligands

- specific, including high resolution power for separations (no unspecific interactions with parts of the mixture to be separated into distinct components)
- biologically inert (no degradation by microorganisms or enzymes)
- hydrophilic, since most chromatographic processes have to be done in aqueous media
- insoluble in aqueous solutions
- mechanically stable
- constant in size, i.e. neither swelling nor shrinking, and flow parameters during the process
- macroporous with a uniform pore distribution
- beaded with uniform bead size to give ideally packed chromatgraphic beds.

Table 2.1. Classification of Solid Supports by Physical Parameters

Parameter	Type of support
Size	
< 10 μm	latices, microspheres
1 μm to 1 mm	chromatographic supports
⩾ 1 mm	solid face supports
Shape	irregular
	spherical
Geometry	particle
	foil (membrane)
	formed macroscopic support (e.g. microtitration plate)
Magnetic behaviour	diamagnetic
	parammagnetic
Mechanical stability	soft
	rigid

Supports for immunosorption techniques may be classified by their physical or chemical properties. Table 2.1. presents a grouping by physical parameters. An example for classification of supports by chemical parameters is given in Table 2.2.

Materials for non-chromatographic methods may also be polyamides (Nylon), cellulose nitrates (nitrocellulose), paper, ferromagnetic metal oxides, and their derivatives and com-posites, respectively.

A selection of supports used for immunoaffinity chromatography is presented in the third row of Table 2.2. which is intelligibly incomplete in view of the innumerable possibilities of matrix variations and the countless manufacturers and distributors. More or less all of the matrices realize the criteria given above and the decision for this or that material depends on the specific separation problem.

In general, for low-pressure and medium-pressure immunoaffinity chromatography the organic (natural and synthetic) media are mostly favoured. For high-performance liquid immunoaffinity chromatography (HPIAC) silica and its modifications are the matrices of choice, especially the recently developed coated media, which have overcome the solubility of silica in neutral to strong alkaline buffer solutions, but some very hydrophilic organic materials are also now available for HPLC or medium pressure chromatography as fast protein liquid chromatography (FPLC).

One reason for the diversity of supports is the circumstance that none of these materials is free from unspecific interactions with biomacromolecules to be separated or the surrounding solute. For instance, most of the support materials give hydrophobic interactions or have charged groups. Therefore, conditions for biospecific adsorption and elution have to be selected, which suppress these interactions. A compromise is to be found, since nonchaotropic salts reduce ionic but elevate hydrophobic interactions while chaotropic salts do the opposite. A more detailed discussion of non-specific ionic and/or hydrophobic interactions between matrix and biomacromolecule, especially proteins, is given in the monography edited by Dubin (1988).

The porosity of the matrix introduces gel permeation effects, which prolongs the washing-out procedure of unbound material (cf. also Chapter 2.4). Some materials may loose parts of their backbone either mechanically (e.g. oligosaccharides entrapped during manufacturing of beaded cellulose) or chemically (e.g. dissolving of silicic acid from silica matrices). Besides a possible destabilization of the matrix these processes may

Table 2.2. Chromatographic Supports for Solid-Liquid-Chromatography

Basic material	Chemical modification or copolymerization, resp.	Examples of commercial supports
I. Supports based on biopoylmers		
Dextrane	cross-linked with bifunctional agents as expoxides; copolymerization of allydextran with methylene-bis-acrylamide	**Sephadex**
Agarose	cross-linked with bifunctional agents as epoxides or 1.3-dibromo-propane;	**Sepharose, BioGel A, Ultrogel**
	copolymerization with acrylamide	**Ultrogel AcA**
Cellulose		**Divicell, Eurocell**
Amylose		**(starch)**
II. Supports based on organo-chemical polymers		
Polyacrylamide	cross-linked with methylene-bis-acrylamide, N-allylamides etc.	**BioGel P**
Poly[N-acryloyl-tris-(hydrxymethyl) aminomethan]		**Trisacryl**
Polystyrene	cross-linked with divinylbenzene	**Eupergit, Wofatit, Styragel and their derivatives**
Poly(hydroxymethacrylate)		**Spheron**
Polyvinylalcohol		
Polyvinylacetate		**Fractogel**
Ethylene-maleic anhydride-copolymers		
Poly(acryloyl morpholine)		**Enzaycryl**
III. Inorganic Supports		
Controlled pore glass, spherical glass	covalently coated with dextranes, glycoles or other hydrophilic polymers	**CPG**
Collodial silica (Kieselgel) glycoles or other hydrophilic	covalently coated with dextrans, polymers	**LiChrosorb, Aquapore, UltroPac, TSK gels**
Clay (Bentonite)		
Alumina		
Controlled pore titania	as silica	
Controlled pore zirconia	as silica	
Nickel oxid	mostly for magnetic sorbents	
Iron oxide	mostly for magnetic sorbents	
Ceramics		
Charcoal	coated with dextran	

counterfeit a leakage (see Chapter 2.2.) of immobilized molecules as antibodies or antigens.

The capacity of an (immuno)affinity sorbent depends on the density of ligands on the surface of the matrix (moles per m^2) and on the specific surface (m^2 per gram), but the analytically determined ligand density need not agree with the observed capacity. This effect may be explained by imagining, that a certain part of the ligands is fixed within the pores of a macroporous material. A relatively large biomolecule cannot now reach this part of the ligand. Pores which are too large may also influence the capacity and the rate of chromatography, since within the lumen of the pores the mass transfer is determined only by diffusion. Diffusion itself is reciprocally proportional to the molecular mass of a molecule. Therefore, during binding or elution the equilibrium between bound and free ligate within the pore is much less disturbed by washing-out of the free component than at the outer surface of the matrix particle.

The way to equalize the rate (speed) of dissociation or association could be the application of very small, nonporous sorbent particles, which realize the high specific surface by reduced particle diameter. In such column packings all reactions are determined by the flux of the mobile phase, diffusion processes are negligible, since the thickness of the solvent part of the stationary phase is small with respect to the matrix particles and the biomacromolecules (theoretical considerations are given e.g. by Eppert (1988)).

Finally, when immunoaffinity chromatography is used on a commercial scale, it should be mentioned that ligands are often very expensive. Therefore, methods have to be included which protect affinity colunms from run down or from accumulation of materials from biological sources. The latter, the so-called fouling, is difficult to reverse, since most of the methods applied for cleaning in place are impossible when biomacromolecules as antibodies are used as ligands.

2.2. Activation of Supports and Immobilization (Coupling) of Affinity Ligands

Similar compromises as described above for supports are to be made when an activation method is to be selected, since no protocol exists which fulfills all criteria for ligand immobilization. Some of the antagonistic requirements which have to be satisfied are:

- The activation reagent should yield a highly reactive intermediate, but this intermediate should not react with constituents of the solvent (buffer) used.
- The activation process should be universal, but the linkage between matrix and ligand should be specific.
- The fixation of the ligand should be strong, but the ligand should not suffer any loss of properties necessary for interaction with the ligate.
- The bond between matrix and ligand should not be split during the chromatographic process but it should be readily cleavable under certain conditions.

Immobilization of ligands may be classified in respect of several characteristics:

- chemical nature of the bond (covalent fixation, adsorption by electrostatic or hydrophobic forces)
- stability of the bond (reversible or irreversible binding, leakage of ligands)
- fixation of the ligand directly to the matrix or immobilization via a molecule of distinct length (spacer)

The following chapter deals mostly with techniques of covalent immobilization. Adsorptive methods as used for the coating of polystyrene surfaces of microtitration plates, blotting methods onto nitrocellulose, polybrene (hexadimethrine bromide, 1,5-dimethyl-1,5-diaza-undecamethylene polymethobromide) coated, polytetrafluoroethylene (PTFE, Teflon) or nylon membranes or covering of microparticles (latices or collodial metal) will be mentioned in Chapter 4 in connection with the description of enzyme immunoassays.

However, there are also some examples of immunoaffinity separations, which use supports where the ligand is bound by ionic and/or other mechanisms or more complex (hydrophobic) adsorption. As an example of the first case, Kataoka et al. (1987) described the separation of IgG^+ and IgG^- vital lymphocyte subpopulations on a support formed by adsorption of immunoglobulin to a polystyrene/polyamine graft copolymer or to a poly(2-hydroxyethyl methacrylate) / polyamine copolymer. They were able to show that in a single step procedure the IgG^+ cells could be obtained at more than 90 % purity with a recovery of 79 to 95 %.

The second type of non-covalent fixation is for instance useful in the preparation of small amounts of highly specific antibodies from polyclonal sera. With this method, neither the preparative purification of the antigen nor a fractionation of antibodies is needed: the protein mixture containing the antigen is separated by sodium dodecylsulfate polyacrylamide gel electrophoresis, and the separated proteins are blotted onto a nitrocellulose or another appropriate membrane by Western blot technique (HALL et al., 1984, OLMSTED, 1988). Areas of this blot containing the antigen of interest are excised and used as an "affinity column" for separation of antigen-specific antibodies, contained in serum or an ascitic fluid. The amount of specific antibodies obtained from blots is sufficient for immunocytochemistry (a protocol is given by HARLOW and LANE, 1988, p. 498).

A third way has been described by MADARA et al. (1990), who also separated antigen(s) in gel electrophoresis, but immobilized the antigens *in situ* with glutaraldehyde and used the polyacrylamide gel as affinity matrix in a minicolumn.

A prerequisite for these methods is the recovery of epitope(s) of the antigen after denaturating electrophoresis by renaturation of the correct three-dimensional structure of the epitope(s) after removal of the detergent. But it should also be possible to use this protocol for sensitive proteins or their epitopes by the application of a non-denaturating electrophoretic system.

In a fourth group, affinity chromatograhy methods can be summarized, in which a not very high specific adsorption mechanism is employed. For example, NGO and KHATTER (1990) described a support in which ligand was synthesized using pentafluoropyridine, dimethylaminopyridine and ethylene glycol and which was successfully used for serum fractionation, including specific adsorption of immunoglobulins.

2.2.1. Activation of Supports for Covalent Fixation

The activation of solid supports for coupling of biospecific ligands may be divided into three types:

- Incorporation of reactive groups into the matrix during synthesis of the support (polymerization)
- Addition of side chains with reactive groups to the matrix by copolymerization of a suitable monomer
- Modification of parts of the matrix molecules by formation of groups able to undergo chemical reactions faster and / or easier then the backbone of the support

Table 2.3. gives a survey of the most common reactions for immobilization of ligands, which are also used for fixation of antibodies and antigens. Reviews of coupling methods are given for instance by GOLDSTEIN (1976), GRIBNAU (1977) and more recently by SCOUTEN (1987). A large number of quick reference surveys on molecular immobilization from the viewpoint of coupled biomolecules (enzymes and other proteins, glycoproteins, polysaccharides) are published by STURGEON and KENNEDY (1980 foll.).

From a chemical point of view there is no difference between activation of, and coupling to, an organic or inorganic support. The most prominent exception is the derivatization of the inorganic support using a functionalized silane bearing amino, hydroxy, carboxy, olefinic or other reactive group. A review of the immobilization of antibodies to inorganic supports, especially to porous glass, is provided by WEETALL and LEE (1989).

Selected References for Table 2.3.

Method No.

1 AXEN, R., PORATH, J., ERNBACK, S. (1967): Chemical coupling of peptides and proteins to polysaccharides by means of cyanogen halides. Nature **214**, 1302-1304

1' KOHN, J., WILCHEK, M. (1984): The use of cyanogen bromide and other novel cyanylating agents for the activation of polysaccharide resins. Appl. Biochem. Biotechnol. **9**, 285-305

2 KAY, G., LILLY, M.D. (1970): The chemical attachment of chymotrypsin to water-insoluble polymers using 2-amino-4,6-dichloro-s-triazine. Biochim. Biophys. Acta **198**, 276-285

FINLAY, T.H., TROLL, V., LEVY, M., JOHNSON, A.J., HODGINS, L.T. (1978): New methods for the preparation of biospecific adsorbents and immobil-

ized enzymes utilizing trichloro-striazine. Anal. Biochem. **87**, 77-90
HODGINS, L.T., LEVY, M. (1980): Affinity adsorbent preparation. Chemical features of agarose derivatization with trichloro-s-triazine. J. Chromatogr. **202**, 381-390

3 NGO, T.T. (1986): Methods of activating hydroxyl groups of a polymeric carrier using 3-fluoro-1-methyl-pyridinium toluene-4-sulfonate. U.S. patent **4**, 582,875

4 BRANDT, J., ANDERSSON, L.O., PORATH, J. (1975): Covalent attachment of proteins to polysaccharide carriers by means of benzoquinone. Biochim. Biophys. Acta **386**, 196-202

5 PORATH, J., FORNSTEDT, N.J. (1970): Group fractionation of plasma proteins on dipolar ion exchangers. J. Chromatogr. **51**, 479-489
SUNDBERG, L., PORATH, J. (1974): Preparation of adsorbents for biospecific affinity chromatography. The attachment of group-containing ligands to insoluble polymers by means of bifunctional oxiranes. J. Chromatogr. **90**, 87-98

6 VREDBLAD, P. (1974): Immobilization of ligands for biospecific affinity chromatography via their hydroxyl groups. The cyclohexaamylose-β-amylase system. FEBS Lett. **47**, 86-89
GELSEMA, W.J., LIGNY, C.L., ROOZEN, A.M.P., WILM, G.P. (1981): Optimal conditions for the coupling of aromatic amines to epoxy-activated Sepharose 6B. J. Chromatogr. **209**, 363-368
MATSUMOTO, I., KITAGAKI, H. AGAI, Y., ITO, Y., SENO, N. (1981): Derivatization of epoxy-activated agarose with various charbohydrates for the preparation of stable and high-capacity affinity adsorbents: Their use for affinity chromatography of carbohydrate-binding proteins. Anal. Biochem. **116**, 103-110

7 AXEN, R., DREVIN, H., CARLSSON, J. (1975): Preparation of modified agarose gels containing thiol groups. Acta Chem. Scand. **B 29**, 471-474

8 BETHELL, G.S., AYERS, J.S., HANCOCK, W.S., HEARN, M.T.W. (1979): A novel method of activation of cross-linked agaroses with 1,1'-carbnyldiimidazole which gives a matrix for affinity chromatography devoid of additional charged groups. J. Biol. Chem. **254**, 2572-2574
BETHELL, G.S., AYERS, J., HEARN, M.T.W., HANCOCK, W.S. (1981): Investigation of the activation of various insoluble polysaccharides with 1,1-carbonyldiimidazole and of the properties of the activated matrices. J. Chromatogr. **219**, 361-372
TSUTSUI, K., MUELLER, G.C. (1982): Affinity chromatography of heme-binding proteins. An improved method for the synthesis of hemin-agarose. Anal. Biochem. **121**, 244-250

9 BORCHERT, A., LARSSON, P.O., MOSBACH, K. (1982): High-performance liquid affinity chromatography on silica-bound Concanavalin A. J. Chromatogr. **244**, 49-56
NILSSON, K., MOSBACH, K. (1981): Immobilization of enzymes and affinity ligands to various hydroxyl group carying supports using highly reactive sulfonyl chlorides. Biochem. Biophys. Res. Comm. **102**, 449-457
NILSSON, K., MOSBACH, K. (1984): Immobilization of ligands with organic sulfonyl chlorides. Meth. Enzymol. **104**, 56-69
KRISAM, G. (1985): Immobilization using organic sulfonyl chlorides. In: DEAN, P.D.G., JOHNSON, W.S., MIDDLE, F.A. (eds.) Affinity Chromatography - A Practical Approach, pp. 52-53

10 CUATRECASAS, P. (1970): Protein purification by affinity chromatography. - Derivatizations of agarose and polyacrylamide beads. J. Biol. Chem. **245**, 3059-1065

11 HEARN, M.T.W., HARRIS, E.L., BETHELL, G.S., HANCOCK, H.S., AYERS, J.A. (1981): Application of 1,1'-carbonyldi-imidazole-activated matrices for the purification of proteins. III. The use of 1,1'-carbonyldiimidazole-activated agaroses in the biospecific affinity chromatographic isolation of serum antibodies. J. Chromatogr. **218**, 509-518
BÜTTNER, W., BECKER, M., RUPPRICH, CH., BOEDEN, H.-F., HENKLEIN, P., LOTH, F., DAUTZENBERG, H. (1989): A novel carbonochloridate for activation of supports containing hydroxyl groups. Biotechnol. Bioengin. **33**, 26-31

12 JAGENDORF, A.T., PATCHORNIK, A., SELA, M.P. (1963): Use of antibody bound to modified cellulose as an immunospecific adsorbent of antigens. Biochim. Biophys. Acta **78**, 516-628
SATO, T., MORI, T., TOSA, T., CHIBATA, I. (1971): Studies on immobilized enzymes. IX. Preparation and properties of aminoacylases covalently attached to halogenoaccetylcelluloses. Arch. Biochem. Biophys. **147**, 788-796

13 GRIBNAU, T.C.J. (1985): 2,4,6-Trifluoro-5-chloropyrimidine activation of Agarose. in: DEAN, P.D.G., JOHNSO N, W.S., MIDDLE, F.A. (eds.) Affinity Chromatography - A Practical Approach, pp. 39-42

14 PORATH, J., LAAS, T., JANSON, J.C. (1975): Agar derivatives for chromatography, electrophoresis and gel-bound enzymes. III. Rigid agarose gels cross-linked with divinyl sulphone (DVS). J. Chromatogr. **103**, 49-62
SAIRAM, M.R., PORATH, J. (1976): Isolation of antibodies to protein hormones by bioaffinity chromatography on divinylsulfonyl Sepharose. Biochem. Biophys. Res. Comm. **69**, 190-196

15 KRISAM, G. (1985): Polyisocyanate activation of hydroxyl group-containing polymers. in: DEAN, P.D.G., JOHNSON, W.S., MIDDLE, F.A. (eds.) Affinity Chromatogrphy - A Practical Approach, pp. 48-52

Table 2.3. Methods for Activation of Frequently Used Matrices and for Coupling of Biomacromolecules and Related Substances (selected examples)

	Support with functional group	Reagent for activation	Reactivative group on support after activation	Biomolecule with reactive group	Coupling product
1	–OH	CNBr	–O–C≡N [a]	NH_2–BM	–O–C(=NH)–NH–BM
	–OH	CNBr	–O –O–C≡NH [b]	NH_2–BM	–O–C(=NH)–NH–BM
1'	–OH	$[(C_2H_5)_3N^+CN]Br^-$	–O–C≡N	NH_2–BM	–O–C(=NH)–NH–BM
	–OH	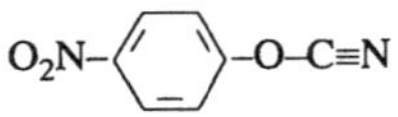	–O–C≡N	NH_2–BM	–O–C(=NH)–NH–BM
	–OH	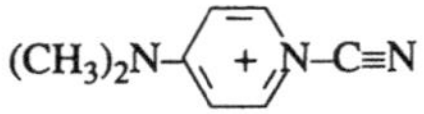	–O–C≡N	NH_2–BM	–O–C(=NH)–NH–BM
2	–OH	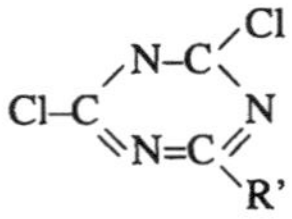	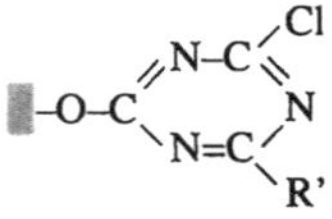	NH_2–BM	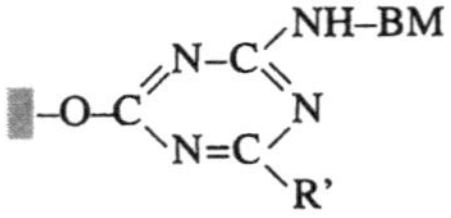
3	–OH	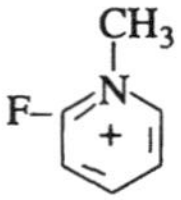	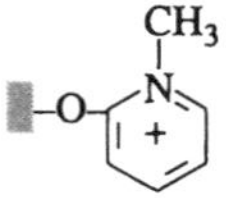	NH_2–BM HS–BM	–NH–BM –S–BM
4	–OH	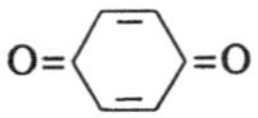	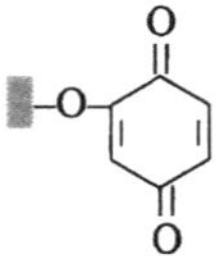	NH_2–BM	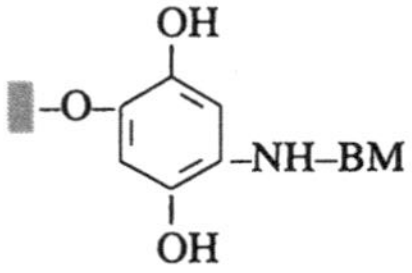
5	–OH	$Cl-CH_2-CH-CH_2$ O	$-O-CH_2-CH-CH_2$ O	HO–BM	$-O-CH_2-CH(OH)-CH_2-O-$BM
	–OH	$Cl-CH_2-CH-CH_2$ O	$-O-CH_2-CH-CH_2$ O	H_2N–BM	$-O-CH_2-CH(OH)-CH_2-NH-$BM
	–OH	$Cl-CH_2-CH-CH_2$ O	$-O-CH_2-CH-CH_2$ O	HS–BM	$-O-CH_2-CH(OH)-CH_2-S-$BM

Table 2.3. Continued from page 36

	Support with functional group	Reagent for activation	Reactivative group on support after activation	Biomolecule with reactive group	Coupling product
6	▮-OH	CH_2-CH . . CH-CH_2 (epoxide rings, -O- bridging)	▮-O-CH_2-CH(OH)- . . -CH-CH_2 (epoxide, -O- bridging)	H_2N-BM	▮-O-CH_2-CH(OH)- . . -CH(OH)-CH_2-NH-BM
	▮-OH	CH_2-CH . . CH-CH_2 (epoxide rings, -O- bridging)	▮-O-CH_2-CH(OH)-OH-CH-CH_2 (epoxide, -O- bridging)	HO-BM	▮-O-CH_2-CH(OH)- . . -CH(OH)-CH_2-O-BM
7	▮-OH	CH_2-CH . . CH-CH_2-S-S-Py (epoxide, -O- bridging)	▮-O-CH_2-CH(OH)—CH-CH_2-S-S-Py	HS-BM	▮-O-CH_2-CH(OH)-CH_2-S-S-BM
8	▮-OH	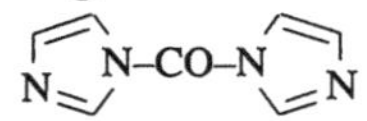	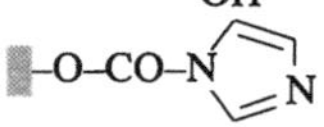	H_2N-BM	▮-CO-NH-BM
9	▮-OH	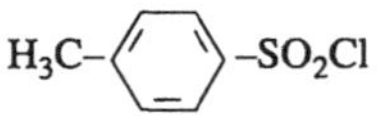	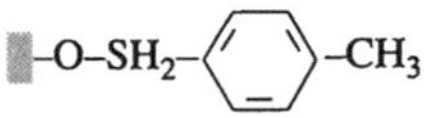	H_2N-BM	▮-NH-BM
	▮-OH	F_3C-CH_2-SO_2Cl	▮-O-SO_2C-CH_2-CF_3	H_2N-BM	▮-NH-BM
	▮-OH	F_3C-CH_2-SO_2Cl	▮-O-SO_2C-CH_2-CF_3	HS-BM	▮-S-BM
10	▮-OH	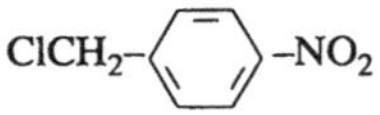	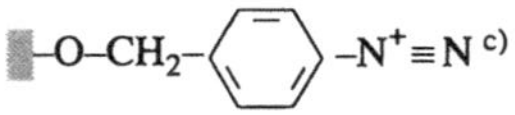	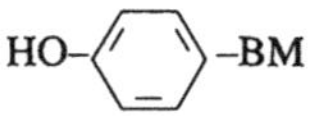	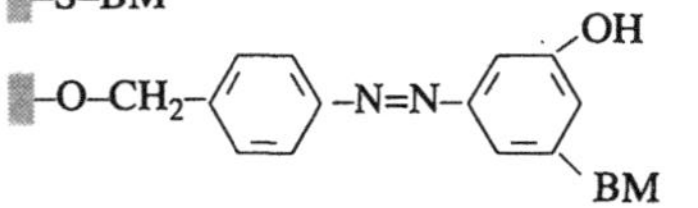
11	▮-OH	Cl-CO-O-R	▮-O-CO-OR	HO-BM	▮-O-CO-O-BM
	▮-OH	Cl-CO-O-R	▮-O-CO-OR	NH_2-BM	▮-O-CO-NH-BM
	▮-OH	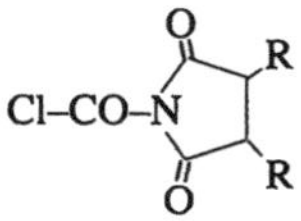	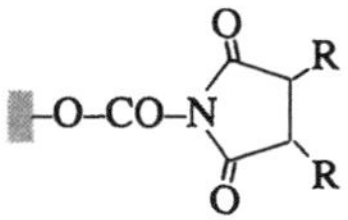	NH_2-BM	▮-O-CO-NH-BM
12	▮-OH	X-CO-CH_2-X	▮-O-CO-CH_2-X	NH_2-BM	▮-O-CO-CH_2-NH-BM
13	▮-OH	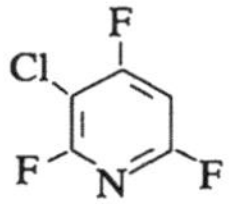	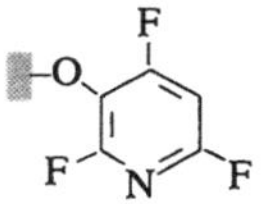	NH_2-BM	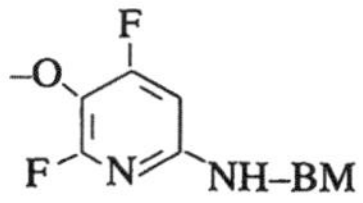

Table 2.3. Continued from page 37

	Support with functional group	Reagent for activation	Reactivative group on support after activation	Biomolecule with reactive group	Coupling product
14	▮–OH	CH_2=CH–SO_2–CH=CH_2	▮–O–C_2H_4–SO_2–CH=CH_2	H_2N–BM	▮–O–C_2H_4–SO_2–C_2H_4–BM
15	▮–OH	O=C=N– . . . . –N=C=O	▮–O–CO–NH– . . . –N=C=O	H_2N–BM	▮–O–CO–NH– . . . –NH–CO–NH–BM
16	▮–OH	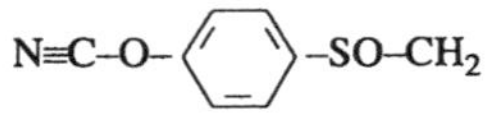	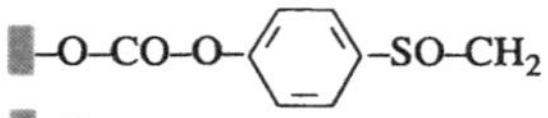	H_2N–BM	▮–O–CO–NH–BM
17	▮–OH	$(RO)_3Si$–C_3H_6–NH_2	▮–O –O–Si–C_3H_6–NH_2 –O	H_2N–BM	▮–O –O–Si–C_3H_6–NH_2=CHC_3H_6CH=NH–BM [d)] –O
18	▮–OH	RO–Si$(CH_3)_2$–CH_2–SH	▮–O–Si–$(CH_3)_2$–CH_2–SH	H_2N–BM	▮–O–Si–$(CH_3)_2$–CH_2– . . –NH–BM [e)]
19	▮–CH–CH– OH OH	($NaIO_4$)	▮–O–CH= . . –CH=O [f)]	H_2N–BM	▮–CH CH– . . N BM
20	▮–CH=O		▮–CH=O	H_2N–BM	▮–CH=N–BM
	▮–CH=O		▮–CH=O	H_2N–BM	▮–CH_2=NH–BM [g)]
21	▮–COOH	Cl–CO–R	▮–CO–O–CO–R	H_2N–BM	▮–CO=NH–BM
	▮–COOH	Cl–CO–R	▮–CO–O–CO–R	HO–BM	▮–CO–O–BM
22	▮–COOH	R'–N=C=N–R"	▮–CO–O–CO–(=NR')NH–R"	H_2N–BM	▮–CO=NH–BM
23	▮–COOH	N-ethyl-isoxazolium-5-(phenyl-3-sulfonate)		H_2N–BM	▮–CO=NH–BM
24	▮–COOH	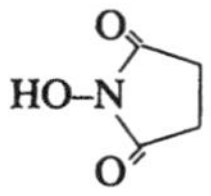	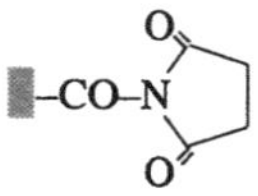 h)	H_2N–BM	▮–CO=NH–BM
25	▮–COOH	1,2–dihydro-2-ethoxy-1-ethoxycarbonyl-quinoline	▮–CO–O–CO–C_2H_5	H_2N–BM	▮–CO=NH–BM
26	▮–COOH	H_2NNH_2 + HNO_3	▮–CO–N_3	H_2N–BM	▮–CONH–BM
27	▮–$CONH_2$	H_2NNH_2 + HNO_3	▮–CO–N_3	H_2N–BM	▮–CONH–BM

Table 2.3. **Continued from page 38**

	Support with functional group	Reagent for activation	Reactivative group on support after activation	Biomolecule with reactive group	Coupling product
28	▮-$CONH_2$	$(OCH-(CH_2)_3-CHO)_3$ [i]	CHO CHO ▮-$CONH-CHCHC_2H_4CH=CC_2H_4CHO$ C_2H_4 CHO	H_2N-BM	CHO CHO ▮-$CONH-CHCHC_2H_4CH=CC_2H_4CHO$ C_2H_4 NH CHO BM
29	▮-NH_2	O=C=N– . . –N=C=O	▮-NH–CO–NH– . . –N=C=O	H_2N-BM	▮-NH–CO–NH– . . —NH–CO–NH–BH
	▮-NH_2	S=C=N– . . –N=C=S	▮-NH–CS–NH– . . –N=C=S	H_2N-BM	▮-NH–CS–NH– . . —NH–CS–NH–BH
30	▮-NH_2	$OCH-C_3H_6-CHO$	▮-$N=CH-C_3H_6-CHO$	H_2N-BM	▮-$NH-C_5H_{10}-NH-BM$ [g]
31	▮-NH_2	—	—	CHO–BM [j]	▮-N=CH–BM
32	▮-$N=NH_2$	—	—	CHO–BM [j]	▮-N=CH–BM
33	▮-NH_2	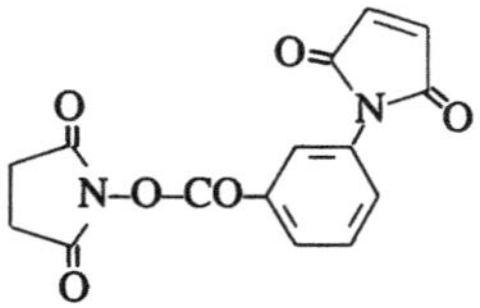	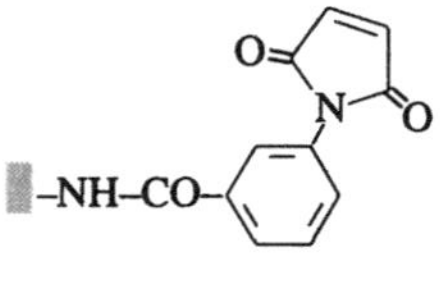	HS–BM	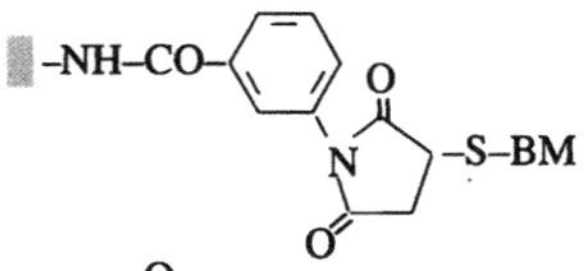
34	▮-SH	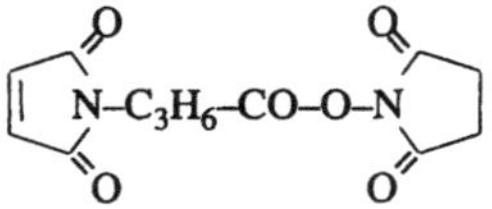	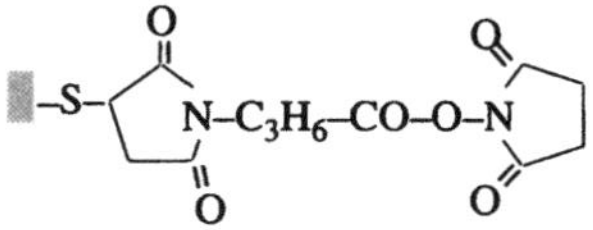	H_2N-BM	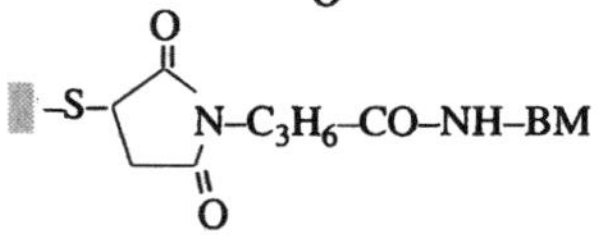

▮, Support; BM, residue of the ligand (e.g. biomacromolecule, spacer); R, R', R", organo-chemical residues; X, halogen.

[a] main reaction product after activation of agarose; [b] main reaction product after activation of dextranes and celluloses; [c] product after reduction and diazotation; [d] coupling of activated support and ligand via glutaraldehyde; [e] second step: addition of N-γ-maleimido-butyryloxy succinimide ester (GMBS) to the SH-group of the support, third step: coupling of antibodies to the obtained active ester; [f] periodate oxidation of carbohydrates; [g] after reduction of azomethins (SCHIFF's bases); [h] by use of carbodiimides; [i] glutaraldehyde trimer; [j] for instance obtained after periodate oxidation of oligosaccharide side chains of glycoproteins

16 Kohn, J., Wilchek, M. (1983) in: Chaiken, I.M., Wilchek, M., Parikh, I. (eds.) Affinity chromatography and biological recognition, pp. 197-207

17 Weetall, H.H., Filbert, A.M. (1974): Porous glass for affinity chromatography applications. Meth. Enzymol. **34**, 59-72
Schössler, W., Boeden, H.-F., Hiepe, F. (1988): A novel procedure for the activation of support materials. in: Kalasz, H., Ettre, L.S. (eds.) Chromatography 87, pp. 381-388

18 Bhatia, S.K., Shriver-Lake, L.C., Prior, K.J., Georger, J.H., Calvert, J.M., Bredehorst, R., Ligler, F.S. (1989): Use of thiol-terminal silanes and heterobifunctional corsslinkers for immobilization of antibodies on silica surfaces. Anal. Biochem. **178**, 408-413

19 Flemming, CH., Gabert, A., Roth, P. (1973): Synthese und Eigenschaften trägerfixierter Enzyme. I. Kovalente Bindung von Trypsin an Dialdehydzellulose. Acta. Biol. Med. Germ. **30**, 177-182
Junowicz, E., Charm, S.E. (1976): The derivatization of oxidized polysaccharides for protein immobilization and affinity chromatography. Biochim. Biophys. Acta **428**, 157-165
Turkova, J., Vajcner, D., Vancurova, D., Stamberg, J. (1979): Immobilization on cellulose in bead form after periodate oxidation and reductive alkylation. Coll. Czech. Chem. Comm. **44**, 3411-3417

20 Weetall, H.H., Filbert, A.M. (1974): Porous glass for affinity chromatography applications. Meth. Enzymol. **34**, 59-72

21 Dean, P.D.G., Johnson, W.S., Middle, F.A. (eds.) (1985): Mixed anhydride activation procedures. Affinity Chromatography - A Practical Approach, p. 44.

22 Engblad, A. (1981): A comparative study of the binding of cartilage link protein and the hyaluronate-binding region of the cartilage proteoglycan to hyaluronate-substituted sepharose gel. Biochem. J. **199**, 297-305
Lyon, M., Phelps, C.F. (1981): A rapid purification of bovine testicular hyaluronidase by chromatography on dermatan sulphate-substituted 1, 6-diaminohexane-sepharose 4B. Biochem. J. **199**, 419-426

23 Patel, A.B., Pennington, S.N., Brown, H.D. (1989): Insoluble matrix-supported apyrase, deoxyribonuclease, and cholinesterase. Biochim. Biophys. Acta **178**, 626-629

24 Cuatrecasas, P., Parikh, I. (1972): Adsorbents for affinity chromatography. Use of N-hydroxysuccinimide esters of agarose. Biochem. **11**, 2291-2299
Frost, R. G., Monthony, J.F., Engelhorn, S.C., Siebert, C.J. (1981): Covalent immobilization of proteins to N-hydroxysuccinimide ester derivatives of agarose. Effect of protein charge of immobilization. Biochim. Biophys. Acta **670**, 163-169

25 Sundaran, P.V. (1974): A new method of coupling proteins to insoluble polymers. Biochem. Biophys. Res. Comm. **61**, 717-722

26 Mitz, M.A., Summaria, L.J. (1961): Synthesis of biologically active cellulose derivatives of enzymes. Nature **189**, 576-577

27 Suttnar, J., Hrkal, Z., Vodrazka, Z. (1977): Affinity chromatography of serum haemopoxin. J. Chromatogr. **131**, 453-457

28 Ternynck, T., Avrameas, S. (1972). Polyacrylamide-protein immunoadsorbents prepared with glutaraldehyde. FEBS Lett. **23**, 24-28

29 Ozawa, H. (1967): Bridging reagent for protein. I. The reaction of diisocyanates with lysine and enzyme proteins. J. Biochem. **62**, 419-423

30 Cambiaso, C.L., Goffinet, A., Vaerman, J.P., Heremons, J.F. (1975): Glutaraldehyd-activated aminohexyl-derivative of sepharose 4B as a new versatile immunosorbent. Immunochem. **12**, 273-278
Glassmeyer, C.K., Ogle, J.D. (1971): Properties of an insoluble form of trypsin. Biochem. **10**, 786-792
Habeeb, A.F.S.A. (1967): Preparation of enzymically active, water-insoluble derivatives of trypsin. Arch. Biochem. Biophys. **119**, 264-268

31 Flemminger, G., Hadas, E., Wolf, T., Solomon, B. (1990): Oriented immobilization of periodate-oxidized monoclonal antibodies on amino and hydrazide derivatives of Eupergit C. Appl. Biochem. Biotechnol. **23**, 123-137

32 O'Shannessy, D.J. (1990) Hydrazido-derivatized supports in affinity chromatography. J. Chromatogr. **510**, 13-21
O'Shannessy, D.J., Wilchek, M. (1990) Immobilization of glycoconjugates by their oligosaccharides: Use of hydrazido-derivatized matrices. Anal. Biochem. **191**, 1-8

33 Crowl, C.P., Gibbons, I., Schneider, R.S. (1980): Recent advances in homogenous enzyme immunoassays for haptens and proteins. in: Nakamura, R.M., Dito, W.R., Tucker III, E.S. (eds.) Immunoassays. A.R. Liss Inc., New York, pp. 89-126

34 Bhatia, S.K., Shriver-Lake, L.C., Prior, K.J., Georger, J.H., Calvert, J.M., Bredehorst, R., Ligler, J.F.S. (1989): Use of thiol-terminal silanes and heterobifucntional crosslinkers for immobilization of antibodies on silica surfaces. Anal. Biochem. **178**, 408-413

2.2.2. Coupling of Ligands

Immobilization of biomacromolecules on solid supports may be divided into two different pathways. Ligands can be coupled (i) directly to the activated support or (ii) via a so-called spacer molecule, which has been bound to the support previously. The latter is followed by a procedure, in which a reactive group of the spacer able to fix the ligand to the matrix is activated.

As shown in Table 2.3. the borderline between cases (i) and (ii) is not very precise since some bifunctional reagents for activation of the support may also serve as (activated) spacers, e.g. bis-oxiranes, glutaraldehyde, triazines, and others.

Application of spacers is necessery when the structure of the ligand which is to interact with the ligate (e.g. antigen and the respective antibody) is too close to the matrix, so that a tight binding in an optimal conformation is not possible. As discussed later, this hindrance was mostly not of importance when antibodies were immobilized, if the fixation occured in a position far from the antigenbinding site(s).

Coupling of relatively small molecules as peptides or haptens to an insoluble matrix should reflect steric interactions between matrix and ligate as well as interactions between a chosen spacer and constituents of the mixture to be separated. Chersi et al. (1989) gave an example for the latter case: they fixed a dodecapeptide (i) via coupling of the peptide with glutaraldehyde to an aminohexyl support, (ii) by coupling directly to the support and (iii) by covalent immobilization to a support containing activated caproic acid. According to case (i) (matrix-$(CH_2)_6$-N=CH-$(CH_2)_3$-CH=N-peptide) the support showed during chromatography of an antiserum much higher unspecific adsorption than the two other supports, which is interpreted as (hydrophobic) binding of serum constitutents to the spacer.

In most cases it is impossible to predict exactly where proteins will be attached to an activated matrix. If antibodies are to be purified on a support containing their protein antigen it may occur that epitopes are too closely attached to the matrix backbone or that the distance between epitope and the matrix is too small for an optimal interaction between antibody (ligate) and antigen (ligand). This is schematically demonstrated in Fig. 2.1.

Hinman et al. (1985) gave an example of such a case. They overcame this problem by coupling

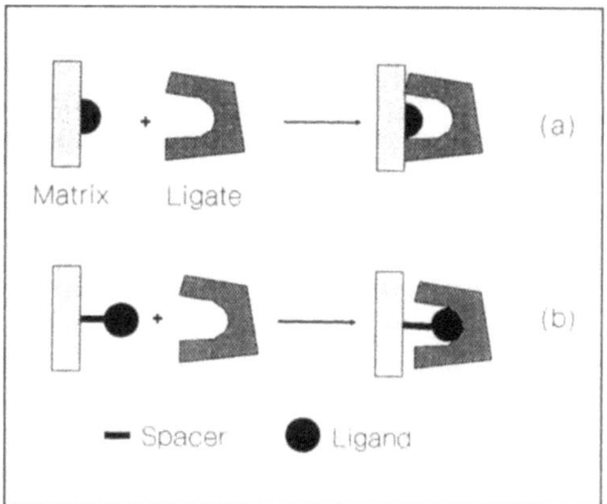

Fig. 2.1. Principle of ligand-ligate interaction.
a) Small ligand and hidden binding region in the ligate. The distance between ligand surface and ligate binding region is too far for interaction. b) Small ligand, immobilized via a spacer molecule, reaches the hidden binding region of the ligate.

a specific acceptor toxin of the acetylchloline receptor to the matrix, followed by affinity adsorption of the receptor to the toxin. They now constructed a combined affinity matrix by covalent fixation of the acetylcholine receptor (antigen) to the toxin with cross-linkers (dimethylsuberimidat or dimethyl 3,3'-dithiobispropionimidat). Despite slight differences between the effects of the two cross-linkers used it was possible to increase the amount of adsorbed specific antibodies twofold, indicating that antibody fractions now reached the antigen which were in part excluded by steric hindrance in consequence of direct connection of the antigen to the support.

A similar approach was made by Sisson and Castor (1990). They omited the random orientation of a coupled antibody by an initial immobilization of protein A to the insoluble matrix followed by an adsorption of IgG to this support and chemical stabilization of the complex by cross-linking the proteins with dimethylpimelimidate. Since protein A binds to the Fc part of an antibody, the antigen-binding sites of the antibody are more or less turned away from the surface of the matrix. The authors reported an at least twofold increase in binding capacity with respect to a support containing immunoglobulin directly bound to the matrix. Further, the stoichiometry of antibody-antigen reactions reached 80 to 100 % of the theoretical value in such columns. But, in general, when an antigen has to be purified, a spacer is mostly not necessary since the large antibody serves a distance molecule as such.

On the other hand, a slight increase of the ratio of moles bound antigen per mole coupled antibody was found by HOFFMAN and O'SHANNESSY (1988), who used hydrazido agaroses with different spacers (Affigel 10-H, Affigel 15-H, Affigel 21-H): The ratio raised from 0.53 to 0.70 mole/mole.

Most of the coupling procedures are based on the reaction of a NH_2-, COOH-, SH- or OH-group as a part of an amino acid side chain of the respective proteinous ligand. A macromolecule as an antibody has a lot of such groups on its surface. In principle, all side chains of a certain amino acid within a protein are able to react in the same manner with the activated support. Considering an immunoglobulin molecule, reactive residues are contained in the Fc as well as in the Fab fragment. Fixation can occur statistically: one part of the immunoglobulin molecule will be bound via the Fc region, another to the Fab: this immobilization will be more or less random also in or nearby the antigen binding region. These different opportunities contribute to the observed relatively low stoichiometry in interactions between an immobilized antibody and a dissolved antigen (or vice versa).

In ideal systems, one antibody should bind two antigen molecules but in reality the ratio between antigen and antibody is less then 1.

For instance, BHATIA et al. (1989) reported a ratio of 0.37 to 0.55, SADA et al. (1986) found a ratio of about 0.5 independently of the use of whole antibodies or Fab fragments (in the latter case the theoretical ratio should be 1:1). Often the ratio is even lower, as discussed above. An increase of this ratio by coupling the antibody in the presence of the respective antigen (protection of the binding region) is mostly impossible, especially when the antigen is a protein which could also become bound to the activated support.

The involvement of the antigen-binding site into the covalent immobilization process could also be a reason for the decrease of the binding constant (increase of the dissociation constant), since fixation suppresses intramolecular movements in the antibody molecule during the interaction process ("induced fit") and/or reduces accessibility of the binding site. An example for such an alteration of the dissociation constant by immobilization of antibodies to different supports is given by DAVIS et al. (1986), as shown in Table 2.4.

Table 2.4. Dissociation Constans of Antibody-Antigen Complexes as Consequences of Different Immobilization Methods. (Data from DAVIS et al., 1986)

Antibody coupled via	K_D [moles/l]
Carbonyldiimidazol activation	1.9×10^{-11}
SCHIFF base after periodate oxidation	1.1×10^{-11}
Isourea after CNBr activation	8.3×10^{-12}
Amide	2.7×10^{-13}
no coupling (control, complex in solution)	7.1×10^{-14}

A reagent specific to arginine residues is presented by DUERKSEN-HUGHES et al. (1987, 1989). The glyoxal group of the reagent 4-(oxoacetyl)phenoxyacetic acid forms a stable, covalent bond with the guanidino group of arginine. Thus, a certain prediction of the locus of fixation in a given protein could be possible.

Another interesting approach to defined fixation of proteins to a chromatographic support was given by HOFFMAN and O'SHANNESSY (1988) and FLEMINGER et al. (1990) (for review see O'SHANNESSY, 1990, O'SHANNESSY and WILCHEK, 1990). Following mild periodate oxidation of the carbohydrate side chain of monoclonal antibodies they bound the immunoglobulin to a carrier (Eupergit C) containing amino or hydrazino groups. Since the oligosaccharide chains are localized mostly in the Fc moity of the IgG molecule (only about 10 % of the normal IgG population contains mannose-rich sugar chains in the Fab fragment (MALAN BOREL et al., 1990), the antigen binding site cannot be hindered by the solid support (the same principle using a heterobifunctional cross-linking reagent was recently described by Zara et al. (1991) for formation of antibody conjugates). For coupling of aldehyde groups (i.e. oxidized carbohydrate side chains of glycoproteins) hydrazino-derivatized supports should be preferred because the hydrazone formed is much more stable to hydrolysis than Schiff base derivatives, which are the reaction products of an aldehyde with a primary amine-containing matrix (O'Shannessy, 1990). These results were also supported by Matson and Little (1988), who examined the parameters for immobilization of monoclonal antibodies via periodate oxidation of the carbohydrate moity of the mabs.

Matson and Little observed a more than threefold increase in binding capacity when the antibody was site-directed immobilized by coupling of aldehyde-containing (oxidized) antibodies to a hydrazido matrix in comparison to a stochastical fixation via NH_2-groups.

Taking into account two binding sites for an antigen in an IgG molecule, Fleminger et al. (1990) found a ratio ranging from 1:1 to 1.7:1 (moles antigen per mole fixed antibody), which provides strong evidence of undisturbed antigen binding.

On the other hand, when the same antibody was fixed to an epoxy-activated support, only 0.15 to 0.76 moles/mol were bound, indicating a fixation of the antibody via amino groups wherever in the Fc as well as in or nearby the binding region of the Fab parts.

A similar approach, useful for polysaccharide supports and oligosaccharide moities of glycoproteins as antibodies, has been presented by Turkova et al. (1990) and Petkov et al. (1990): Carbohydrate side chains of both components were oxidized chemically or with an appropriate enzyme (galactose oxidase or glucose oxidase), then the oxidized protein was coupled via adipinic acid dihydrazide.

Important for the capacity and the chromatographic behaviour of an affinity ligand are the type of activation and the amount of ligand bound per matrix volume (ligand density). Peng et al. (1987) investigated the influence of several activation methods on the ligand concentration. Using cyanogen bromide, tosyl chloride, cyanuric chloride, chromium trioxide or dimethylsulfoxide/carbodiimide as activation reagents of cross-linked cellulose beads, they studied the model system human IgG/goat(anti-human IgG)IgG. Increasing the amount of coupled goat IgG the authors observed a relative decrease of bound antigen (human IgG), but this decrease was not uniform with respect to the different activation procedures applied. Similar experiments were performed by Sada et al. (1986). Antibodies and their $F(ab')_2$-fragments were covalently bound either directly by cyanogen bromide activation or via a spacer to Sepharose or cellulose fibers. A steep drop in binding capacity occurred if the ligand concentration was increased from 0.5 to 5 mg/ml, then the decrease was only slight up to a final concentration of 30 mg of antibody per ml of gel (Fig. 2.2.).

Further, Sada and coworkers found that spacers also influence ligand-ligate interactions. At low ligand densities long-spacered matrices have higher adsorption ratios (moles specifically adsorbed antigen per mole fixed antibody), whereas at high ligand densities this effect is inverted. A definitive interpretation of this effect cannot be given at present.

Despite the problems of directed fixation of antibodies or proteinous antigens, there are two further facts which are much more important: The first is the so-called multipoint attachment, the second is shell formation of immobilized ligands.

Multipoint attachment occurs since a protein mostly has more than one amino acid side chain (bearing e.g. NH_2-groups from lysine and arginine, respectively, or OH-groups from serine, threonine and tyrosine, respectively) which may react at different loci of the activated matrix.

The observation that coupling at elevated pH increases multipoint attachment (Pfeiffer et al., 1987) underlines this conclusion, since at elevated pH more unprotonated NH_2-groups are available for the formation of covalent linkages (the pH value for 1:1 ratio of protonated and unprotonat-

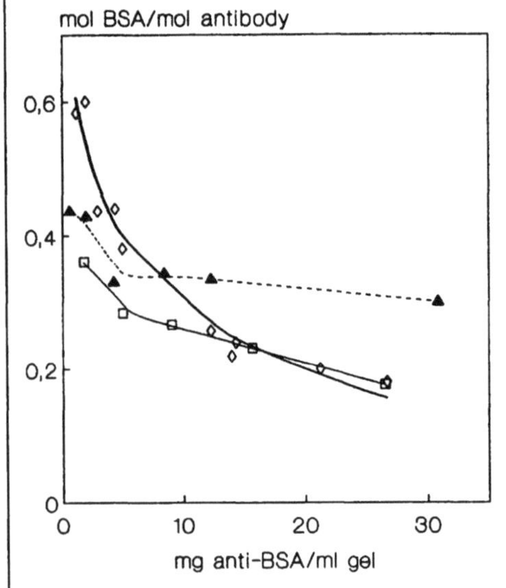

Fig. 2.2. Binding ratio vs. amount of immobilized antibody for different supports. (Data from SADA et al., 1986)
▲ - formyl cellulose, ◇ - CNBr-activated Sepharose, □ - AH-Sepharose

ed NH_2-groups is the pK: lysine α-amino: pK = 9.06, ε-amino: pK = 10.54, arginine α-amino: pK = 8.99, guanidino: pK = 12.48 (DAWSON et al., 1986). Increase of the degree of activation or fixation of all applied ligand molecules will increase the amount of immobilized protein but without adequate enlargement of specific antigen adsorption (PFEIFFER et al., 1987).

Another disadvantage of multipoint attachment could be a mechanical fixation (reinforcement) of the coupled protein. Often, a conformational change occurs during interaction between ligand and ligate and this common new structure is a prerequisite for correct binding. Multipoint attachment diminishes the flexibility of the ligand and therefore decreases the capabilities for specific binding. Interaction forces supported by an induced-fit-mechanism could be weakened. Some observations made on immunoaffinity supports with high ligand density, e.g. decrease of the stoichiometry between ligand and ligate, could be explained in part by a higher rigidity of the fixed antibodies.

On the other hand, multipoint attachment can stabilize a biomacromolecule by protection against denaturation. MOZHAEV et al. (1990) demonstrated, that an enzyme (α-chymotrypsin) maintains its enzymatic activity with higher concentrations of organic solvents, if the number of fixations increases. This effect is valid for reversible as well as for irreversible denaturation. Since elution in immunoaffinity chromatography can also be performed in aqueous mixtures of alcohols or polyols, multipoint attachment could stabilize the conformation of the proteinous ligand.

Multipoint attachment will be favoured especially in cases consisting of a high degree of activation, the use of large ligands and the choice of a matrix with small pore diameter. If the antigen-binding site of an antibody is for example not influenced by steric hindrance by parts of the matrix backbone, multipoint attachment may increase the mechanical stability of the matrix, i.e. by a significant increase of the applicable pressure head of beaded cellulose columns (BOEDEN et al., 1991b), or support a stabilization of the ligand molecule (ZHAO and BELEW, 1986).

Shell formation occurs especially when large molecules react with highly activated supports. It depends on the molecular size of the ligand, the ratio between coupling capacity and amount of ligand available, matrix porosity and reactivity (LASCH et al., 1982). It can be explained by a fast reaction of proteins at the outer surface of the matrix particle resulting in a diminution of pore diameter or a repulsion of further molecules from an activated area. Fig. 2.3. illustrates this effect studied by densitometry of fluorescein-labeled antibodies fixed on two different supports.

The activation reaction need not proceed in every case in the way suggested by the chemical formula. Thus, active esters of spacer molecules do not only react with the ligand to be bound. Side reactions are intensified when the ligand is added weeks after the activation, especially in the case of commercial products.

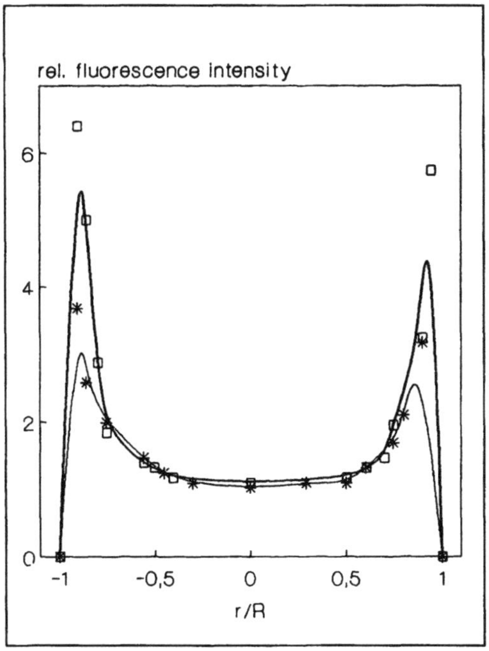

Fig. 2.3. Fluorescence intensity profiles of immobilized fluorescein-labeled antibodies on matrix beads. (Data from SADA et al., 1986)
R - radius of support bead; r - radial position of the fluorescence signal within the bead.
□ - Sepharose particle, * - cellulose bead

An activated group of the matrix reacts not only with NH_2-residues of proteins, it may also react for instance with OH-groups of the matrix which are neighboured. Formulae (I) and (II) (Fig. 2.4.) illustrate this fact, observed with agarose as well as with cellulose supports.

The esters formed (reaction product in formula (I), Fig. 2.4.) and carbonates (in (II), Fig. 2.4.), respectively, diminish not only the content of the expected reactive groups able to fix the ligand, they are also relatively stable during the short "blocking" reaction, which is mostly performed with a moderately alkaline solution of ethanolamine. However, the remaining esters in an affinity chromatographic matrix are reactive enough to undergo an aminolysis by subsequent interaction with the protein solution during the time-consuming passage (loading) of a mixture containing the substance which should be specifically adsorbed. The consequence is a support which, beside the desired ligand, contains other protein species, which may adsorb substances other than those expected. Contamination of the wanted protein species during elution is a consequence, measured for instance as a lower specific activity (biological activity per mass unit of protein) of the product.

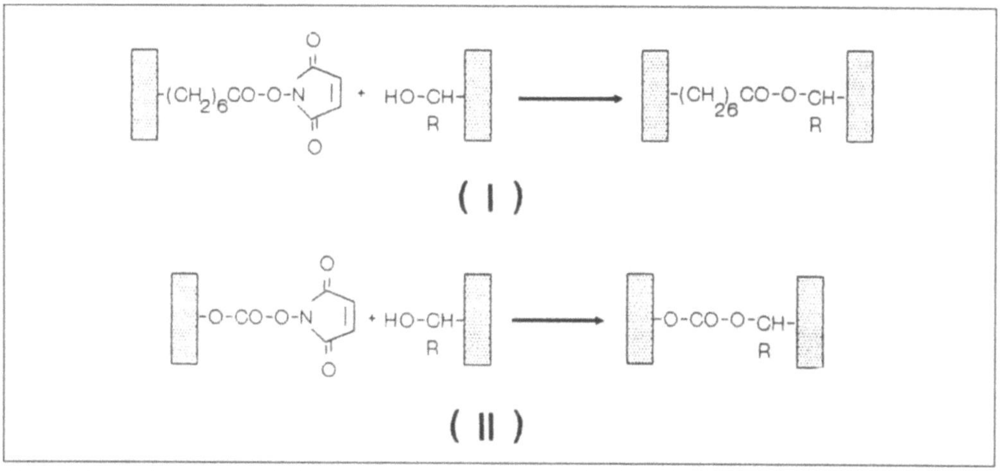

Fig. 2.4. Formation of cross-links in chromatographic supports during the activation process, demonstrated for (I) a spacered activated support (e.g. AffiGel) and (II) a directly activated support.
⊡- matrix backbone

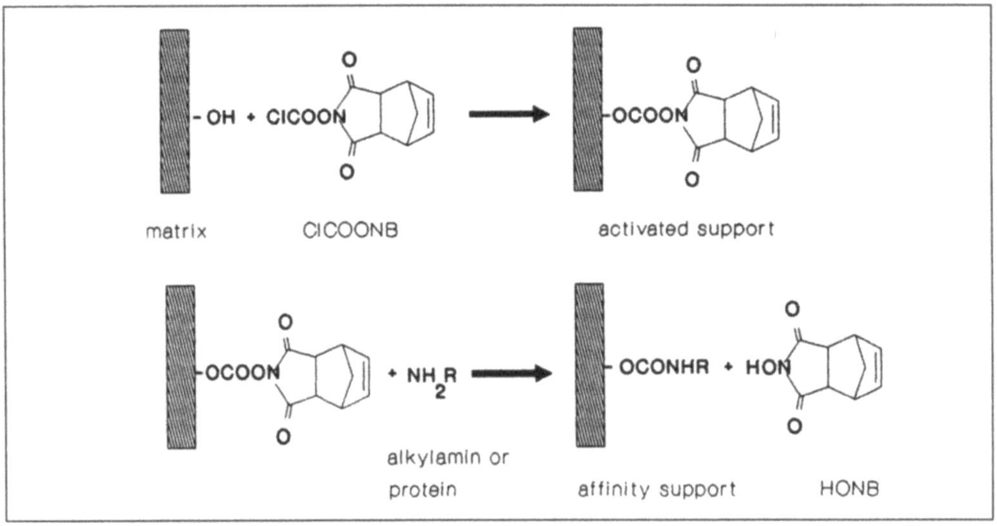

Fig. 2.5. Activation of supports containing OH-groups with ClCOONB and coupling of amines or proteins (acc. to BÜTTNER et al., 1989)
NH_2R - amine or protein, ⊡- support

The formation of carbonates may explain the important increase in mechanical stability of beaded cellulose after activation with N-(chloro-carbonyloxy)-5-norbornene-2,3-dicarboximide (ClCOONB, 5-norbornene-2,3-dicarboximido carbonochloridate) (BOEDEN et al., 1991a,b). Fig. 2.5 schematically shows the reaction path of this interesting activation method (cf. Protocol 2.1.). As discussed above, a subsequent aminolysis (blockade) with 0.5 M ethanolamine, pH 9, does not completely destroy the carbonates formed in a side reaction. The existence of cellulose carbonates after activation with ClCOONB, especially in the case of highly activated supports (> 30 μmoles active groups per ml gel), has been demonstrated by IR spectroscopy (BOEDEN et al., 1991a).

As example of the activation and coupling of antibodies to solid supports not using the well-known cyanogen bromide method (Fig. 2.6.) will be given because experimental details of CNBr activation are often described e.g. by PORATH (1974), DEAN et al. (1985), or HOLTZHAUER (1988), but the activation of polysaccharides as beaded cellulose or other polyols using a carbonochloridate is presented in Protocol 2.1. The application of ClCOONB for activation of supports has the advantages of (i) reproducibility

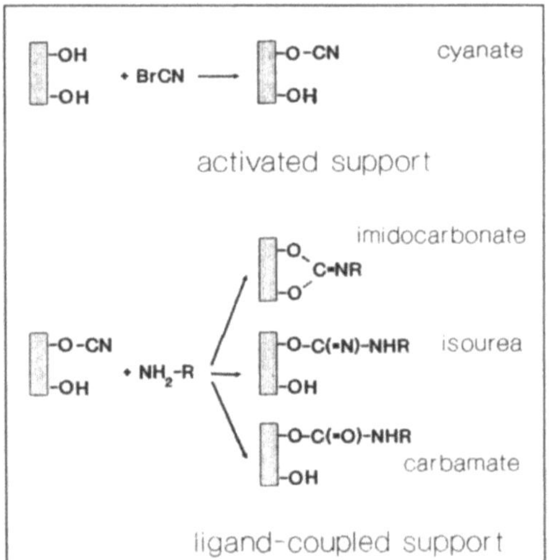

Fig. 2.6. Activation of supports containing OH-groups with CNBr and coupling of primary amines or proteins (acc. to AXEN and ERNBACK, 1971)
NH_2R - amine or protein, ⊡- support

of activation, (ii) handling with non-toxic or very weakly poisonous reagents and products, (iii) coupling of proteins in slighly acidic (pH 5), neutral, or moderately alkaline (pH 9) buffers, and (iv) formation of a chemical bond between the support and an amino group-containing ligand (e.g. protein), which is stable with respect to hydrolytic attack over a broad pH range (BÜTTNER et al., 1989) and (v) which is not charged in aqueous media.

Protocol 2.1.: **Activation of beaded cellulose with N-chlorocarbonyloxy-5-norbornene-2.3-dicarboximide** (ClCOONB)

Method (a): Uncatalyzed activation

Beaded cellulose is transferred to acetone, washed several times with p.a. acetone and filtered on a sintered glass funnel without drying. 100 ml of the moist gel are gently agitated at room temperature with 100 ml of 2.5 to 3 % (w/v) ClCOONB in p.a. acetone in a closed flask overnight. After this, the beaded cellulose is filtered again and washed several times with acetone. The activated support may be stored in an aprotic solvent such as acetone or benzene in the absence of water for several months without any loss of activity.

Method (b): Catalyzed activation

The support is transferred stepwise into an anhydrous solvent (acetone or benzene). The surplus solvent is sucked off. 100 ml of the moist gel are put into a flask; then a solution of 2 g ClCOONB in 60 ml carefully dried solvent is added and the flask closed. After a short mixing period, the catalyst (0.15 g 4-dimethylamino pyridine (DMAP) and 1.5 ml triethylamine in 6 ml of dried solvent) is added dropwise to the agitated mixture over 30 minutes. Shaking is continued for a further 30 minutes, than the gel is filtered off and washed carefully with anhydrous solvent. When strong bases such as DMAP are present, traces of water react quickly with the formed carbonate and the yield of reactive groups is decreased.

After removal of the catalyst by careful washing-out the activated gel can be stored as described for method (a).

Method (b) should be used if HCl formed during activation attacks the matrix, e.g. agarose-derived gels, or OH-groups of the matrix react only slowly under usual conditions.

If a content of activated groups greater than 60 moles per ml gel is needed, the amount of ClCOONB is to be increased.

Determination of content of active groups

Settled activated support is transferred into 5 volumes of cold distilled water and quickly washed with a further 5 volumes of water. The beaded cellulose is filtered by suction on a sintered glass funnel. About 10 mg of the moist gel are weighed exactly into an Erlenmeyer flask and mixed with 0.1 M ammonia to get a total volume of 5 ml. The suspension is stirred for 10 minutes at room temperature, then the absorbance of the supernatant is measured at 270 nm.

For calculation of the content of active groups the absorption of a defined stock solution of ClCOONB (about 50 mM) in 0.1 M ammonia is determined and used as standard or its molar absorption coefficient ($\varepsilon_{280} = 6.4 \times 10^3\ mol^{-1}cm^{-1}$) is used.

Coupling of proteins to activated beaded cellulose

An appropriate amount of activated cellulose stored in an organic solvent is equlibrated with distilled water and filtered under suction. To 1 vol. settled support 1 vol. of an amino group-free buffer (e.g. phosphate, acetate, citrate, bicarbonate, borate, pH 4 to 11) containing 2 to 10 mg protein per ml is added. The mixture is agitated overnight at 4°C or for 2 hours at room temperature. Then the gel is filtered off and the remaining active groups are blocked using an equal volume of 1 M ethanolamine in the coupling buffer. Finally, the support is washed with 10 vol. of 1 M NaCl in 0.1 M acetate buffer pH 4.5, then with 10 vol. of 1 M NaCl in 0.1 M bicarbonate buffer pH 9.0. After equilibration of the gel with an appropriate starting or storage buffer the affinity sorbent is ready for use.

If the coupling yield of proteins should be estimated by UV measurement at 280 nm of the supernatant, the solution has to be acidified to pH

2.5 to eliminate the UV-absortion of the N-hydroxy succinimide derivative.

To avoid interference from other UV absorbing substances, the gel should be washed with water and the protein content is measured using the LOWRY protocol after digestion with 0.1 N NaOH for at least 12 hrs. at room temperature. Low-molecular mass amino group-containing substances can be determined by the KJELDAHL procedure.

The coupling rate depends on the reactivity of the active group of the matrix, its accessibility to the ligand and the temperature. The reactivity of unsymmetric carbonates (reaction products of chlorocarbono esters) or cyanates (from activation by cyanogen bromide) is for example mostly very high. A well-known less reactive group is the epoxy residue.

In general, the accessibility of active groups is not the limiting process, since the pores of most of the supports used are very large with respect to the ligand. Thus coupling is nearly complete after a few minutes, as demonstrated in Fig. 2.7.

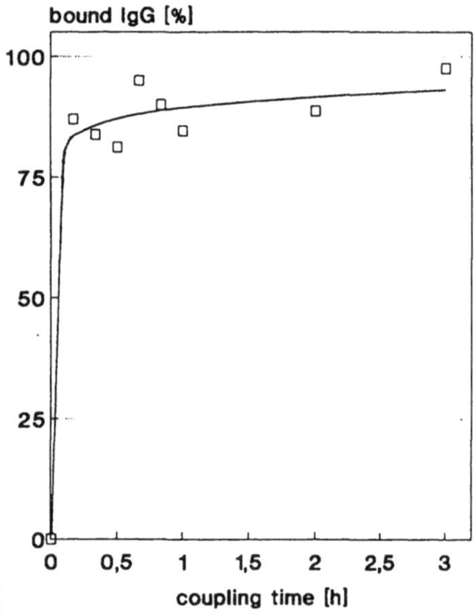

Fig. 2.7. Kinetics of coupling of human immunoglobulin to ClCOONB-activated beaded cellulose (Divicell ONB-Carbonate) at pH 7.2 and room temperature (BOEDEN, unpublished, 1990).
Content of active groups. 30 μmoles per ml wet gel, offered protein concentration. 9.5 mg IgG/ml wet gel.

It should be taken into consideration that the efficiency of the coupling of a biomolecule depends on the pH of the coupling solution. The buffer used for coupling should have a sufficient capacity because in some cases, e.g. in the given example, relatively large amounts of reaction products (N-hydroxy succinimide derivative) occur, which cause a shift in pH, if molarity of the buffer substance is too low or pH is more than 1.5 units away from the pK value of the buffering substance.

On the one hand, for coupling of a protein via NH_2 groups, the pH of the coupling buffer should be weakly alkaline (greater than pH 8), because under these conditions most of the NH_2 groups of a protein are only slightly protonated. On the other hand, hydrolysis of active groups becomes faster and coupling yields are decreased. The latter is caused by competition between aminolysis (= binding of the protein) and hydrolysis (= deactivation of supports). This consideration could be an explanation for the results presented by HEARN and DAVIES (1990), who found a coupling yield of 97 % when IgG was coupled to carbonyldiimidazole-activated Fractogel HW65F at pH 7.0 and pH 8.0, whereas at pH 8.9 the yield declines to 68 %.

After coupling of the specific ligand, blockade of remaining active groups should be performed. Usually, 0.1 to 1 M ethanolamine in a buffer with pH between 7 and 9 is applied. Ethanolamine is preferred, since it does not introduce charged groups into the matrix as glycine for instance does. It is hydrophilic and it is more reactive than e.g. tris(hydroxymethyl) aminomethane (Tris base).

As blocking experiments with ClCOONB-activated cellulose supports have shown, more than 90 % of the active groups were converted at room temperature as well as at 4°C within two hours after addition of the blocking reagent (BOEDEN, private communication). The last ten per cent need up to two hours for completion. The reason could be either the difference in reactivity of the different positions in the carbohydrate unit of the supports (substitution rates of position 2, 3 or 6 in the glucose ring differ up to tenfold (KENNEDY et al., 1985) or the difficult accessibility of active groups in narrow pores of the support. Even though the latter is mostly without relevance for coupling of large ligands, blocking time should be long enough for conversion of all activated positions of the support.

2.2.3. Leakage of Ligands (Bleeding)

A serious problem in affinity chromatography is the loss of bound ligand during the chromatographic process or storage of the wet support, the so-called leakage. The consequences of leakage are contamination of the purified product, which affords additional purification steps, especially in the case of pharmaceutical products (cf. BLOOM et al., 1989), and a decrease of binding capacity. Reasons for leakage could be (i) chemical cleavage of the chemical bond between matrix and ligand or spacer by hydrolysis, aminolysis etc. (cf. e.g. GRIBNAU, 1977, pp. 70-77), (ii) chemical or mechanical cleavage of the backbone of the chromatographic matrix and release of ligands attached to a matrix fragment (KRISTIANSEN, 1978), or (iii) degradation of the ligand, e.g. partial proteolysis of bound proteins (LASCH et al., 1985). Of course, in reality all types of leakage may occur simultaniously in different relationships. Finally, slow elution of strongly adsorbed, but not covalently bound ligand counterfeits leakage.

Data presented by PENG et al. (1986) seem to be a mixture of leakage and retarded washing-out. Strong evidence for the existence of this adsorption phenomenon is given in the paper by LASCH and JANOWSKI (1988). The only way to overcome the apparent release of ligand is an intensive rinsing with an appropriate buffer, which suppresses unspecific interactions between matrix and ligand and which does not alter the properties of the covalently fixed ligand. Further alternating elution cycles with low-and high-pH buffers and medium ionic strengh (0.5 to 1) or a pre-run under affinity chromatography elution conditions can help to overcome this problem.

There is no general rule to prevent leakage, but the main precautions are the choice of an activation method resulting in a relatively stable chemical bond, pretreatment of the support to wash out fragments or very small particles, working in a pH range sparing the matrix (e.g. in slight acidic media in the case of uncovered silica) and inactivation of proteases.

Reduction of leakage is in some cases possible by chemical conversion after the primary coupling step. Thus, the relative easily cleavable azomethin, formed by coupling of an aldehyde (e.g. from glutaraldehyde activation or periodate oxidation of carbohydrates) with a primary amine, can be transformed into the very stable secondary amine linkage by reduction with sodium borohydride (PENG et al., 1986).

GRIBNAU (1977) discussed the leakage problem in detail, providing evidence that small molecules, fixed only via a single bond, are hydrolyzed relatively fast (0.1 % of the ligand bound via cyanogen bromide activation were liberated at room temperature and pH 8 in the first 5 seconds). Reaction products of the hydrolyzed or aminolysed isourea derivative (cf. Fig. 2.6.) formed by coupling of amines and proteins respectively to CNBr-activated supports are amines (proteins) in the pH range from 5 to 10, N,N'-disubstituted guanidine derivatives ($8 < pH < 10$) and N-substitued ureas ($pH > 10$) (GRIBNAU, 1977). Similar results were also obtained by TESSER et al. (1974).

Multipoint attachment increases the stability and reduces leakage, but this effect is superimposed by a facilitation of the hydrolysis, as described by LASCH et al. (1975) and LASCH and KOELSCH (1978). A further disadvantage of multipoint attachment might be the restricted flexibility of biomacromolecules which could diminish interactions between ligand and ligate, as discussed above.

PENG et al. (1986) also investigated the stability of immunosorbents. They found a decrease of capacity during repetitive elution cycles (Fig. 2.8.).

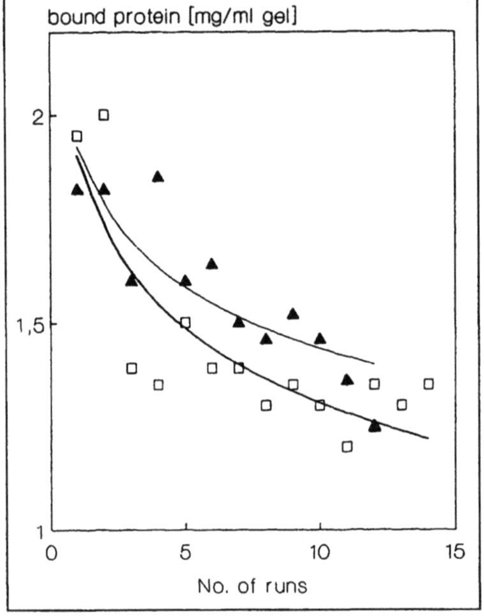

Fig. 2.8. Decrease of binding capacity for antigen of IgG during several reuses of immunoaffinity supports. The antibody was coupled to CNBr (□) and CrO_3 (▲) activated supports, respectively. (Data from PENG et al., 1986).

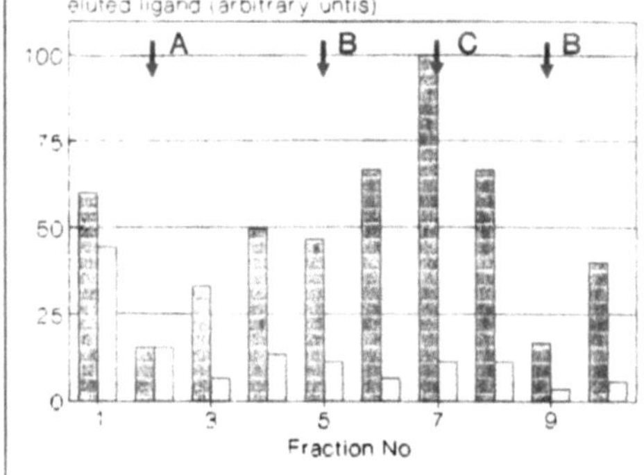

Fig. 2.9. Relative amount of liberated antibody by elution in the presence of the respective antigen (filled bars) or bovine serum albumine as an inert protein (open bars). (Data from PENG et al., 1986).
Arrows indicate the buffer changes for individual chromatographic steps (A, application of sample; B, PBS wash; C, elution with acetic acid/sodium chloride buffer).

This decrease was noticed with different elution media (0.2 M acetic acid/0.15 M NaCl and 4 M NaSCN, respectively) and was explained as leakage of ligand, but inactivation of the ligand could overlay this effect (cf. Fig. 2.13., p. 000).

Using the sensitive ELISA technique, PENG et al. observed too a facilitated loss of fixed antibody when the respective antigen was eluted. Much less antibody was liberated when the column was run under the same conditions but in the presence of a "neutral" protein (e.g. bovine serum albumin) instead of the respective antigen (Fig. 2.9.).

SATO et al. (1987) examined immunoaffinity supports for leakage with respect to storage time and media applied. Generally, the results obtained were similar to those given by PENG et al.

SATO and coworkers reported further that, independent of the neutral buffers used, leakage from CNBr-activated Sepharose columns was significantly higher than from aminopropyl glass beads, that leakage declines during several weeks of storage but is detectable even after 11 weeks. For instance, 0.17 % of the immobilized IgG was releasd after two weeks 16 days later a further 0.06 % were liberated. Whereas a protein solution diminishes the leakage, it is amplifed during the binding of the antigen.

In our laboratory, leakage of [^{14}C]glycine immobilized via ClCOONB (cf. protocol 2.1, p. 47) or CNBr to beaded cellulose (DIVICELL®, Leipziger Arzneimittelwerk GmbH, Germany) and Sepharose, respectively, was studied. Fig. 2.10. demonstrates that under alkaline conditions the urethane formed after coupling of an amine (glycine) to ClCOONB-activated beaded cellulose (Divicell ONB-Carbonate) is much more resistant to hydrolysis than the chemical bond formed after CNBr-activation (BAESELER et al., 1991). This stability is in the same order of magnitude as that of the secondary amine formed after coupling of the amine to epoxy-activated supports.

Table 2.5. Leakage of [^{14}C]glycine from Supports Acitvated by Different Methods. (Data from BAESELER et al., 1992)

Support	Type of linkage	Amount of immobilized glycine [μmoles/ml gel]	Time for release of 1 % glycine at different pH [h]		
			pH 10	pH 8.3	pH 4
CNBr-Seph. 4B	isourea	17	10	40	220
Seph. 4B ONB-carbonate	urethane	20	90	250	630
Seph. CL-6B ONB-carbonate	urethane	10	820	1050	1070
Divicell ONB-carbonate	urethane	24	970	> 1200	> 1200
Divicell Epoxy	sec. amine	13.5	> 1200	> 1200	> 1200

Seph. , Sepharose; ONB-carbonate, active group after activation with N-chlorocarbonyloxy-5-norbornene-2,3-dicarboximide; Divicell, beaded cellulose support

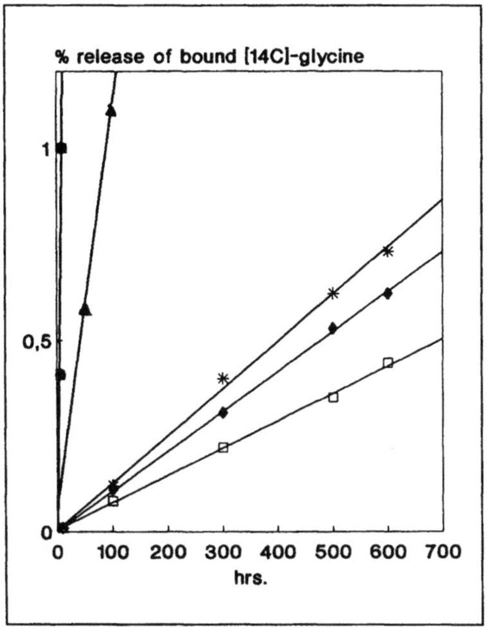

Fig. 2.10. Kinetics of release of immobilized [^{14}C]glycine from different supports in 1 M sodium carbonate buffer, pH 10, at room temperature. (Data from BAESELER et al., 1991).
□ - epoxy-activated beaded cellulose (Divicell Epoxy), ◆ - ClCOONB-activated beaded cellulose (Divicell ONB-Carbonate), ∗ - ClCOONB-activated Sepharose CL-6B, ▲ - ClCOONB-activated Sepharose 4B, ■ - CNBr-activated Sepharose 4B

The difference in stability between Sepharose 4B ONB-carbonate and the Sepharose 6B-CL derivative as demonstrated in Table 2.5. and Fig. 2.10. could be explained by a diminished stability of the Sepharose 4B agarose support, which is not reinforced by an additional cross-linking as in the CL-series. It also seems to be an example of the occurrence of splitting off the matrix-ligand bond (leakage in a narrow sence) combined with a split of the matrix, probably caused by HCl-catalyzed hydrolysis of the agarose backbone. In the latter case ligand bound to fragments of the matrix is released.

Similar results were obtained by FÜGLISTALLER (1989) using different protein A columns (Fig. 2.11.). He observed no leakage of the immobilized protein A during acidic washes with the exception of Affi-Gel A, a N-hydroxysuccinimid-activated agarose support. So it can be concluded that at slight alkaline pH the leakage is preferentially caused by a solvolytic attack on the bond between matrix and ligand, whereas at lower pH other mechanisms could have a higher share in this effect.

It is remarkable, that in accordance with results given by PENG et al. (1986) and SATO et al. (1987), FÜGLISTALLER observed significant leakage in the presence of immunoglobulin.

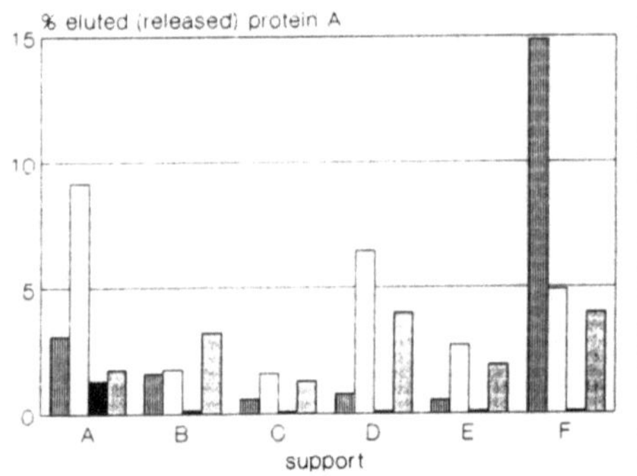

Fig. 2.11. Comparison of protein A leakage from different commercial protein A supports designed A to F in the presence of the specific ligate (+ IgG3) or its absence (- IgG3). Columns were run at pH 8.9 and 4.0, respectively.
(Data from FÜGLISTALLER, 1989, expresed as per cent released protein A of immobilized protein A).
▥; + IgG3, pH 8.9, □ ; -IgG3, pH 8.9, ⬚; + IgG3, pH 4.0, ■ -IgG3, pH 4.0

Whereas PENG et al. discussed their results as a consequence of chemical alteration of the antibody during fixation to the support and of solvolysis, especially in the case of CNBr-activated supports, it could be possible that antibody-antigen interaction may induce a conformation shift of the immunoglobulin molecule. Though the interaction between antibody and antigen is mostly discussed as a static reaction between distinct structures of the antigen and the antibody ("lock-and key mechanism"), during this process some conformational changes could also be induced as a result of binding ("induced fit", DAVIES et al., 1988). This altered structure could be in part less stable to hydrolysis than the unfixed antibody. This hypothesis is supported by the finding that antibodies can act as hydrolytic enzymes (POWELL and HANSEN, 1989), BLACKBURN et al., 1989).

Leakage by proteolysis, which is observed especially when immunoaffinity chromatography is one of the early steps in a purification scheme, can be reduced by chemical modification of antibodies (KONDO et al., 1989). "Activated PEG" (2-O-methoxypolyethyleneglycol-4,6-dichloro-s-triazine, prepared from PEG 5000 or PEG 1900) was bound to antibodies. If the chemical modification of antibodies was done in the presence of the antigen, after fixation to the chromatographic support no change in affinity and capacity was observed but proteolytic attack was significantly reduced.

Thus, leakage is an effect which has to be taken into consideration: but applications of immunoaffinity chromatography have also been reported where leakage was not detectable. And as examples of the durability of immunoaffinity columns, HOCHULI (1990) reported on several hundred reuses of an antibody column for the industrial purification of recombinant interferon without any loss of capacity or specificty, and BAZIN and MALACHE (1986) used an automated laboratory-scale mab purification system for about 1,000 cycles during 18 months.

Because of the excellent selectivity and the possibility of dozens of reuses, immunoaffinity chromatography has become the technology of choice in scaling-up of downstream processing in the purification of pharmaceutical proteins (EVELEIGH, 1982, CHASE, 1984).

Nevertheless, for practical use it is recommended to do a blank run before first application of an immunoaffinity chromatography sorbent to suppress contaminations of the ligate which is to be purified. This run should be done under the same conditions as the following chromatography of the antibody/antigen of interest with respect to loading, washing and elution buffer(s). The fractions got in the blank run may be checked for solubilized ligand to estimate the main part of leakage.

2.3. Adsorption and Desorption of Ligates

In the previous chapter the covalent fixation of ligand to an insoluble matrix was described. For immunoaffinity chromatography the ligand is often an antibody (monoclonal or polylonal or a part of polyclonal preparations) or its antigen-binding fragment(s), but also antigens as proteins, peptides or low-molecular mass haptens are immobilized to catch specific antibodies from immunosera.

The interaction between antibody and antigen is a multi-task phenomenon, during which formation of a covalent chemical bond does not occur. The main forces are electrostatic and hydrophobic interactions, formation of H-bridges and van der Waals bonds, as discussed in Chapter 1.2.4. or by KONDO et al. (1990). It is essential for formation of the highly specific antibody-antigen complex that both parts have the correct three-dimensional structure with the required distribution of electrical charges, polar and apolar areas to realize more than one interaction within a distinct part of the molecules. It may be assumed that covalent attachment of a protein to another molecule, e.g. a macromolecule of the chromatographic support, induces a change in the threedimensional structure of this fixed molecule or of a part of it, since proteins are eminent in a relative flexibility of their geometry.

2.3.1. Adsorption of Ligates

The formation of the antibody-antigen complex between for instance immobilized antibody (ligand) and dissolved antigen (ligate) follows an equilibrium reaction which can be characterized as of the first order by the law of mass action (detailed discussions of the theory and kinetics of affinity chromatography are given by TURKOVA (1978), FAZEKAS DE ST. GROTH (1979), TRUCCO and DE PETRIS (1981), DELISI and HETHCOTE (1982) or KONDO et al. (1990) and of immunochemistry at solid interfaces by NYGREN and STENBERG (1989)). Thus the binding of an antigen by an immobilized antibody (and vice versa) on an immunoaffinity column is dependent upon several factors such as for instance (i) concentration of the antigen in a given mixture, (ii) volume of feedstock loaded, (iii) concentration of immobilized antibody, (iv) its accessibility with respect to the antigen, (v) affinity of the antibody (avidity of polyclonal antibodies, respectively), (vi) efficiency of regeneration of immunoaffinity support after each adsorption/elution cycle and (vii) the degree of fouling of the support.

In general, the following equations may be used for understanding adsorption and desorption processes in immunoaffinity chromatography (for more detailed discussions see Chapter 1.2.):

$$Ab + Ag \underset{K_2}{\overset{K_1}{\rightleftharpoons}} AbAg \qquad (1)$$

$$K_D = K_2 \;/\; K_1 = [Ab] * [Ag] \;/\; [AbAg] \qquad (2)$$

with Ab, antibody; Ag, antigen; AbAg, antibody-antigen-complex; K_D, dissociation equilibrium constant; [Ab], [Ag], [AbAg], concentrations of the respective components; K_1, rate constant for antibody-antigen combination; K_2, rate constant for antibody-antigen dissociation.

As also described in Chapter 1.2., the disssociation constants for antibody-antigen complexes are very low. Mostly they are in the range of 10^{-5} to 10^{-12} moles/l dependent on the nature of the epitope(s) on the surface of the antigen and its interaction with the antibody. For example, TRUCCO and DE PETRIS (1981) described K_D values for the formation of complexes of monoclonal antibodies with viral antigens in the order of 10^{-9} to 10^{-10} moles/l, K_D's of polyclonal antibodies are in the range of 10^{-5} to 10^{-8} moles/l (MURPHY et al., 1976), representing an average of K_D of individual antibody populations.

Experiments to estimate equilibrium data in heterogeneous phase immunoaffinity chromatography suggested a relationship between the molecular mass of the adsorbed antigen and immobilized antibody. SADA et al. (1989) found association constants ($K_A = 1/K_D$) ranging from 1.7 x 10^7 (cytochrome c/anti-cytochrome c) to 5.0 x 10^7 l/mole (IgG/anti-IgG) and pointed out a correlation between molecular mass of the antigen and K_A, but strong evidence for a decrease in K_A with increasing molecular mass is lacking.

The observation that an elution of adsorbed antibodies from immobilized antigens occurs by declining the temperature (e.g. OKUMURA et al., 1977, JATON et al., 1979) could be explained by an increase of the dissociation constant, which as with other equilibrium constants is a thermodynamical parameter.

Discussion of reactions between immobilized antigens or antibodies and soluble antibodies and antigens, respectively, has to consider kinetics in solid/liquid heterogeneous phase systems (NYGREN and STENBERG, 1989). These kinetics are influenced at least by the equilibrium constant K_D of the reaction, by the diffusion rate of the unbound molecules, by the density of fixed molecules on the matrix surface and by the number of binding sites. These aspects should be reflected during the planning of an immunoaffinity chromatography, which means enough time should be provided for binding during adsorption, washing-out of impurities and desorption to proceed with all reaction steps at the molecular level.

Reactions between a large molecule and a small one or between two large molecules need some time to find the best position(s) for correct interaction. In solution, times ranging from 10 seconds to 30 minutes were observed for formation of the antibody-antigen complex (CLAUSEN, 1988, pp. 3-4).

Furthermore, it should be reflected that during a real immunoaffinity chromatography experiment not only the highly specific interactions occur. Diffusion, non-linear flows within the chromatographic bed, gel permeation, ionic and hydrophobic interactions also take part in immunoaffinity chromatography. First, buffers used for adsorption, washing and elution must eliminate the unspecific binding of proteins to the column packing. As manipulation of the buffer composition to decrease one of the unwanted potential interactions may actually enhance other interactions, a careful balance of ionic strength and polarity is required for specific adsorption as well as for desorption. Secondly, the effect of buffer constituents on protein structure, i.e., both the conformation of protein chains and the interaction into oligomeric quarternary structures, must be considered, because chromatographic behaviour of proteins is uniquely dependent on the surrounding solvent, unlike simple, relatively small organic molecules or most other biological macromolecules.

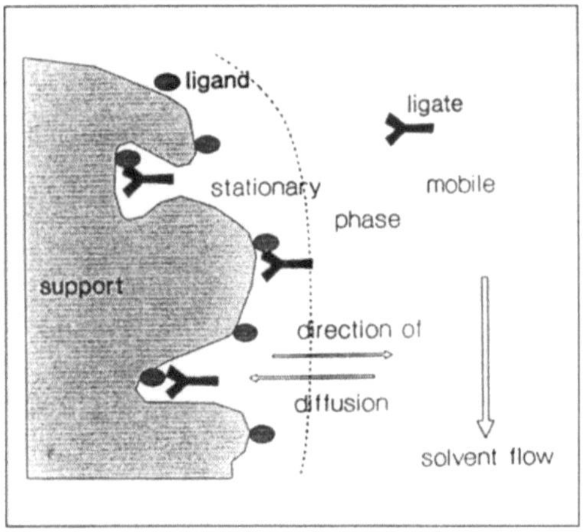

Fig. 2.12. Scheme of transfer of a molecule from the mobile phase via the stationary phase to the ligand at surface of a chromatographic support (matrix).
- - - -, expected theoretical borderline between mobile and stationary phase.

Further, antibodies have to penetrate a certain stationary phase around a given matrix particle to reach the antigen. This process is more or less independent of the flow rate of the (mobile) eluent and is controlled by diffusion phenomena. Since the rate of diffusion is reciprocally proportional to the radius of a molecule (1st FICK's law) and therefore in a first approximation to the molecular mass, large molecules need more time to cross the stationary phase, to enter into caves and to react with their counterparts at the surface of deepenings or pores of the matrix (for a theoretical approach see DELISI and HETHCOTE, 1982). Therefore, it should be mentioned that especially in the case of relatively large and rough matrix particles adsorption is relatively time-consuming and that also the flow rate for washing-out of unbound material should not be taken too high. Fig. 2.12. schematically illustrates these problems.

From the viewpoint of selectivity and association rate an antibody-antigen pair with a low K_D, high assiociation and low dissociation rate constant should be used, but in this case elution affords drastic, in general denaturating conditions.

There are some approaches for finding a compromise between low K_D and easy desorption from an affinity matrix. One opportunity is the alteration of the dissociation (association) relations between a given antibody-antigen pair by chemical modification of the respective proteins. MURPHY et al. (1976) described experiments where the fixed antigen (glucagon) was modified by oxidation, alkylation with 2-hydroxy-5-nitrobenzyl bromide or nitration with tetranitromethane. Whereas from columns containing unmodified antigen the bound antibodies had to be eluted with very strong eluents (e.g. 4 M guanidinium hydrochloride or 0.1 M acetic acid pH 2.2), after chemical modification elution was possible with a simple pH shift from pH 7.4 (phosphate buffered saline, washing buffer) to pH 11 (saline, adjusted to pH 11 with ammonia, elution buffer). This facilitation of elution is also possible by modification of fixed antibodies. In general, this principle of chemical ligand modification should be taken into consideration only if a ligate poorly reconstitutes after the usual elution with strong chaotropic eluents or at high or low pH.

Adsorption of an antigen to its immobilized antibody and vice versa is relatively simple. Normally this step is done in an aqueous buffer of physiological pH and appropriate ionic strengh to avoid (unspecific) ionic or hydrophobic interactions. The most common buffers are phosphate-buffered saline (PBS, 0.04 M Na,K phosphate, 0.14 M NaCl, pH 7.2 to 7.4), saline (0.15 M NaCl), or Tris-buffered saline (TBS, 0.1 M tris(hydroxymethyl)aminomethane, 0.035 M NaCl, 0.01 M glycine, pH 8). Other ions needed for antibody-antigen-interactions such as potassium and calcium are mostly present in sufficient amounts, at least when not using ultra-pure materials. If the protein concentration is too low ($\ll$ 1 mg/ml) and the solution cannot be concentrated, a protective agent such as 0.1 % gelatine may be added. Under these conditions the specific binding between a given antigen and its antibody occurs quickly and selectively. Unbound material is easily removed without a change of the buffer but to further decrease unspecific adsorbed material washings with five or more column volumes should be done with buffers of another composition (higher ionic strength, mild detergents such as Tween 20 in relatively low concentrations (less than 0.1 %), more acidic or alkaline pH etc.).

UV monitoring is the most simple method of controlling loading and removal of impurities, but specific analytical methods such as enzymatic or immunochemical assays should accompany these steps. If UV measurement at 280 nm is used for monitoring, as a rule of thumb it can be taken that impurities are removed and elution can be started if adsorption (calculated for 1 cm light path) is < 0.05.

2.3.2. Desorption Processes

Table 2.6. summarizes elution methods in immunoaffinity chromatography, which will be illustrated by references later on.

The desorption (elution) of the bound ligate from the immunoaffinity matrix is much more difficult. Since the association constant is mostly very high, competitive elution with the unbound ligand is possible only if sufficient free concentrations of the ligand are available to influence the equilibrium. Therefore, the feasibility of a very smooth elution is limited to small, low-molecular mass ligands. A (partial) denaturation of the proteinous constitutents is mostly the only way to recover the adsorbed ligate. To minimize denaturation, which is often a sequence of singular and not very fast intramolecular processes, the duration of the time in which the ligate is in the denaturing medium should be as short as possible. Further, it should be mentioned that during elution at the solvent front of the eluent concentrations of the eluted substance can occur, which exeed the solubility of this substance in the given solvent and cause a precipiation of it, as pointed out e.g. by NIELSEN and WILSON (1987). These formed solids are especially in the case of proteins only partially resolvable during regeneration of the column and could be involved in a

Table 2.6. Principles of Elution Conditions in Immunoaffinity Chromatography (for examples see Table 3.7A.)

Principle		Agent	Type	Action mode
I.	**Chemically**			
I.1	pH shift	d		alteration of electrostatic intra- and/or inter-molecular interactions by reducing positive or negative charges of amino acid residues
I.2	chaotropic	d		denaturation of ligand and/or ligate agents by reducing hydrophobic intramolecular interactions
I.3.	free ligand	nd		competition between free and bound ligand
I.4	competition	nd		competition between ligate and a second antibody for the binding site of the immobilized antibody
I.5	detergent	(d)		suppression of hydrophobic interactions by substitution of hydrophobic counterparts with a soluble detergent
I.6	alteration of complex conformation	nd		use of Ca^{2+}-dependent antibodies
II.	**Physically**			
II.1	electrophoretic	nd		displacement of the equilibrium between bound and dissociated ligate by electromigration
II.2	pressure	(d)		pressure-induced reversible deformation of the antigen-antibody complex
II.3	temperature	nd		increase of K_D by decreasing the elution temperature

d, denaturating conditions; nd, non-denaturating conditions

decrease of yield and recovery of the chromatographic procedure. On the other hand, slight resolution of the precipitate can contaminate the product during a subsequent chromatographic cycle. The irreversible accumulation of proteins on the support, the so-called fouling, could also be amplified by this formation of precipitates.

Development of an elution strategy is an empirical task. First, a decision should be made with respect to the application of the separated protein. Very drastic conditions may be used, if the proteins are isolated for protein chemical purposes. For enzymatic studies or other experiments where the biological activity of a protein is necessary, the elution conditions should be as smooth as possible. A second aspect is the re-use of the column. Since, in the application of denaturing conditions, a part of the ligand is mostly irreversibly denatured during each run, this decrease in binding capacity (and perhaps specificity) should be minimized by the use of a gentle elution protocol. Third, the compatibility and capacity of the buffers applied have to be taken into consideration, which means chemical reactions between components of consecutive buffers should not influence the separation or regeneration processes and that the buffering capacity is really sufficient.

Mostly, no specific elution is possible. Therefore,it should be mentioned that the immobilized and the eluted protein should be in a denaturing medium as short as possible, which means that elution and re-equilibration of the column is to be done quickly and the eluted protein is to be brrought back to physiological conditions by on-line dialysis or at least by pH-compensation by a buffer of high buffering capacity (the pH of the buffer should be close to the pK of the buffering compound and the molarity should be at least twice the elution buffer).

A test protocol for development of elution conditions should start with an acidic buffer pH 3 to 3.5, followed by buffers of lower pH (2.5 to 1.8). If these buffers are not satisfactory, alkaline conditions (pH 10 to 12.5) can be checked. When no pH-shift can or shall be used, increasing ionic

Table 2.7. Buffers and their Composition for Unspecific Elution of Adsorbed Antigens

(main) Component(s) [moles/l]	pH	Composition [g/l]
0.1 M glycine	1.5-2.8	7.507, HCl to pH 1.5 - 2.8
0.1 M glycine, 0.5 M NaCl	2.5	7.507, 29.22
0.1 M sodium acetate, 0.15 M NaCl	1	8.20, 8.77, HCl to pH 1
0.1 M sodium citrate/phosphate	3.0-3.5	21.01 (citric acid), 0.1 M Na_2HPO_4 to pH 3.0-3.5
0.1 M acetic acid/formic acid	2.2	2.0, 2.3
0.5 M acetic acid		30.0
1 M proanoic acid		130.14
0.15 M NaCl/NH_4OH	11.0	8.77, ammonia to pH 11
0.1 M triethylamine	11.5	10.01
2.5 M KSCN	[1]	242.95
0.5 - 3 M NaSCN	[1]	40.54 - 243.21
3 M guanidinium hydrochloride	[1]	286.59
4 M KI, 20 mM Tris-HCl	8.0	664.0, 2.422, HCl to pH 8.0
4 M $MgCl_2$, 10 mM sodium phosphate	7.0	380.84, 0.89 $Na_2HPO_4*H_2O$, pH adjusted to 7.0
5 M LiCl, 10 mM sodium phosphate	7.0	211.97, 0.89 $Na_2HPO_4*H_2O$, pH adjusted to 7.0
6.8 M NaCl	[1]	397.39
6 M urea	[1]	360.36
10 % 1,4-dioxane	[1]	96.7 ml
80 % ethylene glycol	[1]	718.8 ml
80 % ethylene glycol, 20 mM triethylamine	11.5	718.8 ml, 20.24

[1] unbuffered solution, pH not adjusted

strength is achieved by application of salts or organic substances at neutral pH. A rank for increasing elution power could be magnesium chloride (3 → 5 M) < lithium chloride (5 → 10 M) < distilled water < ethylene glycol (25 → 50 %) < dioxane (5 → 20 %) < potassium or sodium thiocyanate (1 → 5 M) < urea (3 → 6 M) < guanidinium hydrochloride (1 → 3 M) < sodium dodecylsulfate (0.5 → 2 %) (according to Harlow and Lane (1988).

The most used method for eluting the biospecifically adsorbed ligate is the application of an elution buffer with relatively high ionic strength (0.1 M) and extreme pH, e.g. 0.1 M glycine-HCl buffer pH 2.5 to 3, 0.2 M citrate buffer pH 2.2 (Weiss and Eisenstein, 1987), 0.1 M formic acid/acetic acid pH 2.5, 1 M acetic acid (e.g. Karlsen et al., 1990) or alkaline buffers with pH > 10.5 (Lim, 1987) (cf. Tables 2.6. and 2.7.). These buffers partially denature proteins and therefore destroy the antigen-antibody interactions.

Another interpretation is suggested by Bartholomew et al. (1983). They found that several monoclonal antibodies to the same antigen (human growth hormone) release bound antigen at different pH. Furthermore, they observed that binding and elution equilibria of a distinct antibody-antigen complex depend on the pH. The authors interpreted their results as a pH-dependent switching of different affine binding sites in the mab's.

Some commonly used buffers for elution are listed in Table 2.7.

The denaturation of antibodies and antigens is only partly reversible, which results in a decrease of capacity at constant ligand density. Hughes and Charm (1979) found that in a device for continuous purification of antigens, during each cycle a decrease in capacity occured, whereas the

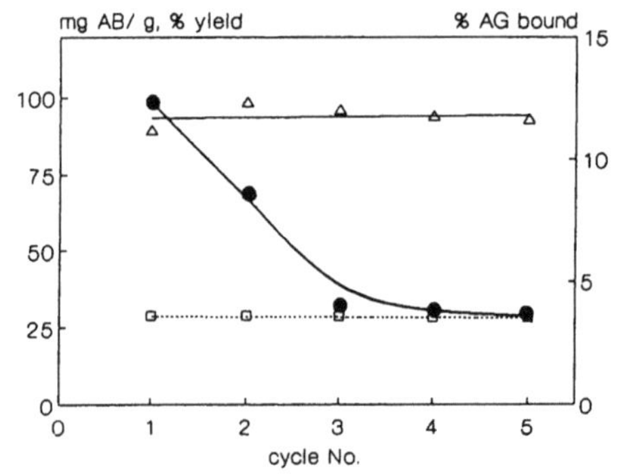

Fig. 2.13. Antibody content, capacity and recovery for continous antigen preparation. (Data from HUGHES and CHARM, 1979)
Δ - Antibody (AB) content in the affintiy matrix [mg/g]; □ - antigen (AG) adsorbed [%]; ● - antigen yielded after elution [%]

antibody content was not significantly influenced (Fig. 2.13.).

Purification experiments with antibody pairs (e.g. human IgG / rabbit (anti human-IgG) IgG) demonstrated that even during skilfull and quick chromatography a variable but sometimes a large part of the eluted material forms insoluble aggregates as a consequence of denaturation or wrong renaturation. The amount of denatured material can be minimized by reducing the duration time in the denaturing buffer as much as possible. Therefore, the eluted fractions should be collected in tubes containing a buffer of physiological pH and a buffering capacity able to neutralize the elution buffer. Moreover, an optimal elution protocol should be started with a buffer of relatively neutral pH and continued by slowly decreasing the pH-value. Using the system interferon/anti-interferon antibodies LIVINGSTON (1975) demonstrated that elution already begins at pH 3.5 (room temperature) and reaches the maximum of 90% at pH 2.6. Similar observations were made when human monoclonal antibodies were purified on protein A or protein G columns (JUNGBAUER et al., 1989).

The following protocol will illustrate a universal procedure for preparing species-specific antibodies.

Protocol 2.2.: **Purification of species-specific immunoglobulin** (according to HOLTZHAUER (1988) p. 106).

Dialyzed immunoglobulin, obtained from 50 % ammonium sulfate saturation fraction of rabbit serum, is coupled to an activated support (cf. Example 2.1). The support should have a relatively low activation degree to get an affinity matrix of about 2 to 5 mg immunoglobulin per ml swollen gel. Then the immunosorbent is equilibrated with phosphate-buffered saline (PBS, 0.136 M NaCl, 0.0027 M KCl, 0.01 M Na, K phosphate, pH 7.2 - 7.4).

The antiserum, directed against whole immunoglobulin or an immunoglobulin class or subfraction (in our example against rabbit whole immunoglobulin), is diluted with PBS to approximately 5 mg protein per ml and loaded onto the column [a]. The volume of the column depends on the capacity of the matrix. As a general rule, the matrix should be used only with 3/4 of the maximal capacity, e.g. if 4 mg/ml biologically active rabbit IgG are immobilized no more than 3 mg of anti-rabiit IgG should be offered per ml of affinity matrix. The flow rate, which depends on the kind of support, should not be too fast. For soft gels it should be in the order of 10 to 20 cm x h^{-1}.

PBS is used to wash out unbound or unspecifically bound material until UV absorption at 280 nm is in the range of the protein-free buffer.

Elution will be performed with glycine-HCl buffer (0.1 M glycine, adjusted with HCl to pH 2.5). The flow rate may be somewhat higher than that of sample application and washing. Fractions are collected into tubes containing 1/2 of the fraction volume of 0.5 M phosphate buffer pH 7.5 to neutralize immediately the acidic elution buffer. When UV absorption of the eluted material drops

[a] A column is preferred because the formation of absorption and desorption equilibria is continous, whereas during a batch procedure these equilibria will be formed only once per step.

to a fifth of its maximal value, elution buffer should be switched to PBS.

Antigen-containing fractions are pooled and dialyzed against PBS. To remove aggregates the dialysate is centrifuged.

Chaotropic salts are also used for elution in immunoaffinity chromatography. These salts destroy the structure of water, which forms a shell around the solved molecule. Nonpolar parts of a molecule (protein) need not be screened from the polar solvent now. The result is a conformational alteration of the molecule (for detailed discussion of the hydrophobic effect see e.g. FRANKS 1975, SRINIVASAN and RUCKENSTEIN 1980, LESSER et al. 1987). The power of an ion/molecule to act as a chaotropic agent corresponds to the HOFMEISTER rank (acc. to PFÜLLER, 1986):

cations:
$(CH_3)_4N^+ < (CH_3CH_2)_4N^+ < (CH_3CH_2CH_2)_4N^+ < (CH_3CH_2CH_2CH_2)_4N^+ < NH_4^+ < Rb^+ < K^+ < Na^+ < Li^+ < Mg^{++} < Ca^{++}$ (< urea) $< Ba^{++} < H_2N{=}C(NH_2)_2^+$ (guanidinium);

neutral substances:
$0{=}C(NH_2)$ (urea) < nicotinamide < methyl-acetamide;
sucrose < fructose < sorbitol;

anions:
$P0_4^{---} < SO_4^{--}\ CL^- < Br^- < CH_3COO^-$ (acetate) $< NO_3^- < ClO_4^- < NO_3^-\ ClO_4^- < CF_3COO^-$ (trifluoroacetate) $< I^- < SCN^- < CCl_3COO^-$ (trichloroacetate) $< CBr_3COO^-$ (tribromoacetate).

Water-miscible organic solvents such as methanol, ethanol, propanol, ethylene glycol, acetonitril, dioxan or polyols also act as chaotropic agents (see e.g. ANDERSEN et al., 1975). For chaotropic elution the most common buffers contain 2 to 6 M guanidinium hydrochloride (JATON et al., 1979), 6 to 7 M urea, 2.5 M sodium thiocyanate (PHILLIPS et al., 1985), 4 M potassium iodide, or 7 M magnesium chloride (WEISS and EISENSTEIN, 1987, KENNEY et al., 1988) (for review see HILL et al., 1986). It should be noticed, that chaotropic substances mostly induce a (partial and possibly reversible) denaturation of a protein, but it is well-known that some such as saccharose or glycerol also act as stabilizers (TIMASHEFF and ARAKAWA, 1989).

A relatively rare, but gentle, method for elution of an antigen is the application of parts of epitope-representing structures (amino acid sequences) of it as competitors to the binding site(s) of immobilized antibodies. This could be the method of choice particulary in the case of very sensitive enzymes or enzymes consisting of several subunits.

Synthetic polypeptides corresponding to immunogenic structures of a protein offer the opportunity for this elution method. This principle was applied for investigation of equilibrium between immobilized antigen (immunogenic peptide) and the corresponding polyclonal antibodies (KONDO et al. 1990).

Recently, an example was given by HUMBERT et al. (1990), who isolated bovine guanylyl cyclase by competitive elution of the enzyme: a synthetic pentadecapeptide corresponding to the C-terminal deduced amino acid sequence of a subunit of the enzyme was used for producing antibodies, which were coupled to Sepharose. After adsorption of the oligomeric enzyme to the immunoaffinity matrix, elution was performed by circulation of a buffer (0.05 M triethanolammonium hydrochloride, 0.175 M NaCl, pH 7.5) containing 0.1 mg/ml of the antigenic pentadecapeptide for 6 hrs. (in this step enrichment was 52fold, yield 7 %).

The same principle was used when elution was performed by application of a second (monoclonal) antibody which competes for the binding site of the first (immobilized) antibody (KIM et al., 1990). This anti-ideotype antibody represents a very smooth eluent even for relatively large molecules such as viral surface antigens, but requires further purification steps to remove the anti-ideotype antibody to get a pure product.

An example of the elution of antigens by detergent is given by NOLLSTADT et al. (1989). Adsorption of the respective antigen to immobilized antibodies and removal of unbound accompanying substances was performed in a buffer containing 0.2 % of the nonionic detergent n-octyl glucoside. Elution was achieved by switching to Tris buffer pH 8.0 supplemented with 0.1 % of the dialysable sulfobetaine detergent Zwittergent 3-12 and 0.035 M lithium diisosalycylate.

Another way to recover an affinity bound ligate is the use of a cleavable spacer molecule which links the ligand to the matrix. Examples of the application of such spacers for affinity chromatography and their cleavage by oxidation of glycolic groups in hydrophilic spacers such as 1,6-diamino-3,4-dihydroxyhexane with sodium periodate or reduction of sulfides as cysteamine derivatives by dithiothreitol are given by MARBURG et al. (1989). The heterobifunctional agent N-succinimidyl 3-(2-pyridyldithio) propionate (SPDP) has also been used for preparation of cleavable immunosorbents (HABEEB, 1981).

The disadvantages of these methods are a irreversible decomposition of the affinity matrix, a partial denaturation of fixed proteins by cleavage of S-S bonds and the still existing antigen-antiboy complex in the eluate, respectively.

PRICKETT et al. (1989) described the purification of a recombinant protein from culture filtrates using a calciumsensitive system. They introduced a short hydrophilic peptide sequence (Flag segment: Asp-Tyr-Lys-Asp-Asp-Asp-Lys (DYK-DDDK)) into the N-terminus of several proteins. A monoclonal antibody bound this peptide in the presence of 1 mM calcium chloride. Elution was performed using 2 mM EDTA in PBS with yields of about 40 %. The authors interpreted their observations as a calcium-dependent alteration of the antibody, but since the amino acids of the fusion peptide are known as calcium chelators it could be possible that the presence or absence of calcium induces a conformational shift in the antigen which results in another structure of the epitope. This alteration also changes the interactions between antibody and antigen. Nevertheless the existence of such molecules offers the possibility of very mild adsorption/desorption procedures in immunoaffinity chromatography.

Mostly, an elution of a bound antigen requires a disturbance of the three-dimensional structure of the binding region of the antibody or the antigen or both if competition for the binding site is excluded. The examples discussed above are given for that disturbance by chemical interactions. High pressure is also able to induce a conformational change, since large molecules are compressible, which causes an alteration of their properties (WEBER and DIRCKAMER, 1983) as well as reaction parameters (LE NOBLE and KELM, 1980). Repeated applications of 200 MPa onto adsorbed antigen-containing immunoglobulin supports yielded in a 90 % recovery of the antigen within several minutes, omitting harsh chemical conditions (OLSON et al., 1989).

A further opportunity for desorption of antigens (antibodies) from insoluble supports is the electrophoretic principle. Even though the dissociation constants of antibody-antigen complexes are very low, it should be mentioned that a distinct part is dissociated. If the soluble part is removed from this balance, a further part must disssociate and so on. A gentle separation of a soluble biopolymer from an immobilized ligand is possible by electrophoretic elution (YARMUSH and OLSON, 1988). This principle was used also for desorption of antigens from antibody-linked matrices under slightly alkaline conditions (10 mM Tris borate, pH 8.2, 4°C, 9 V/cm) employing a membrane trap (SCHULZE-OSTHOFF et al., 1989).

2.4. High-performance Immunoaffinity Chromatography

High-performance affinity chromatography (HPAC) is a subdivision of high-performance liquid chromatography (HPLC) which itself is a part of liquid chromatographic methods. Differences between HPAC and "conventional" affinity chromatography are not great, and therefore most of the statements made in the previous chapters are also valid for HPAC and its special task high-performance immunoaffinity chromatography (HPIAC). Because there is no place for detailed descriptions of HPLC theory and some practical aspects, the reader is referred to the respective reviews, e.g. by LARSSON et al. (1983),

ENGELHARDT (1986), GLÖCKNER (1987), EPPERT (1988), JOHANSSON et al. (1988), OLIVER (1989), WEILE and RENBIN (1989) or GOODING and REGNIER (1990).

The main differences between conventional and high-performance immunoaffinity chromatography are (i) smaller size of HPIAC supports (1 to 10 μm in diameter), (ii) higher pressure (> 1 MPa, 142 psi), (iii) shorter time needed for the whole chromatographic cycle, often half an hour or less, and (iv) higher sensitivity.

A recent survey of the application of HPLC in purification of antibodies is given by JUNGBAUER and WENISCH (1989), who pointed out that ion-exchange HPLC (HPIEC) and its special task hydroxylapatite HPLC are the mostly used principles, especially in isolation of monoclonal antibodies (cf. Chapter 3.1).

There are a lot of similarities between HPIEC and HPIAC, e.g. multi-center phenomena, adsorption/desorption equilibria, diffusion kinetics or accessibilities and densities of ligands. As already pointed out, the theory of HPIEC will not be expressed here in detail. It should be mentioned that some observations made in HPIEC may be used to explain effects in HPAC and vice versa, because mechanisms of ligand-ligate interactions are very similar in ion exchange and affinity chromatography. Theoretical considerations and experimental consequences reflecting basic processes in HPIAC are given by HEARN and DAVIS (1990), JOHNSTON and HEARN (1990), LIAPIS et al. (1989).

Gel permeation chromatographic methods (GPC, respectively size-exclusion chromatography, SEC) are also widely used in investigations of antibody-antigen interactions or purification of protein-protein conjugates (e.g. CARTY and O'KENNEDY, 1988), STEVENS et al., 1988), but this kind of chromatography is also not the aim of this chapter.

Better resolution, a main goal in HPIEC, HPGPC or reversed-phase (hydrophobic interaction) HPLC, is often not necessary in HPIAC because mostly only the high specific adsorption of a component is desired and differences in adsorption/desorption conditions of individual components are not exploited. In general, the goal of HPIAC is a faster separation process than in conventional liquid chromatography (demonstrated e.g. by PHILLIPS et al., 1984a, or SANTUCCI et al., 1988), which is based on the well-known differences in affinity of protein A to immunoglobulin subclasses or immunoglobulins from different animals.

Of course, borderline cases are possible, as for instance in separation of antibodies of different affinity for the same antigen. HPIAC offers the possibility of the preparation of antibody populations which recognize different epitopes from a polyclonal serum. As another example, mouse IgG subclasses may be separated rapidly on a protein A HPLC column by application of a pH gradient starting from pH 6.0 (desorption of IgG1) to pH 4.0 (desorption of IgG2b) (JUNGBAUER and WENISCH, 1989). Protein A matrices as immunosorbents "for honors sake" can be used to distinguish immunoglobulins of different species (KHURANA et al., 1989). Recently, a small non-protein synthetic ligand (AvidAL) has been introduced, that has selectivity similar to protein A or G (BioProbe, Tutsin, California).

As ion-exchange HPLC experiments have demonstrated, small-sized non-porous spherical supports give better resolutions than porous, especially when mixtures have to be separated which are made from molecules with strongly different molecular size (DUNCAN et al., 1987). The height equivalent of theoretical plates (HETP) as unit of column performance depends much less on molecular mass (molecular size and shape) when small-sized non-porous supports are used (DUNCAN et al., 1987). For understanding the equilibirium and dynamic aspects as well as shares of the matrix, experiments with non-porous supports are very suitable (LIAPIS et al., 1989).

Tailing caused by diffusion of components into caves or pores of the support and which is strengthened with increasing flow rates is diminished when non-porous supports are used (schematically demonstrated in Fig. 2.14.). Steeper pH or salt gradients may also be applied in the case of nonporous supports because less time is needed to generate uniform ionic conditions in

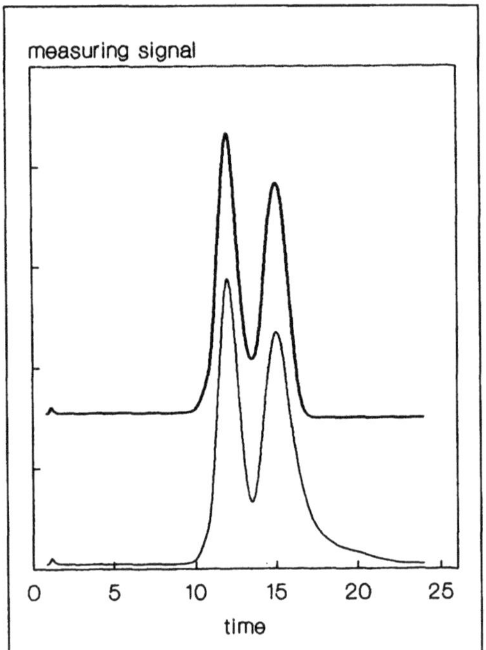

Fig. 2.14. Comparison of HPLC chromatograms with and without tailing.
Runs were performed at porous (lower curve) and non-porous supports (upper curve), respectively (according to DUNCAN et al., 1987).

each (theoretical) bed layer of a column since diffusion or gel permeation processes of small ions as well as of large macromolecules as proteins are suppressed.

Gel permeation effects could also be an explanation for the splitting of a homogeneous antibody population, which was described by HAGE et al. (1986).

Experimental observations and theoretical reflections on the influence of porosity of a given support on the separation of proteins havve been recently published by JOHNSTON and HEARN (1990). Whereas the average pore diameter of a certain support (exclusion limit 5,000,000 dalton, pore diameter 19 nm) is large with respect to the proteins (lysozyme, 14,400 dalton, hydrodynamic radius 2.7 nm, and human serum albumin, 67,000 dalton, 4.5 nm, respectively) significant differences exist in adsorption thermodynamics and kinetics. These distinctions are due to the differences in diffusion behaviour. JOHNSTON and HEARN concluded that protein movements into the porous sorbent can lead to significant restrictions in apparent ligand accessibility.

If porous supports are used, pore size influences further the capacity and specific binding, as demonstrated by HAYASHI et al. (1989). They investigated the influence of the pore size of a diol-coated silica support and found that an optimum exists for the amount of immobilized ligand (antibodies and Fab fragments against natural and recombinant human epidermal growth factor (hEGF)) as well as for the specific binding of antigen (hEGF and its fragments) (Fig. 2.15.). Surprisingly, the absolute amounts of adsorbed hEGF were similar when equal molar quantities of IgG, $F(ab)_2$ or Fab were immobilized. The molar ratios between ligand and ligate were in particular far from the theoretical values (2 for IgG and $F(ab')_2$ and 1 for Fab, respectively).

Most of the coupling procedures applied in low-pressure immunoaffinity chromatography are also possible in HPIAC, especially since supports have recently been developed, which are either hydrophilic organic polymers bearing the same functional groups as supports for conventional chromatography or inorganic matrices which were coated with a tight hydrophilic organic layer or with molecules which prevent silanol groups on the surface from solvatation (e.g. diol or glycophases or with silanes modified silica, purchased by several suppliers, e.g. CLONIS (1989), MAJORS (1989).

On the one hand this coating permits a facilitated activation and coupling of biomolecules as antibodies or antigens and on the other hand it protects the inorganic material from destruction by aqueous mobile phases.

Two methods for preparing affinity columns for HPAC are possible: the support is activated as usual in low-pressure affinity chromatography and coupled with the ligand outside the column; later the HPAC column is filled and used.

Prerequisites for this method are a column filling device and some experience in packing HPLC columns. Furthermore, the best lots of an

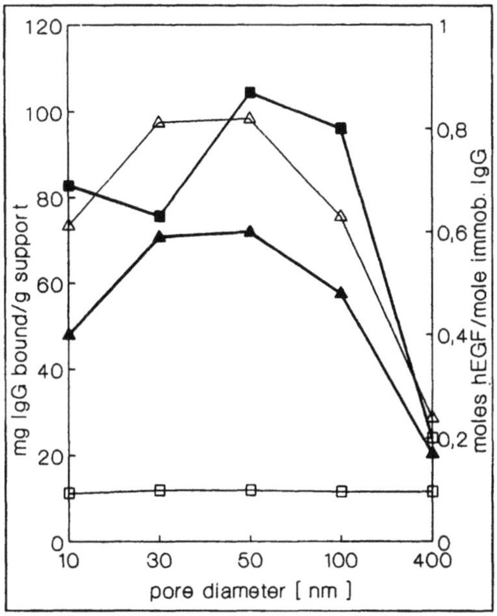

Fig. 2.15. Immobilized amount (mg antibody per g support, ligand density) and molar ratio (moles hEGF adsorbed per mole immobilized IgG, binding capacity) as function of pore size of a macroporous HPLC support.
For supports with low density (sqares), 12.5 mg IgG/g support were added to the activated matix, for high density (triangles), 100 mg/g were offered.
□ - Ligand density for supports with low IgG content, ■ - binding capacity for support with low ligand density, △ - ligand density for supports with high IgG content, ▲ - binding capacity for support with high ligand density (Data from Hayashi et al., 1989)

HPLC support are sometimes not available commercially unpacked.

A number of methods for activation of inorganic supports applicable in HPAC are described in detail in several publications (for instance see Weetall and Lee (1989) or Josic et al. (1988), further experimental details are given by Clonis (1989). The chemistry of the activation and coupling reactions are the same as for organic polymers and are summarized in Table 2.3. Examples of HPAC separations performed on columns, the content of which was prepared by this way, for instance are given by Babashak and Phillips (1988).

The second way utilizes manufacturer-filled ready-for-use columns containing an activated support. Some suppliers offer such columns, e.g. Beckman (Ultraaffinity EP), Merck (Fractogel (carbodiimide-activated)), ChromatoChem (HiPAC Aldehyde activated Affinity Columns), Perstorp Biolytica (SelectiSpher (tresyl-activated)), Whatman (Epoxy PartiSpher). The affinity column is prepared by dissolving the ligand in an appropriate buffer and recycling of this solution through the column for several hours (Santucci et al., 1988).

The use of streptavidin covalently immobilized in HPLC columns for binding of biotinylated antibodies as the biospecific ligands is also an example of this principle (Babashak and Phillips, 1988). The biotin-streptavidin complex has a very low dissociation constant ($K_D = 10^{-15}$ M), which means that this complex cannot easily be dissociated even under extreme pH or in high salt solutions. Thus, elution conditions for the absorbed antigen can be chosen as usual in immunoaffinity chromatography (for a more detailed discussion of applications of the avidin/biotin system in immunochemical systems see Chapter 2.5).

The application of ready-to-use columns need some care in selection of optimal ligand concentration in the binding buffer, buffer composition and speed of solvent flow during the immobilization process.

As pointed out, no general instructions exist for optimal immobilization of a defined protein. When coupling conditions for a given protein should be optimized, it must be taken into consideration that the biological activity of this protein need not be at the highest when coupling yield reaches a maximum. Enzymes and antibodies may suffer from inactivation at pH values where protein immobilization is optimal with respect to the fixed quantity (Taylor, 1985, Hayashi et al., 1989). For example, in a study comparing different activated supports Taylor observed that protein immobilization yield was highest at pH 11 when he bound immunoglobulin G covalently to Separon HEMA 1000, a polyhydroxymethacrylate resin. On the other hand, the ratio between immobilized antibody and adsorbed antigen as an expression of biological activity or immune reactivity was highest when the IgG was coupled in a buffer with lower pH (pH 9). Simlar results were obtained by NAKAMURA et al. (1990). The authors used a tresyl-activated HPLC support, which gave highest antigen binding efficiencies when antibody was coupled at pH 7.6 for one to two hours.

An explanation could be that at high pH (pH 11) most of the lysine or arginine residues are deprotonated, the free NH_2-groups can act as very potent nucleophiles and last but not least the protein exposes a lot of reactive amino acid side chains because it is partially denatured. Immobilization stabilizes this (partially) unfolded state(s) by multipoint attachment and prevents complete renaturation after change to more physiological pH. Using another support (activated glass), he observed differences in both coupling and activity pH depending on the coupling reaction: carbodiimide-activated support (CDI-Glycophase) gave the same discrepancy between optimal coupling and optimal adsorption pH as observed with Separon, whereas the N-hydroxy-succinimide-activated matrix (NHS-Glycophase) yielded affinity supports, where at high pH immobilization proceeds with best results. At this support biological activity is restored completely after switching to pH 7 or lower.

Finally, a method should be mentioned which is a borderline- case between conventional and high performance affinity chromatography. It can be included in HPLC methods because separation times are very short. On the other hand, equipment is quite different from that of usual HPLC. This method was developed from membrane separation processes: synthetic membranes were chemically activated and ligands were coupled to this membrane as usual in affinity chromatography (LUONG et al., 1987, LE et al., 1988). The very thin layer of the membrane disk combined with a relatively large surface which is reached quickly by the solutions enables very fast separations with high resolution. An example of the application of affinity membranes is given by AGRIS et al. (1989), who used protein A-membranes (ProTran) for adsorption of human IgG from whole serum. Buffers for the chromatographic steps were the same as for other immunoafinity methods.

2.5. The Avidin/Biotin System

One of the most useful tools in molecular biology involves the specific binding of the water-soluble biotin (vitamin H) to proteins as the egg white protein "avidin" (BAYER and WILCHEK, 1978; DIAMANDIS and CHRISTOPOULOS, 1991). The biotin molecule can easily be activated (frequently used derivatives are N-hydroxysuccinimido-biotin, biotin hydrazide, photoactivitable biotin (PIERCE, 1990) and coupled to either antigens or antibodies, usually with complete retention of activity. Instructions for the preparation of activated biotin derivatives and their conjugation with protein are given in the relevant literature (e.g. TJISSEN, 1985).

Avidin is a tetramer consisting of four identical subunits having a molecular mass of 15.600 (GREEN, 1975). Each subunit contains a high affinity binding site for biotin with a dissociation constant of approximately 10^{-15} M. In the classical purification method (MELAMED and GREEN, 1963), GREEN and TOMS, 1970) avidin is adsorbed to carboxymethylcellulose at high pH, followed by elution with a stepwise gradient of $(NH_4)_2CO_3$, rechromatography on CM cellulose and crystallization. Moreover, a very simple method using affinity chromatography on 2-imino-biotin agarose or 2-iminobiotin-6-aminohexyl-Sepharose 4B was described by HENEY and ORR (1981).

Proteins with high affinity to biotin also occurs in amphibian eggs and is formed by some microorganisms. Of practical significance is streptavidin produced by *Streptomyces avidinii*, which is unglycosylated, in contrast to the egg white protein. Streptavidin is generally prefered because of certain advantageous properties, e.g. its better accessibility and higher binding specificity. As opposed to avidin, biotin is a low molecular mass substance having the structure shown in Fig. 2.16. The avidin/biotin system is particularly well

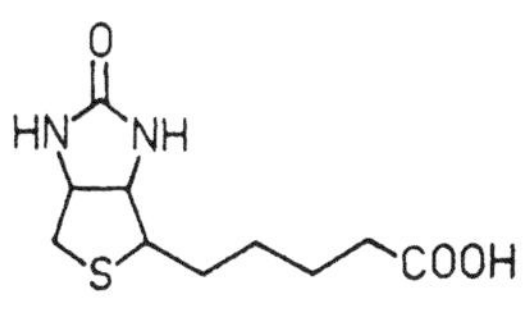

Fig. 2.16. Chemical formula of biotin (vitamin H)

suited for use as a bridging or sandwich system, in association with antigen/antibody interaction.

An application of avidin/biotin reagents has been found to increase the sensitivity and efficiency of numerous immunochemical methods. Some of these uses include:

(i) *Amplification of antibody titers,*

(ii) *Radio-, enzyme- and fluorescent immunoassays:* The application of the avidin/biotin system improves the sensitivity of immunoassays. This is attainable by the variants illustrated in Fig. 4.6. C-E., p. 130 (GUESDON et al., 1979, HSU et al., 1981).

(iii) *Nitrocellulose and nylon transfer blot detection* (STOTT, 1989): Avidin/biotin technology has enhanced the sensitivity of protein detection on Western blots to that of silver staining techniques used for polyacrylamide gels (lower detection limit about 1 ng) (cf. Fig. 4.6. C-E, p. 130),

(iv) *Introducing multiple labels into tissues* (GUESDON et al., 1979, MILIOS and LEONG, 1987) A wide variety of biotinylated primary probes have been used, including antibodies. A tagged avidin detection reagent can be added which would reveal the precise location where the primary probe was bound. The avidin may be labeled with enzymes, fluorescent molecules or with electron microscopy reagents such as ferritin,

(v) *Measurements of antigen concentrations on a single cell* (BAYER et al., 1976),

(vi) *Coupling of antibodies and antigens to solid phase materials* (e.g. agarose): For this purpose avidin is covalently bound on the solid phase (REDEUILH et al., 1985) followed by addition of an antibody/ or antigen/biotin conjugate (LEMOLI et al., 1989; cf. Fig. 2.17.),

(vii) *Separation of substances and purging of samples by avidin/biotin immunoadsorption* (e.g. GRETCH et al., 1987; cf. Chapter 3.2.): A ligand (e.g. an immunoglobulin) that has an affinity for the substance of interest is labeled with a suitable biotin conjugate and incubated with the substance to be separated in a crude mixture. To isolate or deplete this substance (e.g. a protein, receptor, cell), the mixture is passed through an immobilized avidin or streptavidin column which will bind with the biotinylated ligand (cf. Table 3.15A. and Fig. 2.17.).

(viii) *Separation and depletion of cells* (e.g. WORMMEESTER et al., 1984, LEMOLI et al., 1988; cf. also Chapter 3.2.).

The application of the avidin/biotin system in these fields has some advantages compared with conventional methods:

(a) steric hindrance due to the large size of numerous substances can be minimized by the formed spacer arm extending outward from the surface. Frequently, the efficiency of separation procedures, can thereby be improved considerably.

(b) the sensitivity of analytical methods is also improved, generally because of the potential for amplification due to multiple site binding. Moreover, of advantage is that:

(c) Biotinylation has a minimal effect on biological activities of proteins, and avidin derivatives are very stable.

(d) The extraordinarily high affinity between avidin and biotin assures the user of a rapidly formed and stable complex between an avidin conjugate or immobilized avidin and a labeled protein.

The three basic designs employed for *analytical purposes* are the labeled avidin (LAB: GUESDON et al., 1979), the bridged avidin/biotin (BRAB: GUESDON et al., 1979) and the avidin/biotin complex systems (ABC: HSU et al., 1981, PIERCE, 1990). Each is similar in that a biotinylated antibody is bound to an immobilized antigen or primary antibody, but they differ in the manner in which avidin is used in the detection process.

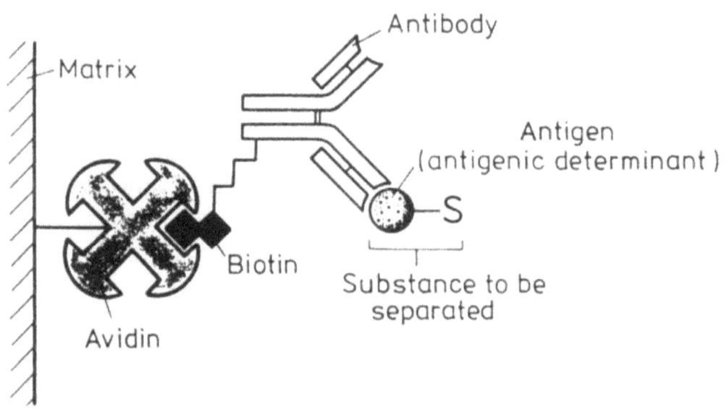

Fig. 2.17. Separation (purification, purging of samples) with aid of immobilized avidin. The antigen or the antigen bearing substance is incubated in a crude mixture with the suitable antibody-biotin conjugate. The complex formed between this conjugate and the substance to be separated is bound to the immobilized avidin or streptavidin as it is shown in the figure. The elution, if required, is often difficult, and suitable methods have to be developed in each case separately (e.g. using an authentic biotin derivative).

(1) *The LAB system* (cf. Fig. 4.6. C, p. 130): When working with antigen bound on a microtiter plate, a primary antibody is added and after washing the specifically fixed antibody is incubated with a biotinylated secondary antibody.

The final step is the addition of the avidin/enzyme conjugate and of a suitable substrate. The intensity of the colour or fluorescence measured should correlate to the concentration of the primary antibody being detected.

(2) *The BRAB system* (cf. Fig. 4.6. D, p. 130): The procedure is essentially the same as developing a LAB complex, except that avidin is not conjugated to an enzyme. This reaction scheme uses avidin as a bridge between the biotinylated secondary antibody and biotinylated enzyme. Due to the multiple biotin binding sites on avidin, more biotinylated enzyme can be complexed to increase the intensity of the substrate colour development.

(3) *The ABC system* (cf. Fig. 4.6. E, p. 130): The ABC system requires, contrary to the LAB and BRAB systems, that the biotinylated enzyme is pre-incubated with the avidin, forming large complexes to be incubated with the biotinylated antibody. The result is a greater concentration of the enzyme on the surface where an analytical reaction takes place, and, therefore, an enhancement of sensitivity.

3. Separation and Purification of Antibodies, Haptens and Antigens

3.1. Purification of Antibodies

On the one hand purification of antibodies is a prerequisite for immunoaffinity purification of antigens and haptens (cf. Chapter 3.2.). On the other, affinity and immunoaffinity chromatographic methods can be used for antibody purification. Both aspects will be discussed in this chapter, but preference is given to problems of antibody purification in general, including also pretreatment of antibody sources and non-chromatographic separation techniques. Because purified antibodies are required for many purposes, appropriate purification procedures have long been of great importance in immunochemistry and protein biochemistry (Nau, 1989 a).

During the last two decades protein separation and purification methods have improved greatly.

Table 3.1. Most Important Techniques for Separation and Purification of Proteins

A. Non-chromatographic procedures	**B. Liquid chromatographic procedures** [a]
■ Precipitation [b]	■ Size exclusion chromatography (gel filtration) [b]
– by salts (e.g. ammonium or sodium sulfate, zinc chloride)	■ Ion exchange chromatography [b]
– euglobulin precipitation (desalting)	– anion exchange
– by organic solvents (e.g. ethanol, acetone)	– cation exchange
– by other organic substances (e.g. Rivanol, caprylic acid)	– mixed mode exchange (e.g. hydroxyapatite, ABx)
– by synthetic organic polymers (e.g. PEG, pluronic polyols, PVP)	■ Hydrophobic interaction chromatography [b]
– isoelectric precipitation	■ Reversed phase chromatography [c]
■ Ultrafiltration	■ Thiophilic adsorption chromatography ("T-gel") [b]
■ Ultracentrifugation	■ Chromatofocusing
■ Liquid-liquid extraction	■ Affinity chromatography [b]
■ Preparative electrophoresis	– dye ligand chromatography
■ Preparative isoelectric focusing [b]	– biospecific affinity chromatography by solid phase bound
	• protein effectors (e.g. enzyme effectors)
	• receptors (lectins, bacterial Fc receptors)
	• antigens or haptens (antibody purification)
	• antibodies (antigen purification)
	■ Covalent chromatography [c]

[a] performed as conventional chromatography, FPLC or HPLC
[b] antibody separation and purification by these methods is described in more detail in this Chapter
[c] not suitable for separation of native antibodies

High performance liquid chromatography has been adapted to protein separation on both the analytical and preparative scale. This was made possible in particular by the development of new solid phase supports (cf. Chapter 2.1.) combining the outstanding attributes of HPLC carriers (e.g. mechanical stability, large flow rate and high resolution power) with the most important properties of classical protein liquid chromatography supports (biocompatibility, large and/or definite pore size, numerous derivatisation possibilities etc.). Equipment for both conventional chromatography and HPLC/FPLC is today available for laboratory use as well as for highly automated industrial scale separation processes. Several new chromatography supports (e.g. spherical hydroxyapatite, BAKERBOND ABx, and thiophilic adsorbents), as well as broad application of affinity supports based on Protein A or G have considerably improved the technical prerequites for antibody purification. But, even with simple precipitation techniques - supposed to be completely superseded by the more modern chromatographic methodes - several surprising results have been obtained using precipitating agents for new purposes (e.g. caprylic acid as a negatively separating agent in antibody purification) or improving pretreatment procedures.

Thus, being confronted with problems of protein separation, one can choose from a great variety of methods (Table 3.1.). Since antibodies are glycoproteins, most of these methods are also available for antibody purification.

Prior to the introduction of hybridoma technology (cf. Chapter 1.3.3.) the situation was rather easy. The only source of specific antibodies was the serum of animals immunized with the appropriate antigen or with the protein-coupled hapten of interest. Since immunoglobulins, especially IgG, represent a major portion of total serum proteins, immune sera satisfy the demands of several applications. In these cases, special efforts in purification are not necessary. However, for most applications (e.g. antibody labeling or immunoaffinity chromatography) at least partially purified antibodies are required. Most freqently, precipitation techniques are used in combination with anion exchange chromatography and result in fairly pure IgG fractions of immune sera (Weir, 1978; Hudson and Hay, 1982). Polyclonal antibodies isolated in this manner satisfy the demands of most in vitro applications. Any further purification, however, is mainly limited by non-specific immunoglobulins and by heterogeneity in specificity and affinity of polyclonal antibodies. Thus, complete separation of antigen-specific antibodies from non-specific immunoglobulins is practically impossible by methods other then immunoaffinity techniques, which are expensive and in the case of labile antigens often not available. However, even polyclonal antibody preparations isolated by immunoaffinity procedures are very heterogeneous in chemical (e.g. pI, hydrophobicity) and immunological properties (affinity, epitope specificity, IgG subclass).

The situation changed with the introduction and broad application of hybridoma techniques for monoclonal antibody production up to industrial scale. With this development, the aim of antibody purification has become increasingly the isolation of individual antibodies with very distinct and constant properties. Isolating monoclonal antibodies from ascitic fluid, the situation is similar to that of immune sera. The monoclonal antibody is one of the main protein constituents of the crude material. Therefore, antibody isolation is relatively easy, in spite of the difficulties involved in removal of non-specific host immunoglobulins, which are present in most ascitic fluids.

But current trends are to prevent animals from hybridoma cell propagation and to favour scaling-up of cell culture for the production of large amounts of monoclonal antibodies (cf. Chapter 1.3.3.). Here the situation is very different from that described above. The monoclonal antibody is only a minor component of a cell culture supernatant among a large bulk of other proteins produced either by the cells themselves or resulting from additives that are necessary for cell growth. This fact requires an adapted purification strategy.

Further new purification problems arose from the development of hybrid-hybridomas that produce bispecific monoclonal antibodies besides the two "parent" antibodies and from gene technical manipulation of antibodies, but also from increasing in vivo application of monoclonal antibodies requiring a higher level of purity. Taking this into account, purification and quality control become more and more the "bottle neck" of antibody production because they require much time and labour and often expensive equipment.

Whereas mammalian cell culture technology has today reached a level of scale and automation that allows a yearly throughput of kilogram quantities, production-scale purification methods for antibodies are still rare and in most cases limited to particular antibodies. Nevertheless, already in 1988, worldwide, there were more than 500 companies and organizations engaged in monoclonal antibody production (Davidson, 1988), and the number is increasing rapidly because of the increasing demands resulting from the broad application of antibodies in medicine and biotechnology.

To date, *in vitro* immunodiagnostic kits (cf. Chapter 4.1.), that require only several grams of antibodies for millions of tests have been the major application area of polyclonal and monoclonal antibodies. However, application of antibodies for immuno-based separation techniques (e.g. immunoaffinity purification of antigens, cf. Chapter 3.2.), *in vivo* diagnosis and especially for therapeutic purposes (e.g radioimmunotherapy, targeting of chemotherapeutic agents or treatment of transplant rejection with anti T cell antibodies (Schlom, 1988; Burchiel and Rhodes, 1983; Cobbold and Waldman, 1984; Klausner, 1986; Ritz and Schlossman, 1982; Goldstein, 1985)) can require gram quantities of pure antibody for a single separation process or for the therapy of a single patient respectively. Thus, a demand of kilogram amounts of antibodies has been predicted for these purposes (Boss, 1986).

Although a large variety of purification procedures is available, it is impossible to find a technique that meets all problems. Nevertheless, one can assume that it is possible today to purify almost any monoclonal antibody to homogeneity (in spite of typical microheterogeneities in pI) using a sequence of several selected purification steps.

However, individual monoclonal antibodies, even of the same IgG subclass, are very similar only in size and shape, but can be very different in chemical (pI, solubility, hydrophobicity and charge density and distribution) and immunological properties (affinity, specificity; KENNEY, 1989). Therefore, a multi-step procedure that is very efficient in the purification of one monoclonal antibody can fail in the case of another. This means, in order to obtain homogeneous antibody preparations, the separation procedure in detail has to be designed for each individual antibody.

However, antibody purities of 90 or even 95 % of total protein can be achieved often using common procedures, even by one-step methods. For many purposes this level of purity is sufficient - immunoaffinity chromatography is one of these.

In contrast, antibodies destined for in vivo application in humans must be essentially pure, at least endotoxins, nucleic acids, pyrogenic viral and bacterial impurities have to be removed completely (BIRCH et al., 1985). Tolerable contamination limits for biotechnological products intended for use in humans are laid down in legal regulations at levels slightly differing from country to country. Regulatory authorities like the Food and Drug Administration (FDA) of the U.S.A. (1987) and the Commission of European Communities (1988) have published proposals for the regulation of monoclonal antibody production and application.

The remarks made above demonstrate that the choice of an appropriate isolation procedure depends on several factors, which have to be considered carefully (SCHMIDT, 1989). Looking for the best-fitting procedure prior to commencing experiments, the operator has to answer at least the following important questions:

A) Concerning the antibody itself:
- Antibodies of which **species** are to be isolated?
- **Polyclonal** or **monoclonal** antibodies?
- Which **class** of immunoglobulins is to be isolated?
- Can **specificity** be used for antibody purification?

B) Concerning the operation:
- From which **source** are antibodies to be isolated?
- Which **pretreatment** is required?
- What are the main **contaminants**?
- What is the final **use** of the antibodies?
- Which analytical **quality control** is required?
- On which **scale** has the purification to be performed?

The last question especially plays an important role concerning cost efficiency. For purification of antibodies on a laboratory scale almost any available method can be taken into consideration and problems can be solved the better the more different methods there are established in the laboratory. The aim of antibody purification should be not to isolate antibodies as pure as possible but **as pure as required** for the desired application. A consideration of this rule is the more important the larger the scale, since each improvement of purity has to be paid for with additional purification steps, lower yield and higher cost.

Nevertheless, even cost-efficient, large-scale production of antibodies for *in vivo* use in humans can be performed if procedures are optimized for individual antibodies and then run computer driven.

The aim of this chapter is to discuss a variety of methods that are useful for antibody separation and purification, on the basis of Table 3.1. Today, most methods are designed for preparation of monoclonal antibodies, but some procedures for isolation of immunoglobulin fractions from immune sera are also mentioned. Most monoclonal antibodies in use are of the IgG class, but purification of IgM and IgA is also of increasing interest. Although in most cases multi-step procedures are required to achieve sufficient purity, the single methods will be discussed and evaluated separately. All methods can be discussed only in general. For detailed protocols the cited references should be consulted. HPLC and FPLC procedures are included in the single sections. To date, most procedures have been developed for laboratory-scale isolation of antibodies, but as far as they are available aspects of scale-up are taken into consideration. The data presented in Tables 3.2. - 3.5. are far from being complete, representing only a small selection from many equivalent procedures.

3.1.1. Pretreatment of Antibody Source

Independent of the antibody source some kind of pretreatment is always advisable. At least cells and debris have to be removed by centrifugation or filtration steps.

The choice of an appropriate pretreatment procedure, however, depends on antibody source. In serum or ascitic fluid the antibody concentration is high enough to omit concentrating measures. As far as antibodies are to be isolated from plasma, fibrin should be removed by chemically induced clotting. Sometimes, especially if heparin has been added, this is advisable also for ascitic fluid, in order to avoid trouble during chromatographic separations. Furthermore, ascites is often contaminated with lipids or with oil (e.g. pristane), which is used to stimulate growth of the ascitic tumor (cf. Chapter 1.3.). Volumes to be handled are mostly small, thus cells, debris, fibrin clots and oil can usually be removed by centrifugation and decantation. Some kind of centrifugation is included in most purification protocols. Several authors find a single low speed centrifugation performed at 1,000 - 6,000 x g to be sufficient, e.g. 20 min. at 1,000 x g (ANNUNCIATO and MARCIANI, 1987), 10 min. at 2,500 x g (PAVLU et al., 1986) or 15 min. at 4,000 x g (BUKOVSKY and KENNETT, 1987), whereas others invest more time in centrifugation using a low speed step (400 - 1,000 x g) for removal of cells and debris, followed by ultracentrifugation for 30 min. at 50,000 x g (DESCHAMPS et al., 1985) or 100,000 x g (BRUCK et al., 1982).

Lipids and oils can be removed more efficiently and without considerable loss of antibody by adsorption onto fumed silica (NEOH, 1986) or Lipidex (DAHLBERG et al., 1980), since separation of these materials from the solution is easier than the decantation of two liquid phases. At least, if HPLC and FPLC are used for further purification, the crude material should be sterile filtered to prevent the expensive columns from bacterial growth and fouling. Furthermore, in so doing a permanent source of pyrogens is excluded. However, it is advisable to use one or even two of the above mentioned methods prior to filtration through 0.45 or 0.22 μm filters, because otherwise lipids and debris would immediately foul the filters.

Cell culture fluids, depending on culture method (cf. Chapter 1.3.), will contain variable amounts of cells and debris. Culture fluids derived from airlift fermentors will be contaminated with large amounts of cells and debris, whereas materials derived from modern compartmented high density cell culture equipment (e.g. hollow fibre reactors) are usually free of cells and debris. If particulate matter represents a problem, the solution must be clarified by centrifugation and/or filtration. The centrifugation and filtration equipment available at that time, especially filtration media but also the theoretical background of the different clarification procedures, have been summarized by BALL (1985). On a laboratory-scale centrifugation can be performed batchwise using conventional rotors of appropriate capacity (up to several litres per run), and decantation can be done per hand. For large-scale systems handling throughputs of 1,000 litres or more per day, this technique is unacceptable but continuous flow centrifugation can solve the problem. Continuous flow rotors are available for conventional centrifuges, allowing flow rates of up to 100 litres per hour, whereas self-cleaning industrial centrifuges can operate at flow rates of more than 1,000 litres per hour. The separation power can be manipulated by altering either the centrifugal force (speed) or the flow rate (BALL, 1985). KENNEY (1986) described a method to improve centrifugation efficiency by flocculation. The main problem in refining of all kinds of culture fluid, however, is the low concentration of the antibody. Thus, prior to purification, the crude material has to be concentrated. Usually this is done by ultrafiltration using membrane filters in

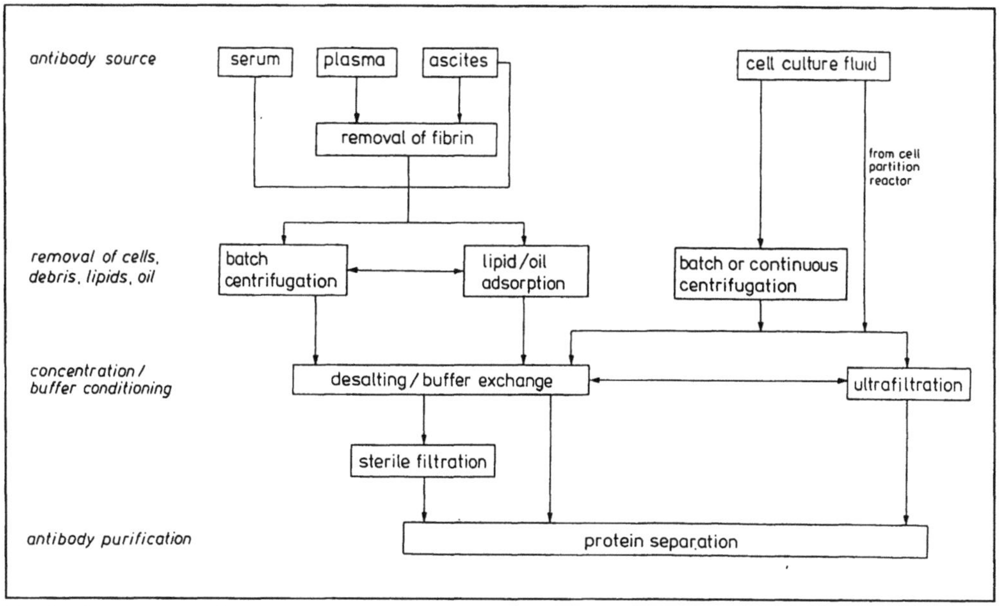

Fig. 3.1. Pretreatment of antibody sources for purification.

tangential flow or hollow fibres, which allow a 50-100 fold concentration of up to 1,000 litres within 1 - 4 hours, and almost quantitative recovery of antibody (Birch et al., 1987; Östlund, 1986). It is advisable to prefer membranes of small pore size (e.g. 10 kD cut-off), since those of larger size (e.g. 100 kD cut-off) do not provide a considerable purification effect but can cause heavy losses of antibody (Scott et al., 1987).

Since both centrifugation and ultrafiltration equipment can be sterilized prior to use, it is advantageous for large-scale processes to use continuous flow centrifuges with effluent being directly applied to the ultrafiltration apparatus. If this can be done on-line to a continuously producing cell culture equipment, the whole complex of cell culture, harvesting, clarification and concentration may be optimized and automated, maintaining sterility throughout all these steps (Kenney, 1989).

Most purification procedures require special starting buffers. Therefore, desalting or buffer exchange are essential. This can be performed easily and without a loss of antibody by gel filtration using a small-pore medium (e.g. Sephadex G-10 or G-25), which also partially removes low molecular weight contaminants. Since this can be performed at any scale up to several thousand litres per hour (Low, 1988), buffer exchange by gel filtration is possible at any stage of pretreatment and purification. It is advisable to use superfine grade gel in order to minimize the dilution factor (Schmidt, 1989). A scheme for pretreatment of antibody sources for purification is presented in Fig. 3.1.

3.1.2. Non-Chromatographic Separation Procedures

Taking into consideration that ultracentrifugation plays a considerable role at most in purification of IgM antibodies, all methods listed in part A of Table 3.1. do not require expensive and sophisticated equipment. Thus, they can be performed in any laboratory. Although tangential flow ultrafiltration does not provide any considerable effect on antibody purification (see above), at least on a

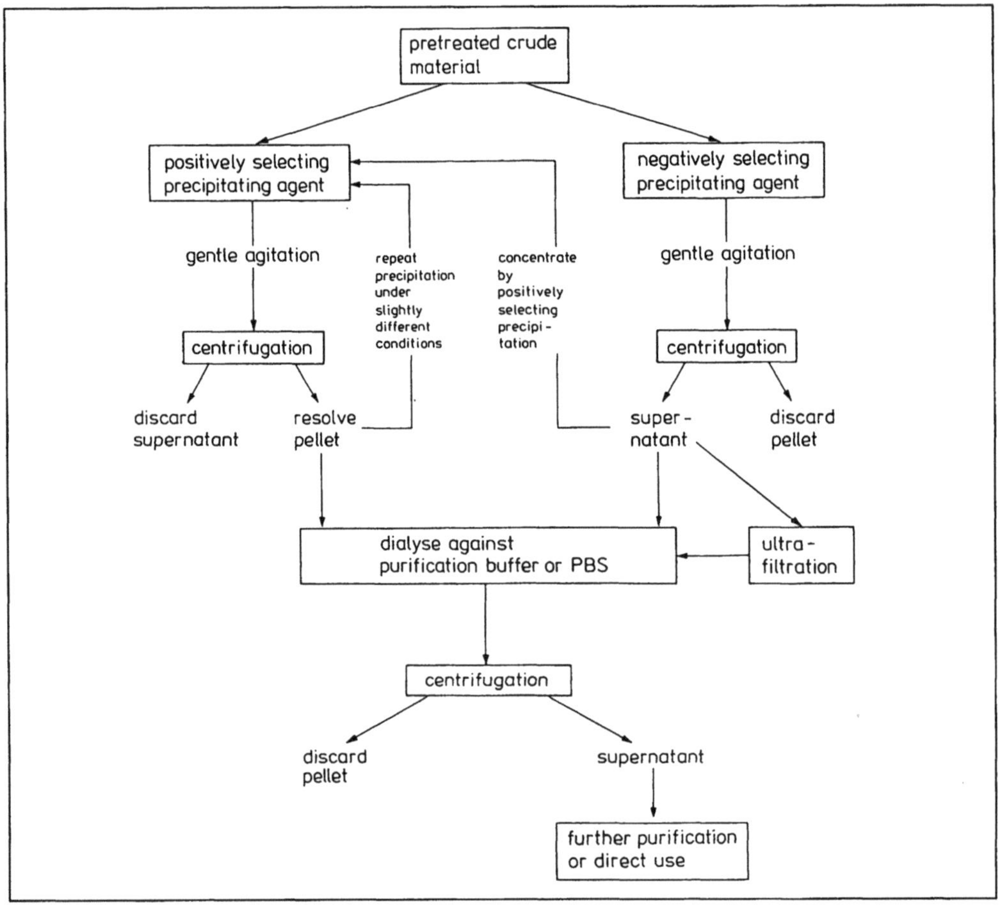

Fig. 3.2. Positive and negative selection by precipitation.

laboratory scale, vertical ultrafiltration using filters of large pore size (100 kD cut-off) can significantly increase the specific activity of monoclonal IgM antibodies with loss being tolerable (NAU, 1989 a).

Most of the non-chromatographic separation methods frequently used are precipitation techniques in various forms. They are not very useful for large-scale antibody purification because of their relatively low separation power, often poor recovery and inconvenience in handling of large volumes of dilute material. Nevertheless, in fractionation of ascites or serum proteins precipitation is often used as the initial purification step, whereas in most cases antibodies purified by precipitation alone do not satisfy the purity demands. Depending on the precipitating agent positive and negative selection of antibodies can be distinguished. By positive selection the antibodies are precipitated and the bulk of other proteins remain in solution, whereas negative selection works in the opposite manner. Salts, desalting, ethanol, acetone and polyethylene glycol select antibodies positively, Rivanol and caprylic acid are negatively selecting agents. Both separation principles can also be used in a purification protocol one after the other (see Fig. 3.2.).

Positively Selecting Precipitation

The advantage of positive selection is that fractionation and concentration of the sample are performed in one step.

As to protein fractionation in general, ammonium sulfate is the most frequently used salt precipitant because of its excellent solubility even at low temperatures but sodium sulfate, zinc chloride and other salts have also been applied.

A classical method for isolation of the immunoglobulin fraction of sera has been described by Hudson and Hay (1989): serum is diluted with an equal amount of PBS and, while permanently agitating, saturated ammonium sulfate solution is added dropwise until a final salt saturation of 45 % is achieved. After one hour of stirring, the cold precipitate is harvested by centrifugation, washed with 45 % saturated ammonium sulfate solution and centrifuged again. The pellet is dissolved in a small amount of PBS and dialysed overnight against 100 vols. of PBS (2 - 3 changes). Insoluble aggregated immunoglobulin is then removed by centrifugation. Similar procedures have been applied successfully as the initial step in purification of monoclonal IgG antibodies from ascitic fluid using 40 % (Burchiel et al., 1984; de Rie et al., 1987), 45 % (Perry et al., 1985) or 50 % (Pavlu et al., 1986) saturation of ammonium sulfate. Purity of the antibodies can be improved considerably if precipitation is repeated at lower salt concentrations but heavy losses of antibody have to be taken into account then. Some authors consider that salt precipitation always reduces the antibody activity (McGregor et al., 1983). Goding (1986), however, suggested a preference for ammonium sulfate precipitation as the initial step in IgM purification too because he often found IgM monoclonals purified by euglobulin precipitation to be partially denatured.

Nevertheless, euglobulin precipitation, i.e. dialysis against deionized water or very dilute buffers, has been applied frequently for purification of human IgM (Weir, 1978), rat IgM and IgG2c (Bazin et al., 1986) and murine IgM and IgG3 (Garcia-Gonzales et al., 1986). The latter dialysed several different defibrinated ascitic fluids twice against 100 vols. of deionized water for two hours at 20°C for IgG3 and for 8 - 15 hours at 4°C for IgM. The precipitate was dissolved in 0.1 M Tris/HCl buffer, pH 8.0 containing 1 mol/l sodium chloride and precipitation was repeated. The preparations were essentially free of albumin and transferrin and more than 90 % of total protein were active antibodies. IgG3 was better purified by this method than IgM. Depending on the lipoprotein content of ascites, the yield was 73 to 90 % for IgG3 and 40 to 90 % for IgM.

A protocol including euglobulin precipitation for removal of IgM, zinc chloride precipitation for removal of IgG and the final precipitation of IgA by ammonium sulfate has been described by Hudson and Hay (1989) for isolation of IgA from human serum. Cripps et al. (1983) have developed a procedure for isolation of IgM (14 % PEG) and IgA (7 % PEG) from normal human serum by polyethylene glycol (PEG) precipitation and immunoaffinity chromatography. The same group (Neoh et al., 1986) has applied PEG precipitation to isolation of murine monoclonal antibodies from ascites. IgM could be isolated successfully from defatted ascites by addition of 4 - 6 % PEG 6000 (purity: > 90 %, yield: > 80 %), whereas for IgG antibodies, which precipitate at 5 - 10 % PEG, this method was not very useful (purity: 30 - 40 %, yield: >70 %). The optimal PEG concentration has to be found empirically for each individual antibody, and for amounts of less than 10 ml ascites considerable losses of antibody have been observed.

Rarely, ethanol (Phillips et al., 1984) and pluronic polyols (Garcia and Ordonez, 1976) have also been used as precipitating agents. McCue et al. (1988) isolated human IgG from effluent III of Cohn plasma fractionation by precipitation with 25 % ethanol using different procedures. They observed considerable losses when immunoglobulins were precipitated at a pH close to their pI. In addition a large-scale procedure for isolation of monoclonal IgM, including ultrafiltration, isoelectric precipitation and gel filtration, provided a yield of only 40 %, with the heaviest losses occurring during the precipitation step (STEINDL et al., 1987). Isoelectric precipitation therefore seems not to be advisable for most immunoglobulins.

Negatively Selecting Precipitation

The advantages of negative selection of antibodies are an improved separation power and a reduced formation of immunoglobulin aggregates during the precipitation process though, usually antibodies are diluted rather than concentrated. Therefore, these methods are not very useful for purification of antibodies from dilute feedstocks and large volumes but they are valuable for isolation of antibodies from ascites or serum.

Rivanol (2-ethoxy-6,9-diaminoacridine lactate) has been used for isolation of IgG from blood plasma already for a long period of time (HOREJSI et al., 1956; SCHULTZE et al., 1965). More recently, Rivanol precipitation followed by gel filtration has been applied successfully to purification of monoclonal antibodies from ascitic fluid that had been dialysed against 50 mM sodium acetate solution (FRANEK, 1986). This method seems to be very efficient for murine IgG1, IgG2a and IgG2b but it cannot be used for IgG3 and IgM. The principle of the action is the formation of insoluble complexes with negatively charged proteins. Thus, albumin is removed efficiently already at Rivanol concentrations of less than 1 %, and many other components of ascites are coprecipitated (e.g. lipids, lipoproteins, IgM and aggregated proteins). Further advantages are that Rivanol is a bactericidal agent and an efficient precipitant of viral particles and nucleic acids (NEURATH and BRUNNER, 1969), and that it can be easily removed from the product by gel filtration. Final monoclonal antibody concentrations of 0.5 - 2.0 mg/ml could be achieved. Exact information on yield is not provided but high purity is documented by PAGE.

Another frequently used negatively selecting precipitant concerning immunoglobulin is **caprylic acid**. Short chain fatty acids have been known to precipitate several serum proteins under slightly acidic conditions (CHANUTIN and CURNISH, 1960). STEINBUCH and AUDRAN (1969) used caprylic acid for isolation of IgG from mammalian sera and the first procedure using caprylic acid for purification of monoclonal antibodies from ascites has been described by RUSSO et al. (1983). Unfortunately, serum or ascitic fluid have to be diluted with 2 - 4 vols. of 60 mM acetate buffer, pH 4.0, to assure optimal conditions for an efficient precipitation of the bulk of serum or ascites proteins. Thus, the antibody preparations obtained are rather pure but very dilute. MCKINNEY and PARKINSON (1987) and REIK et al. (1987) have developed efficient and simple two-step procedures applicable to both serum and ascitic fluid. Bulk proteins are removed by caprylic acid precipitation and then immunoglobulins are precipitated from the supernatant by ammonium sulfate at 45 or 50 % of salt saturation respectively. In both cases highly purified IgG antibodies were obtained, as was demonstrated by PAGE and IEF. Recovery was shown to vary between 50 and 90 % for individual antibodies. The yield does not correlate with IgG subclass. TEMPONI et al. (1988) could demonstrate that neither caprylic acid nor ammonium sulfate precipitation had a significant influence on antibody affinity but purity was considerably improved using the two-step procedure. However, some monoclonal antibodies, especially IgG3, IgA and antiidiotypic antibodies, form an irreversible precipitate with caprylic acid.

Comparing different methods of antibody purification from ascitic fluid, TEMPONI et al. (1989) found the sequential caprylic acid/ammonium sulfate procedure in some cases to result in purities comparable to those obtained with HPLC or immunoaffinity methods with even better recovery rates! Furthermore, this method is rapid and easily applicable for large amounts of ascitic fluid. If gram quantities of murine monoclonal antibodies are to be isolated from ascites, OGDEN and LEUNG (1988) suggested concentrating the supernatant of caprylic acid precipitation by tangential flow ultrafiltration (30 kD cut-off membranes) rather than by ammonium sulfate precipitation. An average purity of 95 % could be achieved by this method, and only 1.5 - 3 hours were required for buffer exchange and

Table 3.2. Selected Non-Chromatographic Methods for Antibody Purification

Antibody source	Precipitating agent(s)	Ig-class/ subclass	Yield [%]	Purity [%] [a)]	Comment	Reference
Murine ascites	dialysis against deionized water, twice	IgG3 IgM	73-90	> 90 40-90	free of albumin and transferrin	GARCIA-GONZALES et al., 1988
Rat ascites	dialysis against 5 mM Tris/HCl, pH7.5	IgG2c	good	n.s.	contain other Ig	BAZIN et al., 1986
Murine ascites	PEG 6000 4-6 % 5-10 %	IgM IgG	> 80 > 70	> 90 30-40	lipids removed by SiO_2 adsorption	NEOH et al., 1986
Murine ascites	Rivanol	IgG		high	IgG in supernatant	FRANEK, 1986
Serum	ethanol	IgG	good	60	heavy losses in activity	PHILLIPS et al., 1984
Serum	45 % $(NH_4)_2SO_4$, twice	IgG	> 50	> 50	yield and purity unsteady	HUDSON and HAY, 1982
Murine ascites	35-50 % $(NH_4)_2SO_4$	various	[b)]			GODING, 1986
Murine ascites	50 % $(NH_4)_2SO_4$	IgG	high	low	insufficient as one-step-method	TEMPONI et al., 1989
Human serum	1. 0.001 M P-buffer 2. zinc chloride 3. 45 % $(NH_4)_2SO_4$	IgA			removal of IgM removal of IgG precip. of IgA	HUDSON and HAY, 1982
Murine ascites	caprylic acid	IgG; not IgG3	> 90	92-98	final ultra-filtration	OGDEN and LEUNG, 1988
Murine ascites	caprylic acid	IgG	high	n.s.	not for IgA and IgG3	TEMPONI et al., 1989
Murine ascites	1. caprylic acid 2. 50 % $(NH_4)_2SO_4$	IgG IgA(?)	50-80	> 90	from acetate, pH 4.8, not IgG3	REIK et al., 1987
Murine ascites	1. caprylic acid 2. 45 % $(NH_4)_2SO_4$	IgG	80-90	high	see above	MCKINNEY and PARKINSON, 1987
Murine ascites	preparative IEF	IgG1	high	high	for lab-scale	ROSEBROUGH, et al., 1986

[a)] related to total protein
[b)] yield and purity depent on individual antibody
n.s. not satisfactory
precip. precipitation

simultanous concentrating of antibodies to a final content of 10-20 mg/ml.

At least for the isolation of murine monoclonal IgG1, IgG2a and IgG2b antibodies from ascites and of IgG fractions from sera, caprylic acid precipitation seems to be a valuable, rapid and inexpensive alternative to the chromatographic procedures but it is not recommended for murine monoclonal IgG3, IgM, IgA and anti-idiotypic antibodies and for isolation of antibodies from culture fluid.

Several selected procedures that are based exclusively on non-chromatographic methods are presented in Table 3.2.

3.1.3. Chromatographic Separation Procedures

Ion Exchange Chromatography

In combination with salt precipitation, ion exchange chromatography in any form is the most frequently used technique for purification of polyclonal antibodies from serum and monoclonal antibodies from ascites. Ion exchange is suitable for all separation problems concerning charged molecules. In the case of antibody purification charge differences (net charge and/or charge distribution on the surface of the molecules) between the antibodies and the main contaminating proteins are utilized for separation. According to separation principles anion, cation and mixed mode ion exchange media can be distinguished.

Anion Exchange Chromatography

Following ammonium sulfate precipitation, conventional anion exchange chromatography on soft gels (e.g. cellulose, dextrans, agarose or polyacrylamide with weakly [e.g. DEAE] or strongly basic [e.g. QAE or QMA] substituents) has been a standard method for purification of immunoglobulins from serum for many years (Levy and Sober, 1960; Garvey et al., 1977; Weir, 1978; Hudson and Hay, 1982; Johnstone and Thorpe, 1982), and similar methods are also efficient for preparative purification of monoclonal antibodies and myeloma cell line immunoglobulins from ascites or culture fluid (e.g. Bruck et al., 1982 and 1986; Manil et al., 1986; Ideyama et al., 1986). Posillico et al. (1987) even routinely isolated monoclonal antibodies of more than 98 % purity from highly concentrated and prepurified culture fluid derived from microencapsulation reactor. Because it is easy to handle and low in cost and requires only simple equipment, soft gel anion exchange chromatography can be performed in any laboratory. Usually, however, due to large particle size and broad particle size distribution, resolution power of soft gel ion exchangers is rather low. Thus, extremely long run times and large amounts of gel and buffers can be required for a satisfactory separation (Nau, 1989 a). High flow rates that are required in production-scale processes to achieve high throughput and rapid regeneration and reequilibration of the columns are impossible with soft gels because high back pressures and poor mechanical stability of the gels can result in column collapse. Furthermore, large changes in bed volume during the separatiom process can require repacking of the columns after each run (Kato et al., 1982). Since the life-time of soft gels is rather short due to chemical and biological degradability, and regeneration and maintainance are very time-consuming, Nau (1989 a) suggested using the relatively inexpensive gels only once.

Usually, antibody recovery obtained by soft gel anion exchange chromatography is relatively low (50 - 80 %) because most matrices tend to bind immunoglobulins irreversibly (Garvey et al., 1977; Kato et al., 1982; Bruck et al., 1986). Although high purity can be achieved, antibody preparations are often contaminated with endotoxins and degradation products of both proteins and matrices (Nau, 1986, 1988 a, 1989c, 1990).

Most of these disadvantages could be overcome by the modern medium- and high-performance matrices. Although charged groups are usually the same as in soft gels, these supports have a definite small particle size, a definite large pore size and a higher protein binding capacity, resulting in a much better resolution power. The HPLC media (particle sizes of 3 - 15 μm) produce the best resolution and are therefore used especially for analytical and semi-preparative purposes, whereas the medium performance supports (silica-based cross-linked soft gels or other polymers of particle sizes between 30 and 100 μm) because of their higher capacity (high density of charged groups) are best suited to the preparative separation of antibodies. The much better chemical and mechanical stability compared with soft gels allows higher flow rates and increases markedly the life expectancy of the columns. Thus, the medium-performance gels especially can be very cost-efficient in large-scale purification of antibodies.

Samples are usually applied to the anion exchange column in low concentrated Tris/HCl (pH 7.0-8.5) or other neutral or weakly alkaline buffers. Sometimes adsorption buffers of a pH up to 9.5 have been used successfully (Danielsson et al., 1988). Under these conditions almost all proteins and indicator dyes contained in an applied solution can bind to the anion exchanger. Thus, the practical capacity available for binding of immunoglobulins would be drastically reduced, if culture fluids or ascitic fluids of low antibody level would be applied to anion exchange without a prepurification (Gemski et al., 1985; Nau, 1988a and 1989b). Therefore, salt precipitation at least is advisable.

After extensive washing with adsorption buffer, antibodies are usually eluted by a sodium chloride gradient in any form. Normally sodium chloride is made up in adsorption buffer for this purpose, but other buffers and pH gradients can also be applied. The mode and slope of the gradient should be optimized for each individual antibody.

Bulk proteins and indicator dyes do not only reduce the capacity of anion exchangers but also resolution, and they can even bind irreversibly to the matrix (Gemski, et al., 1985; Chen et al., 1988; Nau, 1988a, 1989b). Antibodies can be the better separated from albumin the higher their pI, whereas removal of transferrin by ion exchange is always difficult since its pI is similar to that of most immunoglobulins (Deschamps et al., 1985).

Although several more or less efficient one-step procedures for purification of monoclonal antibodies by anion exchange chromatography from ascites (Clezardin et al., 1985; Gemski et al., 1985; Annunziato and Marciani, 1987; Danielsson et al., 1988) and from serum-free culture medium (Stocks and Brooks, 1989) have been described, this technique because of its limited capacity, seems not to be very useful as the initial step for purification of monoclonal antibodies from culture fluid, in particular if the culture fluid is supplemented with serum. However it can be very efficient if it is used in multi-step procedures after ultrafiltration and/or salt precipitation (Burchiel et al., 1984; Burchiel, 1986; Pavlu et al., 1986; Bruck et al., 1986; Scott et al., 1987; Chen et al., 1988; Jungbauer and Wenisch, 1989) or cation exchange chromatography (Scott et al., 1987; Danielsson et al., 1988) or as the final purification step for complete removal of endotoxins and nucleic acids (Nau, 1988a, 1989a).

Radial streaming anion exchange chromatography (Zetaprep, LKB) allows an easy scale-up and rapid throughputs (Jungbauer et al., 1988) but it has a poor concentrating effect. However, this technique followed by cation exchange HPLC is capable of purifying even monoclonal antibodies of low pI, which are difficult to separate from albumin (Jungbauer et al., 1987; Jungbauer and Wenisch, 1989).

Anion exchange chromatography is also a useful method for separation of antibody fragments from complete antibodies (Clezardin et al., 1985; Demignot et al., 1989).

Although retention has been discussed to correlate with IgG subclass of monoclonal antibodies (Deschamps et al., 1985), this seems to be an over-simplification. Retention properties of monoclonal antibodies can vary from not binding at all up to eluting even later than the strongly bound albumin. Thus, method development is often complicated.

Immunoglobulins other than IgG are usually worse purified by anion exchange chromatography, although under certain buffer conditions some IgM monoclonals could be eluted as fairly pure preparations later than the albumin peak (Nau, 1989 a).

The most ***important advantages*** of anion exchange chromatography concerning antibody purification are:

1) The soft gel matrices are inexpensive and easy in handling and do not require sophisticated equipment.
2) Good chemical and microbiological stabilities of medium- and high-performance gels allow convenient cleaning-in-place.
4) Satisfactory life expectency of medium- and high-performance matrices
5) A vast variety of different anion exchange supports are commercially available for both

HPLC and conventional liquid chromatography.
6) Almost complete removal of pyrogenic and nucleic acid contaminants from antibody preparations is possible.
7) Fairly pure IgG fractions can be isolated from salt precipitates of sera.

General ***disadvantages*** are (those common only to soft gels are not considered here):
1) The method is not suitable in the presence of large amounts of contaminating proteins, i.e. not as the initial purification step.
2) Retention properties of individual antibodies are very different.
3) Indicator dyes can disturb separation.
4) Good purification is more or less limited to the IgG class.
5) Large-scale performance cannot easily be predicted from analytcal HPLC results.

Cation Exchange Chromatography

Cation exchange has been used less frequently for purification of antibodies than anion exchange but also this method is of value, at least in multi-step procedures (e.g. BURCHIEL et al., 1984; KATO et al., 1984; CARLSSON et al., 1985; KEYNES, 1986; SCHWARTZ et al., 1986, SCOTT et al., 1987; JUNGBAUER et al., 1987; MALM, 1987; NAU, 1988a).

Nevertheless, several authors have also tested the usefulness of cation exchange chromatography as a single-step procedure (BURCHIEL, 1986; MENOZZI et al., 1987; DANIELSSON et al., 1988). After comparative HPLC studies on antibody purification from ascites using equivalent columns of a strong anion exchanger (Mono-Q), a strong cation exchanger (Mono-S), a chromatofocusing support (Mono-P) and a hydrophobic interaction medium (Alkyl Superose HR), DANIELSSON et al. (1988) reported cation exchange to be the method of choice for purification of all monoclonal antibodies of a pI greater than 7.2 because these antibodies are efficiently adsorbed under mild conditions and elute essentially pure in a yield of more than 80 %, whereas for antibodies of lower pI other methods provide better results. In an ideal case, due to its high pI of 7.5, a monoclonal IgG antibody could be purified by strong cation exchange chromatography to almost homogeneity with a recovery of 80 % (EHRNSTRÖM and GUSTAVSSON, 1988). MENOZZI et al. (1987) described a one-step procedure for isolation of monoclonal antibodies from culture fluid using mass cation exchange on AMF Zetaprep 250 SP. After adsorption and washing at pH 5.5 antibodies could be eluted free of albumin and transferrin by a sodium chloride gradient at pH 8.0. Recovery was 89-90 % but this method provided only a poor concentrating effect. Thus, a final concentration step (e.g. salt precipitation) is required. Also BURCHIEL (1986) reported cation exchangers to be capable of providing antibodies in high yield and purity, and he also observed a very strong dependence of both purity and recovery on the pI of individual monoclonal antibodies.

Usually, samples are applied to cation exchange columns in low concentrated buffers at weakly acidic pH, and pH has to be chosen the more acidic, the lower the pI of the antibody of interest. But the lower the adsorption pH, the more other components of the sample are bound, and capacity is considerably reduced. At a pH of less than 5.0 chromatography of serum or ascites gives already trouble: isolation of antibodies from cell culture fluid, however, is impossible under those conditions or limited to extremely low sample loads (KATO et al., 1984; SCHWARTZ et al., 1986; BURCHIEL, 1986).

Furthermore NAU (1988a, 1989 a) has reported that even antibodies which should bind strongly to cation exchangers, can be inhibited from binding by other sample components and that in most cases a certain portion of antibody is found in the flow through. Several authors observed that at an adsorption pH of less than 5.0 contaminating proteins are often bound stronger than the antibodies themselves (CARLSSON et al., 1985; BURCHIEL, 1986; KEYNES, 1986; SCHWARTZ et al., 1986; NAU, 1989 c). The low pH that is often required for a satisfactory adsorption has been discussed as reducing the yield of active antibodies but CARLSSON et al. (1985) could demonstrate for 15 different *in vitro* produced monoclonal antibodies, including IgG1, IgG2a, IgG2b and IgA (pI range: 5.2 - 8.3), that even incubation of culture fluid at pH 3.0 for three hours did not result in a measurable loss of activity.

Adsorption and elution conditions can be varied in a wide range and have to be optimized for each individual antibody. On the one hand, this complicates method development but on the other it improves the general chances of antibody purification by this method.

Normally, antibodies are eluted from cation exchangers by both switching to neutral or weakly alkaline pH and increasing of ionic strength. MENOZZI et al. (1987) achieved good results, eluting monoclonal IgG antibodies by 0.2 M Tris/HCl, pH 8.0, but applying a 0 to 0.5 M sodium chloride gradient made up in 0.1 M Tris/HCl, pH 8.0, purity of the antibody preparations could be further improved. Most authors elute antibodies by salt gradients made up in either adsorption buffer (DANIELSSON et al., 1988) or in buffers of higher pH (MENOZZI et al., 1987), whereas MALM (1987), in order to reduce the elution volume, preferred to optimize a single-step elution buffer for each individual monoclonal antibody. He obtained his best results with antibodies that could be eluted at relatively low pH and low salt concentration in opposite flow direction.

As already discussed for anion exchange, contaminating proteins that are bound to the matrix often markedly decrease resolution and coelute with the antibodies (e.g. CARLSSON et al., 1985; BURCHIEL, 1986; KEYNES, 1986; SCHWARTZ et al., 1986; NAU, 1989 c). Nevertheless, a three-step procedure including desalting by Sephadex G-25, cation exchange chromatography on SP-Sephadex G-50 and gelfiltration on Superose 6MB developed by CARLSSON et al. (1985) was adapted to serum-supplemented media by MALM (1987). He used S-Sepharose FF instead of SP-Sephadex and Sephacryl S-200 for gel filtration. Optimizing both adsorption and elution conditions, recovery for most monoclonal antibodies was more than 90 % in the cation exchange step and the main contaminant albumin could be removed completely. Purity and recovery were shown to decrease with increase of serum content of the medium and bovine immunoglobulins could not be completely removed. A great advantage of this procedure is that all chromatography media can be easily sanitized by cleaning-in-place with 0.01 - 0.1 M NaOH. ÖSTLUND et al. (1987) have demonstrated that this procedure can provide final purities of more than 95 % at rapid throughputs. For isolation of monoclonal antibodies from m^3-amounts of perfusion culture fluid SCOTT et al. (1987) have followed two different separation sequences, both of which include cation exchange chromatography (A: ultrafiltration - salt precipitation - cation exchange; B: ultrafiltration - cation exchange - anion exchange). In both cases purities of more than 90 % were achieved, but monoclonal antibodies of low pI could not be purified by either of these procedures. A method for the isolation of gram amounts of monoclonal antibodies, even of low pI, from large volumes of culture fluid (JUNGBAUER et al., 1987; JUNGBAUER and WENISCH, 1989), including cation exchange chromatography, has been presented in the previous section. Strong cation exchange followed by size exclusion chromatography is also valuable for purification of monoclonal IgM antibodies from ascites (EHRNSTRÖM and GUSTAVSSON, 1988).

The advantages and disadvantages of cation exchange are similar to that of anion exchange. However, cation exchange is generally applicable for initial separation but contrary to anion exchange it seems not to be capable of separating low pI antibodies from albumin and transferrin.

Mixed Mode Ion Exchange Chromatography

Though **hydroxyapatite** is the correct name (BERNARDI, 1971) of a liquid chromatography medium introduced by SWINGLE and TISELIUS, 1951) for application in protein separation, the term "hydroxylapatite" is also often used. This material has been applied in the purification of numerous polypeptides and proteins (e.g.

Tiselius et al., 1956; Bernardi, 1971, 1973; Bernardi et al., 1972; Hirata et al., 1984).

For some thirty years it has been known that hydroxyapatite chromatography is capable of separating human serum proteins, including immunoglobulins (Hjerten, 1959) but because of the heterogeneity of immunoglobulins - resulting in broad elution peaks and incomplete purification (Hjerten, 1959; Kawasaki et al., 1985) - it did not at any time play a considerable role in preparation of polyclonal antibodies. For monoclonal antibodies and myeloma proteins the situation is rather different. Smith et al. (1984) have isolated immunoglobulins and even free light chains from culture medium of lymphoblastoid cells as well as a monoclonal antibody from culture fluid. One of the first hydroxyapatite HPLC procedures for monoclonal antibody purification was reported by Juarez-Salinas et al. (1984).

Today, one can assume that hydroxyapatite chromatography in both conventional and HPLC modes is one of the most important methods for purification of monoclonal antibodies and myeloma proteins. Purification procedures for monoclonal antibodies of all murine immunoglobulin classes and IgG subclasses and of other species have been described (Juarez-Salinas et al., 1984, 1986 a); Brooks and Stevens, 1985; Stanker et al., 1985; Bukovsky and Kennett, 1987; Iino, 1988; Yamakawa and Chiba, 1988; Ahn and Choi, 1989 a,b; Harshman, 1989). However, independent of class and subclass a number of monoclonal antibodies cannot be purified by either of these modes.

The exact separation mechanism of hydroxyapatite is still under investigation. Obviously, the interaction between hydroxyapatite and proteins is essentially electrostatic but some kind of specific complex formation is being discussed as a component of interaction too (Bernardi and Kawasaki, 1968; Bernardi, 1973; Gorbunoff, 1984 a,b; Gorbunoff and Timasheff, 1984). The function of hydroxyapatite as a mixed mode ion exchanger is based on interactions between calcium and phosphate groups of hydroxyapatite with carboxyl and amino groups of the proteins respectively. Thus, differences in surface charge of individual proteins are responsible for protein selection. Normally, proteins with higher pI are more strongly adsorbed and elute later than those with a lower pI but in accordance with a zwitter ion mechanism Smith et al. (1984) suggested that charge distribution rather than net charge is responsible for selection.

Because there are substantial differences in pI and charge distribution of individual monoclonal antibodies, even of the same IgG subclass, it is understandable that a wide distribution of retention times has been observed, with murine IgG1 showing the widest range.

Most hydroxyapatite procedures so far described for the isolation of monoclonal antibodies differ in details only. Usually, the clarified antibody source (ascites or culture medium) is diluted (usually 1:10) or buffer exchanged with 10 mM sodium phosphate buffer, pH 6.8 (starting buffer). Caution! Some monoclonal IgM antibodies precipitate under these conditions. The solution is applied to the hydroxyapatite column equilibrated with starting buffer. In order to prevent the column from fouling and corrosion a small precolumn filled with hydroxyapatite or Sephadex G-10 should be used, also in conventional mode, and pH values below 5.5 have to be strictly avoided. High back pressure in the conventional mode can be easily avoided using a column geometry of a length not more than twice the diameter. All unbound proteins are washed out with two to three bed volumes of starting buffer and antibodies are eluted by a stepwise or linear gradient of 10 to 300 mM sodium phosphate, pH 6.8. For most antibodies, however, a gradient up to 200 mM is more efficient. UV monitoring usually shows two more or less well separated peaks, the second of which normally contains the antibody. Resolution can be improved by applying a flatter gradient, running the elution at a smaller flow rate or altering the column geometry. Yield is more than 80 % in most cases but purity depends on the individual antibody; purities of more than 95 % can be observed and in rare cases, no purification effect at all. Columns can easily be regenerated by 0.5 M sodium phosphate, pH 6.8, or 1M sodium chloride (at least 3 bed volumes), and reequilibrated with starting buffer (at least 6 bed volumes). If not counterindicated by the further use of the antibodies, all buffers should be complemented with a bactericidal agent (e.g. 0.02% sodium azide) and 0.01 mmol/l calcium chloride.

Although applicable as initial or even single purification step, because of its relatively low capacity, hydroxyapatite is better used after salt precipitation, ion exchange or protein A chromatography (Brooks and Stevens, 1985; Juarez-Salinas et al., 1986; Yamakawa and Chiba, 1988; Tarditi and Mariani, 1990).

After several runs back pressure can increase but usually this does not markedly affect resolution power. However, repacking of open columns with a replacement of the top of the matrix is recommended after 20-25 runs. The life expectancy of HPLC columns can be much longer (as demonstrated by Josic et al., 1988) than critically noted by several authors (e.g. Pavlu et al., 1986; Nau, 1989 a).

Hydroxyapatite chromatography can also be used as the final step in large-scale purification of monoclonal antibodies from culture medium, one reason being to remove DNA (von Wedel, 1987).

It is important to mention that, better than most other separation media, hydroxyapatite is capable of separating monoclonal antibodies from host immunoglobulins or IgG idiotypes from each other (Juarez-Salinas et al., 1986 a). Furthermore, bispecific antibodies can be separated from monospecific antibodies and nonsense combinations contained in hybrid hybridoma derived ascites (Karawajew et al., 1987, 1988; Tarditi and Mariani, 1990; Robins et al., 1990).

The often critically noted long separation times and poor resolution of irregularly shaped hydroxyapatite could be improved considerably by the development of spherical or bead-shaped HPLC supports but problems in part also result from the separation principle itself and, thus, are hardly open to influence.

More recently also agarose-encapsulated hydroxyapatite (IBF BIOTECHNICS) has been successfully applied to purification of bispecific monoclonal antibodies (Robins et al., 1990).

The most ***important advantages*** of hydroxyapatite chromatography can be indicated as:
1) relatively strong binding of most immunoglobulins
2) easy handling
3) mild running conditions
4) relatively low cost
5) capability of purifying bispecific monoclonal antibodies and IgG idiotypes.

Disadvantages are:
1) low capacity
2) shorter life expectancy than several other media
3) limited variability of procedures
4) often broad elution peaks and dilute preparations
5) tendency to bind immunoglobulins nonspecifically and irreversibly
6) fragility.

More recently J.T. Baker's **Bakerbond ABx** appeared on the market. This silica-based chromatography support, which has been developed specifically for antibody purification, is available for batch techniques and conventional liquid chromatography (40 μm Prepscale ABx) as well as for HPLC/FPLC (5 or 15 μm particle size). It can be applied in both analytical or preparative runs and application on an industrial scale should not be a problem. A hydrophilic polymeric coverage eliminates nonspecific binding of proteins, thus providing excellent recovery of mass and immunological activity of antibodies. ABx functions as a weak cation exchanger and a mild anion exchanger supported by weak hydrophobic interaction (Nau, 1986, 1989 a, b). Best resolution can be obtained with the spherical or spheroidal HPLC matrices, whereas the irregularly shaped Prepscale carrier provides the highest capacity of up to 1 mole equivalent (mEq) per gram, compared to 0.5 mEq/g of the 5 μm support.

ABx has outstanding affinity-like adsorption properties for immunoglobulins. Although at present there are only a limited number of references, ABx has been reported to be capable of isolating pyrogen-free monoclonal antibodies of all classes and IgG subclasses of many species

(NAU, 1986, 1988 a, 1990, 1989 a-c). Because most of the proteins that are present in common antibody sources (e.g. albumins, transferrins and proteases) as well as the frequently used pH indicator dyes, phenol red and phenolphthalein, do not bind to ABx, extremely high sample loads are possible and a high level of purity can be obtained - often in a single chromatographic step. Ross et al. (1987) applied ABx chromatography to purification of several mouse and rat monoclonal antibodies from ascites and achieved in all but one case purities of more than 95 % in a single chromatographic step. They also observed that ABx is capable of efficiently separating light chain variants of a monoclonal IgG antibody. Multiple forms of immunoglobulins, antibody classes, subclasses, conjugates and fragments were also resolved by ABx. Thus, under optimized conditions isolation of bispecific monoclonal antibodies from ascites or culture fluid is possible too. Very high recovery of mass and immunological activity of antibodies has been reported more than once (NAU, 1986, 1989 a,b ; Ross et al., 1987; CHEN et al., 1988).

In contrast to hydroxyapatite, running conditions can be varied within a wide range and for each buffer combination the binding and elution properties of an individual antibody are different. Although this renders mobile phase optimization rather difficult this should not be perceived as a disadvantage because the variability of the method improves the chances of purifying "problem" antibodies. Even under suboptimal conditions purity of antibodies after ABx chromatography is usually more than 70 %.

Although often used for antibody elution in early investigations, according to recent manufacturers product information phosphate buffers should be avoided if possible. After investigation of some forty monoclonal and polyclonal antibodies and several albumins, transferrins and proteases under identical conditions on an analytical ABx HPLC column, NAU (1989 b) reported retention times of 16-68 min. for murine monoclonal antibodies (all IgG subclasses, IgM, IgA and IgD), 22-37 min. for polyclonal IgG of five species and only 3 min. (void) for albumins, transferrins and proteases of different species.

The high sensitivity and capacity of ABx allow even isolation of very low concentrated monoclonal antibodies from serum-supplemented culture medium without a concentration step. In contrast to most other separation media, Prepscale ABx can be used for batch isolation of monoclonal antibodies from ascites or culture fluid (NAU, 1988b, 1989b).

Optimal adsorption of antibodies to ABx is achieved at low ionic strength and weakly acidic pH. Under these conditions some antibodies (especially highly sensitive monoclonal IgM) can precipitate or lose activity (NAU, 1988a, compare hydroxyapatite). For purification of such antibodies, adsorption has to be performed at higher ionic strength and / or pH but usually this results in a lower capacity. Nevertheless, excellent results have also been reported for ABx purification of IgM monoclonals (CHEN et al., 1988; NAU, 1988 a, 1989 c, 1990).

Although the bulk remains unbound, some forms of α_2-macroglobulin, albumin, transferrin and proteases can bind to ABx and coelute with antibodies. Furthermore, host immunoglobulins of ascites for the most part cannot be separated from monoclonal antibodies. Nevertheless, purities achieved with a single ABx HPLC step can sometimes be higher than those obtained by selected multi-step procedures using other HPLC media (CHEN et al., 1988, NAU, 1988a, 1989c, 1990).

ABx purified monoclonal antibodies often still contain nucleic acids and lipopolysaccharides. To make such preparations suitable for in vivo use, these contaminants have to be removed by subsequent anion exchange or hydrophobic interaction chromatography steps. As also observed for other affinity-like separation media (especially in the presence of large amounts of contaminating proteins) a certain portion (usually less than 5 %) of antibody is often found in the flow through, although the column is not overloaded.

Though buffer conditions are very variable, suitable standard procedures are provided by the manufacturer (NAU, 1988b, 1989b) for isolation of antibodies from ascites, culture fluid or serum and for batch extraction respectively, which should be used in initial experiments. In all cases ABx is equilibrated with a 10-25 mM 2-(N-morpholino)-ethane sulfonic acid (MES) buffer, pH 5.6 (buffer A). Samples are diluted with 10-35 mM MES, pH 4.0, to give a final pH of ≈ 5.6. After sample application all unbound material is removed by extensive washing with buffer A. The elution conditions depend on the antibodies. For purification of murine monoclonal antibodies from ascites for instance, a linear gradient 100 % buffer A ⟶ 100 % buffer B (1 M sodium acetate, pH 7.0) is recommended, whereas for isolation of polyclonal IgG from serum ammonium sulfate gradients are preferred. In most cases individual modification will improve results.

Most ***important advantages*** of ABx are:

1) Preferential binding of all immunoglobulins (purification of monoclonal and polyclonal antibodies as well).
2) Very high capacity and low irreversible binding of proteins.
3) Long life expectancy (more than 1,000 hours of use).
4) Vast variety of running conditions.
5) Suitability for both chromatography and batch extraction.

Disadvantages of ABx are:

1) Lipopolysaccharides and nucleic acids can bind to ABx and often coelute with antibodies.
2) A certain (small) amount of antibody remains unbound.
3) A long time and large amounts of buffer are required for equilibration and reequilibration (up to 20 bed volumes).

From the current point of view Bakerbond ABx chromatography seems to be one of the most influential methods for the purification of polyclonal and monoclonal antibodies, but it should not be glorified as being the only universally applicable technique.

Table 3.3. shows several selected chromatographic one-step procedures for antibody purification from different sources.

Size Exclusion Chromatography

This separation method is based on differences in molecular size (and to a less extent in shape) between individual proteins that result in different migration rates within the size exclusion (gel filtration is a synonym) media. Media are provided for many different molecular weight ranges by many companies for both conventional liquid chromatography and HPLC.

For separation of antibodies, media of relatively large pore size are recommended, those which provide the best possible resolution between immunoglobulins (molecular mass 150 kD) and the main contaminating proteins (50-75 kD). The differences in molecular weight are large enough to remove completely small amounts of albumin and transferrin as well as aggregated immunoglobulins from antibody preparations. However, contaminants of equal or similar molecular weight (e.g. host immunoglobulins in ascites or bovine immunoglobulins in serum supplemented culture fluids) cannot be separated from monoclonal antibodies.

Because the resolution power of all size exclusion media in general is rather poor, satisfactory resolution can usually be obtained only if the volume of the applied sample is less than 5 % of the gel bed volume. Thus, capacity is very low (e.g. less than 1 % of that of Bakerbond ABx) and too high protein concentrations can disturb the separation or even destroy size exclusion media by irreversibly clogging the pores (BURCHIEL, 1986). Furthermore, gel filtration does not have any concentrating effect but often results in a considerable dilution of the products. For these reasons size exclusion chromatography is all but unsuitable for initial purification of antibodies from any source, despite, perhaps, isolation of IgM monoclonals from high antibody level ascites. Recently a more or less successful method for purification of murine IgM and IgG monoclonal antibodies from ascites by use of Sepharose 6B has been described (DIAZ et al., 1989).

However, size exclusion chromatography can provide excellent results if it is used in multi-step

Table 3.3. Selected Chromatographic One-Step Procedures for Purification of Antibodies (without biospecific affinity chromatography)

Antibody	Matrix	Sample buffer	Elution	Yield	Purity	Reference
Mouse ascites or culture fluid	BioGel HT (BIORAD)	0.01 M Na-phosphate pH 6.8	step: 0.12 M Na-phosphate; gradient: 0.12-0.3 M Na-phosphate	70-80 %	free of albumin	BUKOWSKY and KENNETT, 1987
Mouse ascites	BioGel HT (BIORAD)	0.01 M Na-phosphate pH 6.8	gradient: 0.01-0.3 M Na-phosphate, pH 6.8	high	depends on antibody	STANKER et al., 1985
Mouse ascites	BioGel HTP (BIORAD)	0.01 M Na-phosphate pH 6.8	gradient: 0.01-0.15 M Na-phos-	separation of bispecific antibodies		KARAWAJEW et al., 1988
Mouse ascites	spherical hydroxyapatite (HPLC)	0.01 M Na-phosphate pH 6.8	gradient: 0.01-0.3 Na-phosphate	> 95 %	depends on antibody	YAMAKAWA and CHIBA, 1988
Mouse or rat ascites	Bakerbond ABx (J.T. BAKER)	0.01 M MES, pH 5.6 (buffer A)	B: 1.0 M NaOAc, pH 7.0, gradient: 100 % A - 35 % B	depends on antibody	95-99 %	ROSS and KOPROWSKI, 1987
Ascites or culture fluid	Bakerbond ABx (J.T. BAKER)	0.01 M MES, pH 5.6 (buffer A)	B: 1.0 M NaOAc, pH 7.0, gradient: 100 % A - 100 % B		> 99 %	CHEN et al., 1988
Culture fluid	Bakerbond ABx (J.T. BAKER)	0.01 M MES, pH 6.0	gradient: 0-0.25M KH_2PO_4, pH 6.8	high	> 90 %	CRANE, 1987
Mouse ascites	Bakerbond MAb (J.T. BAKER)	0.01 M KH_2PO_4, pH 6.8 - 6.4	gradient: 0.01-0.125 M phosphate	> 95 %	> 95 %	CRANE, 1987
Mouse ascites or papain digest	Mono-Q (PHARMACIA)	0.02 M tri-ethanolamine/HCl, pH 7.7	gradient: 0-0.035 M NaCl in adsorption buffer; 0-0.25 M KH_2PO_4, pH 6.8		traces of transferrin	CLEZARDIN et al., 1985
Ascites	DEAE Toyopearl (TOYO SODA)	0.02 M Tris/HCl pH 8.0	gradient: 0.03 M NaCl in adsorption buffer	87-91 %	free of proteases	ANNUNZIATO and MARCIANI, 1987

Table 3.3. Continued from page 84

Antibody	Matrix	Sample buffer	Elution	Yield	Purity	Reference
Culture fluid	AMF Zetaprep 250 SP (LKB)	culture fluid adjusted to pH 5.5	gradient: 0-0.5 M NaCl in 0.1 M Tris/HCL, pH 8.0	≈ 90 %	10-15 fold enriched	Menozzi et al., 1987
Culture fluid	QAE-Zetaprep (LKB)	0.05 M Tris/HCl, pH 8.0	steps: 0.01; 0.15, 1.0 M NaCl in adsorption buffer	> 90 %	transferrin not removed	Jungbauer et al., 1988
Mouse ascites	Mono-S (Pharmacia)	0.02 M NaCl in 0.05 M MES, pH 6.0	gradient: 0.02-1.0 M NaCl in adsorption buffer	> 80 %	depends on pI	Danielsson et al., 1988
Mouse ascites	Mono-Q (Pharmacia)	0.02 M bis-tris-propane, pH 9.5	gradient: 0-1.0 M NaCl in adsorption buffer	> 80 %	depends on pI	Danielsson et al., 1988
Mouse ascites	Alkyl-Superose (Pharmacia)	2.0 M $(NH_4)_2SO_4$ 0.1 M Na-phosphate, pH 7.0	linear decreasing salt gradient	> 80 %	high; traces of albumin	Danielsson et al., 1988
Mouse ascites	Mono - P (Pharmacia)	0.025 M tri-ethanolamine, pH 8.3	polybuffer, pH-gradient: 8.3 - 5.0	> 80 %	insufficient	Danielsson et al., 1988
Mouse ascites or culture fluid	thiophilic adsorbent "T-gel"	0.5 M K_2SO_4 (solid added)	0.05 M Na-phosphate, pH 8.0	> 90 % for IgG, less for IgM	depends on antibody source	Belew et al., 1987
Ascites, culture fluid or serum	thiopilic HPLC adsorbent (self-made)	0.5 M Na_2SO_4 in 0.05 M $(NH_4)_2SO_4$, pH 8.0	0.1 M citrate pH 3.0	IgG: 85-90 % IgM: ≈ 70 %	almost homogeneous	Nopper et al., 1989
Mouse ascites	DEAE AffiGel Blue (Biorad)	0.025 M NaCl in 0.02 M Tris/HCl, pH 7.2	gradient: 0.02-0.1 M NaCl in adsorption buffer	75-90 %	> 90 %	Bruck et al., 1986

MES morpholinoethane sulfonic acid
NaOAc sodium acetate

procedures for final purification of antibodies rather independent of antibody source after a concentration step (PARHAM, 1983; BROOKS and STEVENS, 1985; CARLSON et al., 1985; JUAREZ-SALINAS et al., 1986 b; BAZIN et al., 1986; MALM, 1987; STEINDL et al. 1987; SCOTT et al., 1987; HWANG et al., 1988; HASSL and ASPOCK, 1988; CHING et al., 1989). SCOTT et al. (1987) used size exclusion chromatography in a process-scale procedure only after they had achieved high antibody concentration and a purity level of 90 - 95 % by other methods. The procedure followed by MALM (1987) which includes cation exchange and gel filtration is also useful for large-scale purification of monoclonal antibodies from serum-supplemented cell culture fluids. STEINDL et al. (1987) have purified monoclonal IgM from 150 l of culture fluid by ultrafiltration, isoelectric precipitation (heavy losses) and gel filtration on Sephacryl S-300 to almost homogeneity (40 % yield). Murine monoclonal IgM antibodies could also be purified from ascites and culture fluid by a method combining strong anion exchange and size exclusion FPLC (CLEZARDIN et al., 1986). A two-step procedure described by HASSL and ASPOCK (1989) using hydrophobic interaction chromatography and gel filtration resulted in essentially pure IgY from chicken egg yolk. SCHMIDT (1989) has demonstrated the excellent resolution of the new Superdex™ 200 prep grade (PHARMACIA), which was specifically designed for final antibody purification. One procedure, including ultrafiltration, cation exchange and a final gel filtration on this medium, resulted in a IgG2a monoclonal antibody preparation essentially free of albumin, transferrin and antibody dimers.

A good prepurification provided, size exclusion chromatography is not limited to monoclonal antibodies.

The ***advantages*** of size exclusion chromatography are:

1) Complete separation of albumin, transferrin and aggregated immunoglobulins from antibody preparations is possible.
2) Physiological running conditions can be used.
3) Buffer exchange and final purification can be performed in one step.

The main ***disadvantages*** are:

1) very low capacity
2) Resolution is rather poor and depends on sample volume and protein load.
3) Pores often tend to clog at high protein load.
4) The method often requires long run times and large columns resulting in high cost.

Although there are other separation procedures that provide better resolution and extremly higher capacity, one can expect gel filtration to remain of importance as an excellent method for the final purification of antibodies.

Hydrophobic Interaction Chromatography

Concerning antibody purification the separation principle of this technique is based on differences in hydrophobicity between antibodies and other components of the sample. Hydrophobic residues (or regions) of the proteins interact with the hydrophobic substituents of the matrix (usually alkyl or phenyl groups), resulting in a more or less strong adsorption of the proteins to the matrix. This selection principle is totally different from those of ion exchange and size exclusion chromatography. Thus, hydrophobic interaction chromatography, together with thiophilic adsorption chromatography (see next section), substantially expands the method repertory available for isolation of antibodies.

Other than reversed phase chromatography, which is almost unsuitable for antibody purification because of irreversible binding and denaturation of immunoglobulins, hydrophobic interaction procedures do not necessarily include organic solvents. The adsorption process is promoted by high salt concentrations. Usually, antibody samples are applied to hydrophobic interaction columns in buffers of a pH close to 7.0 (e.g. 25 mM phosphate buffer, pH 7.2) containing 0.7 - 2.0 mol/l of ammonium sulphate, with optimal salt concentration depending on both chromatography medium and antibody. These conditions are not harmful to antibodies but the higher the salt concentration the more different substances are adsorbed to the matrix, resulting in a heavy decrease in capacity available for the binding of antibodies. Elution is usually performed by a gradient of decreasing salt concentration. Serum proteins, DNA and lipopolysaccharides elute very early and are therefore well separated from immunoglobulins, which elute relatively late. Nevertheless, individual antibodies can elute over a wide range of the gradient. Thus, optimization of adsorption and elution conditions is required for each individual antibody in order to achieve optimal capacity and high resolution.

Although DANIELSSON et al. (1988) have estimated hydrophobic interaction chromatography to be as efficient in one-step HPLC purification of murine monoclonal IgG antibodies as cation exchange, usually it is not sufficiently specific to be used as a routine one-step procedure. Because of the relatively low capacity, it should not be used for initial separation of ascites proteins and it is absolutely unsuitable as the initial step in large-scale purification of monoclonal antibodies from culture fluid.

However, in multi-step procedures hydrophobic interaction chromatography can conveniently be used after methods producing antibody samples of high ionic strength (e.g. ion exchange, ABx, hydroxyapatite or affinity methods) because these samples can often be applied directly to the hydrophobic interaction column without the need of time-consuming dialysis or excessive dilution (NAU, 1989, a).

Hydrophobic interaction chromatography has been reported as being even capable of separating murine monoclonal IgG antibodies from bovine immunoglobulins (NAU, 1989 a). This is particularly important if antibodies are to be isolated from serum-containing culture fluids.

With the improvement of hydrophobic interaction media and optimization of running conditions, hydrophobic interaction chromatography will also play an increasing role in multi-step purification of antibodies on larger scales.

Thiophilic Adsorption Chromatography

Although it has been applied rarely up to the present, thiophilic adsorption chromatography must not be underestimated as being a method for the purification of polyclonal and monoclonal antibodies with an almost universal application.

Divinyl-sulfonyl activation has long been known as a method for coupling of ligands to chromatographic supports (SAIRAM and PORATH, 1976). Investigating several aliphatic residues coupled to divinyl-sulfonyl Sepharose, PORATH et al. (1985) found the 2-mercapto-ethanol derivative (T-gel) to have a preferential affinity for immunoglobulins and α_2-macroglobulin. Similar to hydrophobic interaction, the adsorption process is promoted by high salt concentrations (e.g. 0.5 M potassium sulfate). However, PORATH (1987) was able to demonstrate that the separation principle differed from that of hydrophobic interaction. Presumably, the thioether group - in close vicinity to the sulfonyl group - is responsible for the outstanding adsorption properties of T-gel (therefore the term "thiophilic"):

Sepharose-O-CH_2-CH_2-SO_2-CH_2-CH_2-S-CH_2-CH_2OH

Based on these data, BELEW et al. (1987) developed a simple and efficient procedure for the isolation of murine monoclonal antibodies from ascites or culture fluid which is capable of purifying all subclasses of IgG as well as IgM by a single chromatographic step. Solid potassium sulfate is added to the antibody source to give a final salt concentration of 0.5 mol/l. This solution is clarified by centrifugation at 2,000 x g for 5 min. and applied to a T-gel column equilibrated with 50 mM sodium phosphate buffer, pH 8.0, containing 0.5 mol/l potassium sulphate (adsorption buffer). After extensive washing with adsorption buffer until all unbound material is eluted, antibodies are eluted with 50 mM potassium phosphate buffer, pH 8.0, without salt. Usually, recoveries of 85 % or more have been achieved by this method, and purity of several antibodies was comparable to that obtained by immunoaffinity chromatography using immobilized antigen. After more

Table 3.4. Selected Multi-Step Procedures for Purification of Antibodies (without affinity chromatographic methods)

Antibody source	Sequence of purification steps	Comments	Reference
Murine and rat ascites	A) 50 % $(NH_4)_2SO_4$ precipitation; anion exchange HPLC (various media) B) 50 % $(NH_4)_2SO_4$ precipitation; cation exchange HPLC (various media) C) 50 % $(NH_4)_2SO_4$ precipitation; size exclusion HPLC (various media)	yield: high purity: > 80 % yield and purity high if pI > 7.0 resolution depends on protein load	Burchiel, 1986
Murine ascites	Rivanol precipitation; size exclusion chromatography (Sephadex G-100)	high yield and purity without pretreatment	Franek, 1986
Murine ascites	50 % $(NH_4)_2SO_4$ precipitation; DEAE AffiGel Blue chromatography	yield: 75-90 % purity: 90-95 %	Bruck et al., 1986
Murine ascites	40 % $(NH_4)_2SO_4$ precipitation; anion exchange (DEAE Sephacel); 30 min. 56°C	yield: 50-70 % purity: > 99 %	de Rie et al., 1987
Culture fluid	A) ultrafiltration; 40 % $(NH_4)_2SO_4$ precipitation; cation exchange (S-Sepharose FF) B) ultrafiltration; cation exchange; anion exchange C) A) or B) followed by size exclusion chromatography	1000 litre-scale see above homogeneous antibodes	Scott et al., 1986
Serum-free culture fluid	cation exchange (SP-Sephadex); size exlusion FPLC (Superose 6B)	yield: 45-90 %, traces of albumin, transferrin	Carlsson et al., 1986
Culture fluid with serum	cation exchange (S-Sepharose FF); gel filtration (Sephacryl S-200 HR)	yield: 50-90 %, free of albumin and transferrin	Malm, 1987
Ascites or cluture fluid	anion exchange FPLC (Mono Q); size exclusion FPLC (Superose 6)	tandem columns, very useful for IgM	Clezardin et al., 1986
Culture fluid	ultrafiltration; isoelectric precipitation; gel filtration (Sephacryl S-300)	for IgM on large-scale; yield: 40 %, high purity	Steindl et al., 1987
Murine ascites	50 % $(NH_4)_2SO_4$ precipitation; defatting; A) anion exchange HPLC (Mono Q) B) hydrophobic interaction HPLC (TSK Phenyl 5PW) C) hydroxyapatite HPLC (BioGel HPHT)	comparative study yield: > 90 %, high purity yield: > 75 %, high purity worse resolution	Pavlu et al., 1986
Murine ascites	$(NH_4)_2SO_4$ precipitation; hydroxyapatite HPLC (BioGel HPHT)	purity: 90-95 % for IgG useful also for IgM	Crane, 1987
Goat anti-rat IgG serum	protease inactivation; anion exchange (QA-52, Waters); cation exchange (SE-52, Waters)	yield: 97 % 65 % of total protein is active IgG	Schwartz et al., 1986
Culture fluid	ultrafiltration; anion exchange (DEAE-Sepharose FF); cation exchange FPLC (Mono S)	free of transferrin, final concentration up to 27 mg/ml	Jungbauer and Wenisch, 1989
Murine ascites	50 % $(NH_4)_2SO_4$ precipitation; hydroxyapatite HPLC (BioGel HPHT)	separation of IgG idotypes	Juarez-Salinas et al., 1986
culture fluid	ABx; hydrophobic interaction (HI-Propyl); anion exchange (MAb); ABx (all Bakerbond)	therapeutic grade monoclonal antibodies	J.T. Baker firm information

Table 3.4. **Continued from page 88**

Antibody source	Sequence of purification steps	Comments	Reference
Ascites or culture fluid	variable sequences of anion exchange cation exchange and size exclusion using Trisacryl and Ultrogel resins (IBF)	therapeutic grade, conditions depend on individual antibodies	SERVA News 1/1989, pp. 2-3
Serum	2.5 M $(NH_4)_2SO_4$ precipitation; dye ligand chromatography (Remazol Yellow GGL-Sepharose)	yield: > 88 %, highly pure IgG	WORTHINGTON et.al., 1987
Murine ascites	dye ligand chromatography (AffiGel Blue); gel filtration (ACA-22)	yield: 30-60 %, homogenous IgM	JOHNSON et al., 1987

than 100 runs a significant loss in capacity or selectivity of the column was not observed. Thus, a long life expectancy of T-gel columns can be assumed.

The most important ***advantages*** of thiophilic adsorption chromatography are:

1) The method probably seems to be applicable to immunoglobulins of all classes and subclasses of several species.
2) Adsorption and desorption can be performed conveniently under non-denaturing conditions.
3) Scale-up should not be a problem.
4) Dialysis steps can be omited.
5) Long life expectancy and convenient regeneration of columns.

Disadvantages:

1) The matrices are not yet commercially available.
2) Short experience.
3) No separation of host or serum immunoglobulins from monoclonal antibodies.

More recently NOPPER et al. (1989) have developed a very efficient silica-based thiophilic HPLC adsorbent, containing a structure of two thioether groups equidistant to a sulfonyl group:

$$\text{Si-O-Si-}C_3H_6\text{-O-}CH_2\text{-CHOH-}CH_2\text{-S-}C_2H_4\text{-}SO_2\text{-}C_2H_4\text{-S-}CH_2\text{-}CH_2OH$$

With this adsorbent the best results were obtained using 0.5 M sodium sulfate containing 50 mmol/l ammonium sulfate, adjusted to pH 8.0 for adsorption and washing and 0.1 M citrate buffer, pH 3.0 for elution. Very high yield (> 95 %) and excellent purity could be achieved with murine monoclonal IgG antibodies: for an IgM monoclonal this method was not as efficient (68.5 % recovery).

Since all reagents required for the preparation of this adsorbent are rather inexpensive, the method will probably find broad application in large-scale purification of antibodies.

Some selected multi-step procedures for preparation of high purity antibodies without use of biospecific affinity methods are presented in Table 3.4.

Miscelaneous Methods

Dye ligand chromatography is based on affinity of proteins to certain dyes. Because albumin has a high affinity to Cibacron Blue F3GA, immobilization of this dye to anion exchangers could considerably improve separation of antibodies from albumin (BRUCK et al., 1982, 1986; HRKAL et al., 1989). JOHNSON et al. (1987) obtained homogeneous monoclonal IgM antibodies by a two-step procedure including AffiGel Blue (BIORAD) and acrylamide-agarose gel chromatography, though the yield was only 30 - 60 %. A large-scale isolation of 99.5 % pure IgG and albumin from human plasma (50 l) by Blue Trisacryl (isolation of albumin) and DEAE

Trisacryl (binds all remaining proteins but IgG) has been reported by SAINT-BLANCARD et al. (1982). Immunoglobulin fractionation from serum was also possible with some 90 % recovery by chromatography on Remazol Yellow GGL-Sepharose using pH and salt gradients for elution (WORTHINGTON et al., 1987).

The following methods are not frequently used and are suitable for laboratory-scale only but can be valuable for special questions.

Isoelectric focusing (IEF), based on pI differences of proteins, is valuable for both analytical and preparative purposes. Microheterogeneities in pI of myeloma proteins, have been discussed as resulting from glycosylation and deamination after biosynthesis of the protein part (AWDEH et al., 1970). Such microheterogeneities are also typical of monoclonal antibodies and thus IEF pattern of monoclonal antibodies can be used as a control for stability of clones (HAMILTON et al., 1987). In special cases preparative IEF can be an alternative to chromatographic purification of antibodies (ROSEBROUGH et al., 1986; EGEN et al., 1988). Even separation of high affinity antibodies of polyclonal sera from those of lower affinity was possible by preparative IEF (ENDO et al., 1985).

Immunoglobulin fractionation could also be achieved by **chromatofocusing**, which is based on the same selection principle (ENDO et al., 1985; GALLO et al., 1986). Although this technique was estimated not to be useful as a routine method (DANIELSSON et al., 1988), it can provide a very high resolution. For instance, JUNGBAUER et al. (1990) were able to separate isoproteins of monoclonal antibodies by applying a very narrow pH gradient on a Mono-P column (PHARMACIA).

Isotachophoresis, although in some cases providing high yield (SCHMITZ et al., 1988), plays a subordinate role in antibody purification.

Affinity and Immunoaffinity Chromatographic Methods

These methods, which are based on a ligand-ligate interaction (cf. Chapter 2.3.), theoretically provide the highest selectivity. Concerning antibody purification a distinction can be made between immunoaffinity chromatographic and not immuno-based affinity chromatographic techniques.

Affinity Chromatographic Purification of Antibodies by Not Immuno-Based Methods

Although **Jacalin** (jackfruit lectin), which has a strong affinity to human IgA1 and also weakly binds IgA2, IgM, IgD and IgE, has been estimated as being a valuable tool for preparation of at least IgA and IgD antibodies (KONDOH et al., 1987, AUCOUTURIER et al., 1989) and **Concanavalin A** can be useful in IgM purification, bacterial immunoglobulin receptors (because of their interaction with the Fc region also known as Fc receptors) play by far the most important role in affinity purification of antibodies.

When **Protein A** of *Staphylococcus aureus* was isolated for the first time (VERWEY, 1940), its later outstanding role in immunochemistry could not be foreseen. But immediately after the first use of Protein A for affinity chromatographic purification of immunoglobulins (HJELM et al., 1972) it gained widespread application in this field. Protein A matrices are today provided by various companies. Because of its excellent binding properties to IgG of many species and its outstanding stability at low pH and high temperatures and in several denaturing agents (e.g. 4 M urea, 4 M thiocyanate, 6 M guanidine hydrochloride; GODING, 1978; LINDMARK et al., 1983), Protein A is an ideal tool for antibody purification. Indeed, Protein A chromatography is capable of providing high purity antibodies with very good yield in a single step, and the development of the Protein A matrices was a breakthrough in antibody purification technology.

Although Protein A can bind a wide spectrum of IgG antibodies, its affinity to individual antibodies is very different, and immunoglobulins of other classes are bound rather weakly or not at all. For instance, affinity to murine IgG is much lower than to human IgG, which is bound very strongly. Nevertheless Protein A chromatography is one of the most frequently used methods in purification of murine monoclonal IgG antibodies. Several authors have reported affinity as depending strongly on the IgG subclass, allowing even separate isolation of IgG subclasses from serum (e.g. KRONVALL et al., 1969; EY et al., 1978; GODING, 1978; SEPPÄLÄ et al., 1981; SARVAS et al., 1983), whereas STEPHENSON et al. (1984) did not observe a subclass typical elution pattern of murine monoclonal antibodies.

After the initial investigations and even in a recent paper (NAU, 1989a) it has been pointed out that a major drawback of Protein A matrices is not to bind murine IgG1 and several rat monoclonals. However, with improved knowledge of the mainly hydrophobic nature of interaction between Protein A and the Fc part of IgG (DEISENHOFER, 1981) and about parameters affecting the adsorption of antibodies, i.e. pH, salt concentration, temperature (GOLDRING et al., 1988) purification of most murine monoclonal IgG1 antibodies also became possible by Protein A. Binding of antibodies to Protein A is increased at pH > 8.0 (EY et al., 1978; DELACROIX and VAERMAN, 1979; ROUSSEAUX et al., 1981) and/or high salt concentrations (e.g. FREDRIKSSON et al., 1986; ÖSTLUND, 1986). TU et al. (1988) have reported adsorption of weakly binding monoclonal antibodies to be improved at low temperature (4°C) and efficient elution of those antibodies to be possible by simply increasing temperature to 37°C without a change in pH.

In the initial studies, elution of the antibodies from Protein A columns had been performed at pH values of less than 3.0, which often resulted in losses of biological activity of pH sensitive antibodies. However, it was possible to demonstrate that by far most monoclonal antibodies elute already at much higher pH: the weakly bound IgG1 usually at pH 6.0 - 7.0, IgG2a at pH 4.5 - 5.0 (rarely lower), the rare IgG3 at pH 4.5 - 6.0, and only the tightly bound IgG2b can require pH of less than 4.0 (EY et al., 1978; STEPHENSON et al., 1984). Thus, most antibodies can be purified under rather mild conditions.

Today, antibody samples are usually applied to Protein A columns in 0.1 M phosphate or Tris buffers, pH 8.0 - 8.5, containing (or not) various concentrations of salt (usually sodium chloride), and antibodies are eluted by sodium citrate buffers of pH depending on the antibody that is to be purified (2.8 - 7.0). Several firms provide ready-to-use adsorption and elution buffers (e.g. PIERCE's MonoPure™). It seems to be advisable, however, to optimize the conditions for each individual monoclonal antibody, at least if large scales have to be considered.

By a different binding site Protein A is also capable of binding Fab and $F(ab')_2$, which can be used for purification of these fragments (YOUNG et al., 1984). The binding of immunoglobulins other than IgG has been reported to be mediated exclusively by this site (INGANÄS, 1981).

Although purity of antibodies obtained by Protein A chromatography is usually more than 95% of total protein, which is satisfactory for many purposes, and also viruses and nucleic acids can be almost completely removed (LEVY et al., 1984), at least for antibodies destined for in vivo use additional purification steps are required (LEE et al., 1986) to remove remaining pyrogens and leaked Protein A. This can be accomplished by anion exchange or gel filtration (KENNY and CHASE, 1987; DUFFY et al., 1989; BLOOM et al., 1989).

According to IgG binding, bacterial immunoglobulin receptors have been classified into five types (MYHRE and KRONVALL, 1981; reviewed by BOYLE and REIS, 1987) but until now beyond Protein A (type I) only Protein G (type III) and a receptor of human group U streptococci (neither of these classes) have been applied to antibody purification. Protein G has been reported as binding IgG of all subclasses of many species (especially mouse and rat) much better than Protein A (BJÖRCK and KRONVALL, 1984; ÅKERSTRÖM et al, 1985; ÅKERSTRÖM and BJÖRCK, 1986). However, most determinants recognized on the Fc of IgG by Proteins A and G seem to be identical or overlapping, whereas Fab determinants are more different (ELIASSON et al., 1989).

Protein G chromatography carriers are now available from several companies, even as recombinant products with further improved properties but until now they have been much more expensive than equivalent Protein A matrices. The stronger affinity of Protein G need not necessarily result in better purification of antibodies, as was demonstrated by JUNGBAUER et al. (1989). The protein derived from human group U streptococci has extremly high affinities to rat and mouse IgG and to all murine IgG subclasses (CHHATWAL and BLOBEL, 1987) but it is not yet available commercially.

Since separation power of affinity methods is fairly independent of sample volume, they are most suitable as the **initial** step in antibody purification from any source. In order to protect the expensive affinity columns from fouling, however, feedstocks should be sterile filtered, and the use of a precolumn is required. Performance of fouled Protein A columns can be restored by guanidine hydrochloride or other appropriate cleaning-in-place methods (KENNEY, 1989).

If carefully handled, the life expectancy of Protein A columns can be rather long, e.g. a Protein A Sepharose column could be used for more than 100 cycles for commercial purification of monoclonal antibodies from culture fluid in an automated process with batch sizes of up to 300 grams of antibody (KENNEY and CHASE, 1987). A further advanced-scale procedure, capable of purifying up to 4 grams of monoclonal antibody per cycle at almost quantitative yield using a 500 ml Protein A Sepharose column, has been described by LEE et al. (1986). Both groups have reported a subsequent ion exchange step to result in antibody preparations that are essentially free of detectable contaminants.

Small particle high performance matrices available with both Proteins A and G are advisable for analytical purposes and laboratory-scale antibody purification. However, for economic reasons the less expensive medium performance supports (larger particle size) should be preferred for larger scales, these providing almost as good resolution.

As the most ***important advantages*** of affinity chromatography on immunoglobulin receptor columns the following can be pointed out:

1) capable of purifying almost all IgG antibodies
2) very high specificity
3) suitable for large volumes of very dilute feedstocks, and therefore ideally suitable as initial purification step
4) good chemical stability of the ligand (cleaning-in-place)

Disadvantages that should be mentioned, are:

1) high cost of the matrices
2) leakage of ligand, although mostly minimal.

Immunoaffinity Chromatographic Purification of Antibodies

Immunoaffinity chromatography, although providing a very high specificity, need not necessarily be considered as the most efficient method of antibody purification because it requires large quantities of either highly purified antigens or purified antibodies specific to the antibody of interest. Thus, enormous cost can arise already from preparation of the immunosorbents, which are usually not commercially available.

Antigen-antibody interaction in most cases is as strong (cf. Chapter 1.2.) as to require harsh elution conditions, e.g. extremes of pH and/or ionic strength or even detergents or chaotropic agents. These conditions can be harmful to both immunosorbents (leaking of the ligand or altering of its spatial structure) and antibodies (altering of spatial structure or even chemical modification, resulting in considerable losses of immunological activity). Taking into consideration that until now most immunoadsorbents have been prepared on the base of polysaccharide soft gels, and that these as well as the ligands themselves are subject to biodegradation, life expectancy of the columns is limited and the antibody preparations are often contaminated with digestion products and endotoxins. Thus, further purification steps are often required, at least if antibodies are destined for *in vivo* use. Most immunosorbents require permanent refrigeration, and an efficient cleaning-in-place is practically impossible. Furthermore, the capacity of immunoaffinity columns is relatively low. These disadvantages together make immunoaffinity chromatography not very suitable for large-scale purification of monoclonal antibodies added to which there exist more economical methods. It is much more important for purification of antigens on various scales (cf. Chapter 3.2.).

On a laboratory scale, however, immunoaffinity chromatography is a valuable method for purification of antibodies from any source because in this case the advantage of extremely high specificity outweighs the disadvantages discussed above.

Although great expense is neccessary to raise antibodies against the antibody species of interest, the use of such antibodies as ligands in immunoaffinity purification of monoclonal antibodies is advantageous, especially if it is hardly possible to purify the desired antibodies by other methods. CORMONT et al. (1986) have reported a successful procedure for purification of monoclonal and polyclonal murine IgM antibodies with the use of rat monoclonal anti-mouse IgM antibodies as immunoaffinity ligand. The purity level achieved at a yield of more than 90 % (from ascites) can hardly be obtained by other procedures. More recently, a similar method of extremely high specificity (no cross reactivity with either IgA or IgE) has been described by MONESTIER et al. (1989).

Since more than 95 % of all rat monoclonal antibodies belong to the κ light chain type, murine anti-rat κ monoclonal antibodies could be used almost universally for immunoaffinity purification of rat monoclonal antibodies from cell culture fluid and ascites (BAZIN et al., 1984 a, b). Under special conditions, using a murine monoclonal anti-rat κ 1a antibody, rat myeloma proteins of all classes and subclasses (from serum) and monoclonal antibodies (from ascites) could be isolated in high purity and with almost quantitative recovery (BAZIN et al., 1984 b). In all these cases, immunosorbents had been prepared from activated Sepharose and antibody elution was performed at pH 2.8.

The most important advantage of using immobilized antigen for antibody purification is that only antigen-specific antibodies are recognized. This means that monoclonal antibodies can be separated from host immunoglobulins of ascites and from bovine immunoglobulins of serum-supplemented cell culture medium, and in the case of polyclonal antibodies antigen-specific antibodies can be isolated free of non-specific immunoglobulins.

Protein antigens are not used very frequently for immunoaffinity purification of antibodies (e.g. STANISLAWSKI and COEUR-JOLY, 1972; VOCKLEY et al., 1984; KEENAN, 1988) because purification of the proteins is often more difficult than purification of the corresponding antibodies. For sterical reasons it is sometimes advantageous to couple only a limited amount of protein antigen to the matrix (AITHAL et al., 1988). Immobilization of synthetic peptides instead of intact protein antigens can allow separation of different specific antibody populations (DAY and HASHIM, 1984) but it can also be an alternative in purification of monoclonal antibodies, if the corresponding protein is unstable or not available. Peptides usually require coupling via a spacer.

By special activations also DNA (KITAGAWA and SASAKI, 1987), oligo- and polysaccharides (JEFFREY et al., 1975; KOZEL and HERMERATH, 1988) and lipopolysaccharides (GIRARD and GOICHOT, 1981) have been coupled via a spacer to Sepharose and used for purification of specific antibodies.

Most frequently, however, immobilized haptens are used as immuno-affinity adsorbents for purification of hapten-specific antibodies required for analytical or diagnostic purposes (e.g. ALI and JACOB, 1984; FORMSTECHER et al., 1986; TANIMORI et al., 1987; BOUZERNA et al., 1988; SAMUEL and ABUKNESHA, 1990). Most of the low molecular compounds can easily be synthesized or isolated from a natural source. Therefore, preparation of the immunosorbents is not such a difficult problem.

Usually, antibody samples are applied to immunosorbent columns under physiological conditions. Unbound substances are washed out with PBS or a similar buffer, containing (or not) small amounts of a detergent (for removal of non-specifically adsorbed proteins), and the antibodies are then eluted by lowering pH to 2.8 or even lower. However, elution by alkaline pH (LIM, 1987), by buffers containing low concentrations of an

Table 3.5. Selected Affinity and Immunoaffinity Chromatographic Procedures for Purification of Antibodies

Antibody source	**Affinity adsorbent**	**Adsorption from**	**Elution**	**Comments**	Reference
Human milk	Jacalin-Sepharose 4B	0.2 M NaCl, in 0.005 M phosphat	0.2 or 0.5 M galactose or 1 M NaOAc in PBS	separation of sIgA1 and sIgA2	Kondoh et al., 1987
Culture fluid (mouse mab)	Protein A-Sepharose 4B	0.1 M phosphate, pH 8.0	0.1 M citrate pH 6.0 pH 4.5 pH 3.5	 most IgG1 most IgG2a and IgG3 some IgG2b yield > 95 %	Stephenson et al., 1984
Culture fluid (mouse mab)	Protein A-Sepharose 4B	0.1 M phosphate, pH 8.4	0.1 M citrate pH 4.5	large-scale up to 4 g per run	Lee, et al., 1986
Mouse ascites	Protein A-Sepharose	0.1 M phosphate, pH 8.1, at 4°C	switch to 37°C or 0.1 M citrate pH 5.5 or 3.5	low temperature improves binding	Tu et al., 1988
Mouse ascites	Protein A-Sepharose	PBS, pH 8.0	0.1 M citrate, steps pH 6.0;	high yield and purity of IgG2a	Levy et al., 1984
Mouse ascites or serum	Preotein A-Sepharose	PBS, pH 8.0	0.1 M citrate, stepwise decrease of pH	IgG1: pH 6.0-7.0 IgG2a: pH 4.5-5.0 IgG2b: pH 3.5-4.0	Ey et al., 1978
Papain and pepsin digests of antbodies	Protein A-Sepharose Cl 4B	PBS, pH 7.4	0.1 M citrate stewise decrease of pH	isolation of Fab or $F(ab')_2$ using Fab- site of Protein A	Young et al., 1984
Culture fluid of human mab	Protein A-Superose,	0.1 M phosphate/0.2 M citrate pH 9.0;	pH steps: 6.0 - 3.0	yield 70-76 % sharp elution	Jungbauer et al., 1989
	Protein G-Sepharose FF	0.1 M glycine/NaOH, pH 9.0	pH steps: 6.0 - 3.0	yield: 50-70 % broad elution	
Culture fluid (rat mab)	Protein G-Agarose (Genex)	clarified source	0.1 M glycine/HCl, pH 2.5	rat IgG1 and IgG2a with good yield, both mab's were not separable by Protein A-Sepharose	Monestier et al., 1989

Table 3.5. Continued from page 94

Antibody source	Affinity adsorbent	Adsorption from	Elution	Comments	Reference
Culture fluid	Selecti Spher-10 Protein G (HPLC) (Perstorp)	0.05 M phosphate, pH 6.0 (A)	gradient: 100 % A - 100 % B B: 0.05 M glycine/ HCl, pH 2.2	purity: > 95 % yield: 80-100 % capacity: 2-5 mg/ml gel	Ohlson et al., 1988 a,b
^{125}I labeled mouse IgG and subclasses	"Protein U" Sepharose 4B (self-made)	neutral pH	0.1 M glycine/HCl pH 2.0	test application; recovery: > 80 % for all IgG subclasses	Chhatwal and Blobel, 1987
Culture fluid (rat mab)	mouse-anti-rat æ mab-Sepharose 4B	clarified, wash with PBS	0.1 M glycine/ HCl in 0.15 M NaCl, pH 2.8	yield: > 75 % useful also for very contaminated antibodies	Bazin et al., 1984a
Mouse ascites or culture fluid	rat anti-mouse-IgM-Sepharose 4B	clarified source	0.1 M glycine/ HCl in 0.15 M NaCl, pH 2.8	yield: > 90 % from ascites yield: > 50 % from culture fluid	Cormont et al., 1986
Culture fluid (monoclonal mouse IgM)	rat mab anti-mouse IgM-Sepharose 4B	clarified source	0.1 M glycine/ HCl, pH 2.5	no cross reaction with IgA and IgG, used routinely for IgM purification	Monestier et al., 1989
Goat anti-serum to lacto-N-difucohexaose	lacto-N-difuco-hexaose-I Sepharose	PBS	free lacto-N-difucohexaose	40 % $(NH_4)_2SO_4$-precipitation and dialysis before; yield: 90-95 %	Jeffrey et al.,
Rabbit-anti-hormone antiserum	hormone-divinylsulfonyl-Sepharose	clarified serum, wash: 0.1 M Tris/HCl/ NaCl, pH 7.6	0.5 or 1.0 M NH_4OH, at 4°C	for antibodies to several hormones, high yield and purity	Sairam and Porath, 1975
Rabbit anti-melittin antiserum	melittin-Sepharose	load and wash with borate saline, pH 8.4	0.1 M glycine/ HCl, 0.075 M NaCl, pH 2.7		Kaetzel and Dedman, 1987
Culture fluid of human anti-DNA mab	DNA-Sepharose 4B (with spacer)	0.01 M Tris/ HCl, pH 8.3 0.003 M EDTA	5 % DMSO, pH 10.7 in 0.5 M NaCl	yield: > 90 % (≈ 1 mg from 100 ml culture fluid)	Kitagawa and Sasaki, 1987

Table 3.5. Continued from page 95

Antibody source	**Affinity adsorbent**	**Adsorption from**	**Elution**	**Comments**	Reference
Rabbit anti-dexamethasone serum	dexamethasone coupled to Ultraffinity EP column (BECKMAN) (HPLC)	PBS (dissolved and dialyzed $(NH_4)_2SO_4$-precipitates)	citrate/phosphate/borate buffer, pH 3.1 containing 20 % acetonitrile	yield: 30-39 % harsh conditions because of the high affinity of the mab's	FORMSTECHER et al., 1986
Culture fluid (mouse mab)	*S. typhi* endotoxin-Sepharose 4B	PBS at 4°C (dialyzed salt precipitates)	0.1 M glycine/NaOH, pH 11.0 at 25°C	yield: 38 % IgM	LIM, 1987
Rabbit antiserum to S82 peptide (of myelin)	S82-AH- and S82-CH-Sepharose 4 in tandem use	PBS (after salt precipitation and anion exchange	3 M $MgCl_2$	yield: total: ≈ 37 % S82-CH-S.: ≈ 30 % S82-AH-S.: ≈ 7 %; high affinity mab are not eluted	DAY and HASHIM, 1984

Purity of the antibody preparations was essentially high in all cases.

Table 3.6. Haptens Purified by Immunoaffinity Chromatography

Hapten	**Source** (material)	**Adsorbent** (protein/gel)	**Elution conditions**	**Comment**	**References**
Carbohydrate Glcα1-6Glcα1-4 Glcα1-4Glc (as [^{3}H](Glc)4-ol)	human urine	a) mab bound to **1** (1.2 mg/ml) or b) mab adsorbed to **11** (14.4 mg/ml)	0.2 M Na-acetate, pH 2.5, 10°C or temperature gradient: 4 - 37°C	for analytical determination the hapten was radioactively labeled by ^{3}H	LUNDBLAD et al., 1984
Blood group A-active oligosaccharides	human new born faces	murine mab (IgM type) adsorbed to silica coated with a hydrophilic phase + ConA	isocratically with TBS, pH 8, or by a temperature gradient		DAKOUR et al., 1987
2-amino-3-methylimidazo [4.5-f] quinoline (IQ); 2-amino-3.8-dimenthylimidazo [4.5-f]quinoxaline (MIQx)	heated meat products	IQ-recognizing mab bound to **1**	methanol (recovery ≈ 80 %)	IQ and IQMx are identified as carcinogenic substances; quantified by HPLC	TURESKEY et al., 1987
Aflatoxins, derivatives and metabolites	human and rat urine	mab (IgM type) against aflatoxin B_1 bound to **1**	50 % DMSO in PBS	quantified by RIA and HPLC	GROOPMAN et al., 1985
Gibberellins (methylesters): GA_1, GA_3-GA_5, GA_7, GA_9	immature soybean and pea seed	ab bound to: a) **1** (35 mg/ml) or b) carbodiimidazol-activated Fast Flow Sepharose CL 4B	methanol	columns reusable more than 500 times	DURLEY et al., 1989
2.4-dinitrophenol (DNP)	DNP-BSA conjugate (27 moles DNP/mol BSA)	anti-DNP murine mab bound to Sepharose	0.1 M DNP	DNP removed by ion exchange chromatography	ESHAR et al., 1980

Adsorbent materials (numbering used in Chapter 3.2):
1 = CNBr-activated Sepharose 4B (PHARMACIA), **2** = CNBr-activated Sepharose CL B6 (PHARMACIA), **3** = protein-A Sepharose CL 4B (PHARMACIA), **4** = glutaraldehyde-activated amino hexyl Sepharose 4B (PHARMACIA), **5** = Affi-Gel 10 (BIORAD), **6** = Affi-Gel 15 (BIORAD), **7** = glutaraldehyde-activated Ultrogel AcA22 (LKB), **8** = Blue A Matrex Agarose (AMICON), **9** = applied solid phase material not or not exactly specified, **10** = CNBr-activated Sepharose CL 4B (PHARMACIA), **11** = protein-A Sepharose 4B, **12** = Bio-Gel P-6 (BIORAD), **13** = CNBr-activated Sephadex G-200 (PHARMACIA), **14** = Dynabeads M-450 (DYNAL)

organic solvent (FORMSTECHER et al., 1986; KITAGAWA and SASAKI, 1987) or by electrodesorption (PRUSIK and KASICKA, 1985) can provide also good results. In most cases, in spite of the harsh elution conditions, both purity of the antibody preparations and recovery are more than 90 %. A prerun under elution conditions is always advisable in order to reduce leakage of ligand during elution of the antibodies.

High performance immunoaffinity chromatographic procedures for antibody purification are still rare (FORMSTECHER et al., 1988) and will probably not become as important as other HPLC methods.

Table 3.5. presents a small collection of procedures for antibody purification, which are based mainly on affinity and immunoaffinity chromatographic methods.

Table 3.7A. Enzymes and Other Proteins Separated and/or Purified by Immunoaffinity Chromatography

Antigen	Source	Adsorbent[a)] (protein/gel)	Elution conditions[b)]	Recovery, purification	Comment	References
Acid elution						
human fibroblast interferon $\beta 1$	C40 cell line	mab bound to agarose-polyacrylhydrazide (7 mg/ml)	50 mM citric acid/HCl, pH 2	82% 400 fold	prepurified by Sepharose-Blue (PHARMACIA)	CHERNAJOWSKY et al., 1984
Brain tissue factor (apoprotein)	human brain	goat anti-tissue factor bound to **6** (10 mg/ml)	0.1 M glycine, 0.1 M NaCl, 0.1 M Triton, pH 2	90% 2400 fold	corresponds immunologically to the rabbit brain tissue factor	RAO, 1988
Interferon	human leukocytes	ab bound to **4** (14 mg/ml)	9 M ethane diol, 0.1 M citric acid, 0.3 M NaCl, pH 2	5000 fold	one-step procedure	SECHER and BURKE, 1980
Chorio-gonadotropin	urine of pregnant woman	mab bound to **1**	pH gradient elution, (pH 7.2-2.5)	97.3% 97 fold	cf. Protocol 3.2.	KAISER unpublished
Transglutaminase	human erythrotes	mab bound to **5** (9.3 mg/ml)	0.1 M acetic acid 150 mM NaCl, 1 mM EDTA, pH 2.6	74% 120 fold	eluted fractions immediately neutralized	LEE et al., 1986
α_1-acid glycoprotein	normal or inflamed rat serum	rabbit ab bound to **1**	0.2 M glycine HCl, pH 2.6	80%	contains 0.6% serum albumin	DRECHOU et al., 1989
Mycobacterium antigen	*Mycobacterium avium*	mab bound to **1**	2 M urea, 1 M acetic acid	0.77%	subsequently dialyzed	ABE et al., 1989
Transforming growth factor	*Echerichia coli*	mab bound to **4**	0.1 M Na-acetate pH 3.5	n.g[c)]	purification controlled by HPLC	WINKLER et al., 1986
Contracture inducing insect toxins	Scorpion venoms	rabbit ab against *Androctonus australis H.* venom coupled to **10** (0.05 μmole/g)	0.53 M formic acid, pH 2.05	1% related to the venom	subsequently purified by RP-HPLC	DEDIANOUS et al., 1987
Tetanus toxin	*Clostridium tetani*	a) equine ab (19.9 mg/ml **10**) or b) murine ab (1.25 mg/ml **10**	a) 0.1 M HCl, b) 0.1 M citric acid/HCl, pH 3	a) 64% b) 80%	step b) requires an addition of Sephadex G-15	SHEPPARD et al., 1987

Table 3.7A. Continued from page 98

Antigen	Source	Adsorbent[a)] (protein/gel)	Elution conditions[b)]	Recovery, purification	Comment	References
α-L-iduronidase	human liver	two columns with different mab's bound to **5**	50 mM Na-citrate, 2 M NaCl, pH 4	n.g.	prepurified with **8**	Clemens et al., 1989
Alkaline elution						
DNA-polymerase α-DNA-primase	human placenta	anti-human DNA-polymerase mab bound to **1** (3 mg/ml)	10 % glycerol, 1 M KCl, pH 11.3 - 11.5	123 fold	prepurified by phosphocellulose chromatography	Podust et al., 1989
C3b inactivator	human plasma	mab bound to **1**	0.05 M diethylamine, pH 11.5	1900 fold	prepurified with an IgG column	Hsiung et al., 1982
ALkaline phosphatase	intestinal content of calves	rabbit ab bound to **4**	50 mM triethylamine/HCl, pH 11.4	65 % 847 fold	subsequently purified by DEAE-cellulose	Schwenzer et al., 1987
α-fetoprotein	umbilical cord	mab bound to **1** (4.3 mg/ml)	0.05 M NH_3, 0.5 M NaCl	68.3 %	cf. Protocol 3.1.	Kaiser and Micheel, 1991
Antitumor acidic glycoprotein	*Streptococcus pyogenes* extract	ab bound to **1** (10 mg/g)	lysine/KOH, 0.14 M KCl, pH 11	n.g.	eluate immediately neutralized	Yoshida et al., 1989
Archidonate 12-lipoxigenase	porcine leukocytes	mab bound to **1**	20 % glycerol, 50 mM diethylamine, pH 10.4	5 % 51 fold	prepurified by precipitation and ion exchange chromatography	Yokoama et al., 1986
Other elution conditions (high ionic strength, chaotropic ions, polyalcohols etc.)						
Adenosine deaminase	human thymus	mab bound to **3** and crosslinked by dimethyl suberimidate	a) 4 M, b) 6 M urea	47 % 320 fold	-	Philips et al., 1987
Glycogen synthase	rat skeletal muscle	mab bound to CNBr-activated Sepharose	4 M $MgCl_2$, glycerol	25 % 517 fold	prepurified by DEAE cellulose and precipitation	Baldwin et al., 1989
High density lipoprotein subclasses	prepurified high density lipoprotein	mab bound to 4 (subclass 2: 0.36 mg/ml; subclass 3: 0.15 mg/ml)	3 M SCN^-	n.g.	adsorption under batch conditions	James et al., 1989

Table 3.7A. Continued from page 99

Antigen	Source	Adsorbent[a] (protein/gel)	Elution conditions[b]	Recovery, purification	Comment	References
Human growth hormone (hGH)	lysate of hGH-producing *Escherichia coli* or pituitary extract	mab bound to **1** (7 mg/ml)	stepwise with 1 M, 2 M and 4 M KSCN	n.g.	subsequently purified by ion exchange chromatography (cf. Protocol 3.3.)	JÒNSDÒTTIR et al., 1986
Myelo-peroxidase	human myeloid leukemia HL-60 cells	mab bound to **2**	3 M $MgCl_2$, pH 8	38 % 1500 fold	subsequently dialyzed against 10 mM Tris/HCl	HUR et al., 1989
Nitrate reductase	*Nicotiana plumbaginifolia* seeds	a) maize nitrate reductase mab and b) *N. plumbaginifolia* mab against ribulose 1.5-bi-phosphate carboxylase; (bound to **7**; 4 mg/ml)	1 M KCl, 10 % glycerol, 50 mM HEPES, pH 7.5	53 % a) 2615 fold b) 21025 fold	two-step procedure	MOREAUX et al., 1989
Phospho-lamban	canine sarcoplamatic reticulum	mab bound to **5**	10 % glycerol, 2.8 M $MgCl_2$, pH 7.5	70 %	prepurified by an IgG column	SUZUKI et al., 1987
Tyrosinated detyrosinated and nontyrosinable tubulin	beef brain microtubuli	mab (anti-Tyr-tubilin) bound to **1** (5 mg/ml)	a) 0.1 M b) 0.8 M KCl/PEM, pH 6.65	n.g.	labeled $[^3H]$Tyr	PATURLE et al., 1989
C1 inhibitor	human plasma	IgG anti-C1 inhibitor bound to **1** (1 mg/ml)	0.5 M NaCl/PBS pH 7	61 % 785 fold	prepurified by ion exchange and metal chelate chromatography	PROGRAIS et al., 1987

[a] numbering of adsorbent materials see Table 3.6., [b] cf. also Table 2.6., [c] n.g. = not given

Table 3.7B. Purging of Sample Solutions from Antigens by Immunosorption

Depleted substance	**Source**	**Adsorbent*)** (Protein/gel)	**Comment**	**References**
Factor VII	Citrated human plasma	rabbit ab against human factor VII bound to **1** (2.5 mg/g)	column regenerated with 0.1 M glycine/HCl, pH 2.5	TAKAMIYA et al., 1986
Mistletoe lectin I	murine tumor cell glycoprotein fractions	rabbit anti-mistletoe lectin I ab bound to **1** (7mg/3g)		WALZEL et al., 1989
Plasmodium antigen	*Plasmodium falciparum* culture medium	anti-human horse serum proteins bound to **10** (2 mg/ml)	column regenerated with 3 M KSCN	THELU et al., 1989

*) numbering of adsorbent material see Table 3.6.

Precipitation techniques will remain of importance as a rapid tool for antibody enrichment, at least on a laboratory-scale. HPLC methods will dominate in the laboratory-scale preparation of antibodies and for analytical purposes because of excellent resolution and very short run-times whereas medium-performance procedures, because of lower cost and higher capacity, will be preferred for larger scales. Summaries of information on antibody purification by HPLC or FPLC procedures have been provided by among others PERRY et al. (1985), BURCHIEL (1986), CRANE (1987), KEYNES (1988), EPSTEIN et al. (1988), JUNGBAUER and WENISCH (1989) and valuable surveys on pilot-up to production-scales, as far as data were available, were given by ÖSTLUND (1986), ÖSTLUND et al. (1987), KENNEY (1989) and SCHMIDT (1989). Economical industrial production and purification of kilogram amounts of monoclonal antibodies will be accomplished through the use of highly optimized and automated on-line processes.

3.2. Positive and Negative Selection of Free and Structure-bound Haptens, Antigens and Receptors

Poly- and monoclonal antibodies have already been applied for many years: (a) to separate and to isolate the complementary haptens and antigens, inclusively receptors and antigen-bearing particles of biological origin as membrane fragments or other cell debris, viruses and cells by immunosorption in analytical or in preparative scale for further studies (positive selection), or (b) to purge (deplete) sample solutions and suspensions respectively from certain unwanted contaminations (negative selection). In case (b) further studies with purged (depleted) material is intended.

For immunosorption procedures the required antibody is bound to the solid phase material (e.g. beads) by one of the usual methods or the immunosorbent is prepared in some other manner (cf. Chapter 2.2.). Moreover, immunoprecipitation techniques are also applied, especially for routine analysis in medical diagnostics. Further possibilities include the application of microparticles and paramagnetic solid phase supports as well as a combination of the highly stable avidin-biotin complex with the antigen-antibody reaction (cf. Chapter 2.5.). The increased application of immobilized antibodies in liquid chromatography techniques was stimulated initially by the following factors:

(1) From the theoretical point of view it is possible to produce antibodies against any biomacromolecule or biosubstance (cf. Chapter 1.3.) and to immobilize them without appreciable loss of their biological recognition ability (cf. Chapter 2.2.),

Table 3.8. Receptors Purified by Immunoaffinity Chromatography

Receptor (= R.)	**Source**	**Adsorbent** (protein/gel)[*]	**Elution conditions**	**Recovery, purification**	**Comment**	**References**
Opiate R.	hybrid cell line	mab bound to **1**	0.02 M PBS	n.g. [a]	cell surface protein cross-linked before	CARR et al., 1987
γ-interferon R.	human cell line	mab bound to **5**	0.2 M glycine/HCl, 1% Triton X-100, pH 2.2	n.g.	subsequently purified on rhuIFN-γ coupled to 5[b]	AGUET and MERLIN, 1987
β_2-adrenergic R.	prepurified mammalian lung membranes	a) auto-ab bound to **3** or b) mab 10% bound to **3**	a) 2% SDS, 5% mercaptoethanol, glycerol, b) 10 μM (-)-propanolol	n.g.	eluate of step b) radiolabeled with ^{125}I	FRASER and VENTER, 1982
Prolactin R.	rat liver membranes [c]	mab bound to **5** (40 mg/25 ml)	5 M $MgCl_2$	52% 1072 fold	prepurified by benzamidine Sepharose 6B	OKAMURA et al., 1989
Murine $\alpha\beta$ T cell R.	T cell hybridomas (cell lysate)	mab bound to Sepharose 4B **(9)**	50 ml diethylamine, pH 11	n.g.	cf. GOODMAN et al., 1988	KUBO et al., 1989
Human uterine progesterone R.	human uteri	mab against rabbit receptor bound to **5**	50 mM $(NH_4)_2CO_3$, pH 10.8	n.g.	purified was the R.-stereoid complex	VU HAI et al., 1989
Fc γ R.	pretreated myelinated and unmyelinated human nerves	F(ab')$_2$ fragments of mab against placenta Fc Receptor bound to **1** (1.5 mg/ml)	0.1M Tris buffer, pH 11	n.g.	immediadiately neutralized and dialized against PBS	VEDELER et al., 1989

[*] numbering of the adsorbent material see Table 3.6.
[a] n.g. = not given, [b] rhuIFN-γ = recombinant human interferon γ, [c] crude microsome Triton X-100 solubilized receptor.

(2) Antibodies may also be generated against low molecular substances (cf. Chapter 1.3.),
(3) Monoclonal antibodies with a relatively high antigen or hapten specificity required for immunosorbent techniques can frequently be obtained in sufficient amounts by currently available methods (cf. Chapter 1.3.).

Haptens, Antigens and Receptors

Among the immunoaffinity chromatographic techniques published in the relevant literature, the separation and purification of various kinds of proteins are now being most extensively developed. Against this, the purification of haptens by

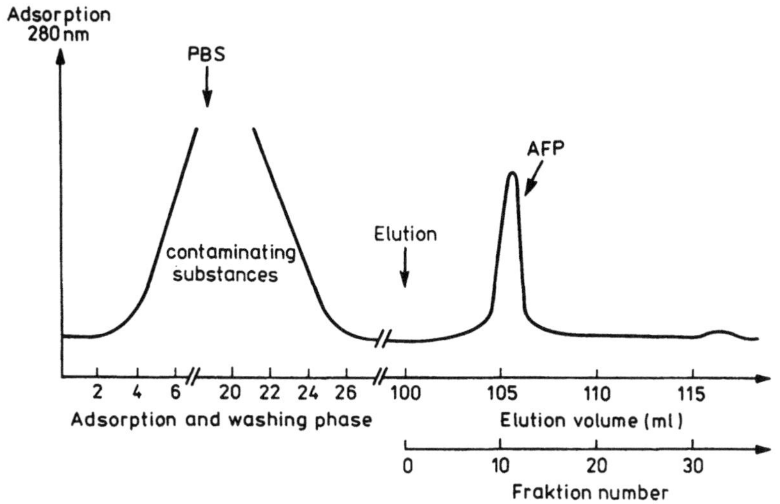

Fig. 3.3. Elution diagram of AFP. Details are given in Protocol 3.1. (page 103).

the immunosorption procedure is of only a little importance, since fewer expensive methods (e.g. gel permeation, hydrophobic, ion exchange chromatography) can be used advantageously for this purpose. Frequently, for proteins, especially those used in medical therapy, a high degree of purity (e.g. the absence of pyrogenic and viral activities in the final product) and stability (e.g. by purging from proteolytic contaminations) is required. This can be achieved by, for instance, combination of the immunoaffinity chromatographic step with additional purification procedures such as filtration and precipitation techniques etc.

Although such procedures have become increasingly important only in the last few years with the availability of numerous specific monoclonal and polyclonal antibodies respectively, a surprising number of substances have already been isolated or removed from sample solutions by immunosorption methods and it can be assumed with justification that unlimited possibilities for an ever broader application of these techniques will remain in the future.

In the following tables (Table 3.6., 3.7A., 3.7B. and 3.8.) examples are shown of haptens, proteins and receptors which were separated and purified respectively by immunosorption from materials of different origin (Table see p. 97–102).

An insight into the general sequence of such procedures is provided in the enclosed protocols (Protocol 3.1., 3.2. and 3.3.):

Protocol 3.1.: **Purification of the tumor marker α-fetoprotein (AFP)** (alkaline elution, Kaiser and Micheel, 1991).

16 ml of collected umbilical cord serum is applied to a column (0.5 x 10 cm) filled with the monoclonal antibody coupled to CNBr-activated Sepharose 4B (13 mg/3 g gel) by one of the usual methods (cf. Chapter 2.2.). The optimal flow rates are 4 ml/h for all steps.

After washing with 80 ml PBS (pH 7.2), the AFP is desorbed by 25 ml of an unbuffered alkaline solution of 0.5 M ammonia containing 0.5 mol/l NaCl; effluent is controlled spectrophotometrically at 280 nm and fractions of 0.5 ml are collected separately in tubes. The elution diagram obtained is shown in Fig. 3.3.

To remove traces of immunoglobulins, the fractions 5-15 of the chromatographic procedure are given to a second column (1 x 5 cm) filled with 3 ml murine specific goat antibodies bound to the same matrix followed by washing with PBS. The flow through fractions containing the purified AFP are pooled and stored at -20°C. The sequence of this procedure is summarized in Table 3.9.

Table 3.9. Purification of α-Fetoprotein (AFP) from Serum

Step	Protein[a] (mg/ml)	AFP[b] (µg/ml)	Recovery (%)	Purification (fold)
Serum	10	60	100	1
Eluate	0.52	290	93.7	1116
IgG-free AFP	0.25	245	68.3	1960

determined by: [a] protein assay according to LOWRY et al., (1951), [b] radioimmunoassay

Protocol 3.2.: **Purification of the tumor marker human choriogonadotropin (HCG)** (acidic elution, KAISER, private communication).

1200 ml filtered urine from pregnant woman (2nd or 3rd month of pregnancy) is applied to a pre-column containing 5 ml Sephadex G10. The effluent is immediately given to an affinity column (15 x 35 mm) containing the specific monoclonal antibody bound to 15 ml CNBr-activated Sepharose CL-4B.

Table 3.10. Purification of Human Choriogonadotropin from Urine

	IU	IU/ml	Recovery (%)	Purification (fold)
Urine	22200	18.5	100	1
Product	21600	1800	97.3	97

Subsequently, the gel is washed with 500 ml PBS to remove unspecifically adsorbed substances followed by the elution of the adsorbed HCG with 50 ml buffered solution using an acidic pH gradient (solution 1: PBS, pH 7.2; solution 2: 0.2 mol/l glycine + HCl, pH 2.5). The effluent of the affinity column is monitored spectrophotometrically at 280 nm; the optimal flow rate for all steps is 20 ml/h. All fractions containing HCG are neutralized immediately, pooled, concentrated by membrane filtration and stored at -20°C. Finally, the affinity column is regenerated for a subsequent purification step by equilibration with approximately 100 ml PBS. The sequence of this procedure is summarized in Table 3.10.

Protocol 3.3.: **Purification of human growth hormone (hGH)** (elution by chaotropic ions) (JÓNSDÓTTIR et al., 1986)

mabs of IgG1 subclass are bound to CNBr-activated Sepharose 4B; approximately 7 mg/ml gel). 1 ml of crude pituitary extract or lysate of recombinant *E. coli* (containing 1.5 mg protein) is applied to 5 ml of immunosorbent using a K 16/20 column (PHARMACIA). The binding capacity is 0.45 mg hGH per ml adsorbent as measured by adsorption and elution of purified pituitary hGH traced with iodinated hormone (15,500 cpm) in a column containing 1 ml immunosorbent.

After 15 minutes of incubation 15 ml PBS is added as washing buffer and subsequently the bound hGH is eluted stepwise with 1 M, 2 M and 4 M KSCN at pH 7.4, 15 ml of each. As established spectrophotometrically at 277 nm, most of the hGH is eluted in the 2 M fraction, which moreover contains various contaminations of lower and higher molecular weight. The fractions are dialyzed against PBS and concentrated in collodium bags.

Homogeneous 22 kD hGH is obtained through an additional ion exchange chromatography on DEAE-Affi-Gel Blue (BIO-RAD). To remove the non-hGH contaminations, which are usually substances leaking from the adsorbent (e.g. Ig), and, finally, to obtain an extremely pure 22 kD hGH, a gel filtration (e.g. with AcA 54 Ultrogel, LKB) can be performed.

All steps are carried out at 4°C, and the preparations are stored at -20°C until further application.

Recombinant Proteins

In the case of recombinant proteins, the yield of the final product can sometimes be increased by

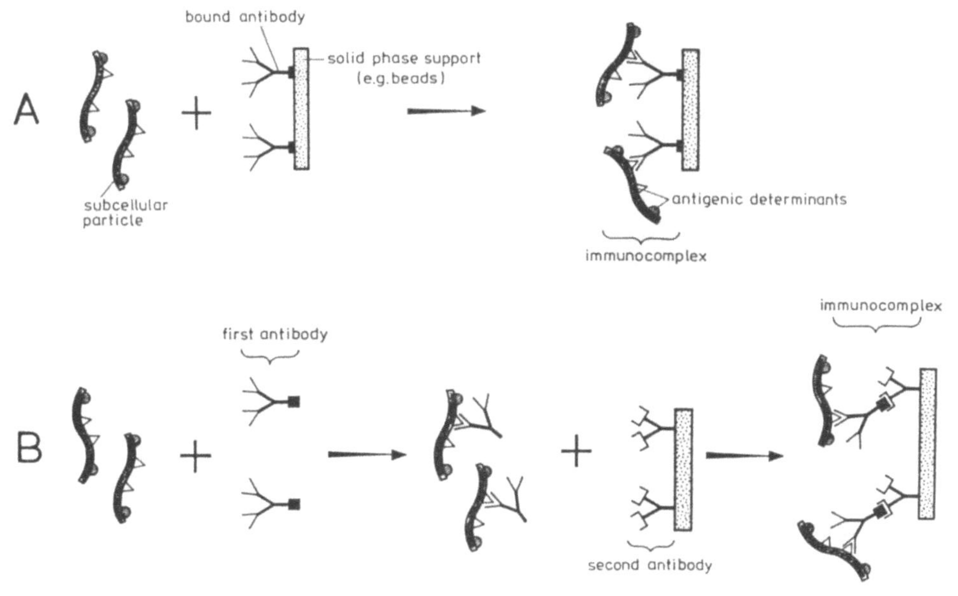

Fig. 3.4. Schematic representation of the direct (A) and indirect binding (B) of antigen bearing subcellular particles to an immunosorbent.
(A) The antibody specific for an antigenic determinant on the subcellular particle is bound to the solid phase material (e.g. microspheres). This immunosorbent is used to adsorb the appropriate cell debris.
(B) The antibody specific for an antigenic determinant acts with the subcellular material forming an immunocomplex. A second antibody specific for the Fc-region of the first one (or a bacterial immunoglobulin receptor or crosslinked *Staphylococcus aureus* cells) is bound to the solid phase carrier. This immunosorbent is also able to bind the immunocomplex formed before.
Another possibility - not represented here - is to treat the second solid phase bound biomolecule with the first one, and to incubate this immunosorbent subsequently with the sample solution containing the antigen-bearing subcellular particles to be purified.

expressing them as part of a larger fusion protein. Examples are the fusion of the desired protein to an oligo- or polypeptide sequence. The particular disadvantages of this approach, however, are: (a) that the fusion protein products may fail to fold properly into the native active state and (b) that it is often difficult or impossible to remove the additional amino- or carboxy-terminal sequence from the desired protein product.

These problems can be circumvented, e.g. by fusion to a short hydrophilic peptide such as Asp-Tyr-Lys-Asp-Asp-Asp-Asp-Lys, which is engineered onto the N-terminus of a protein using short oligonucleotides (Hopp et al., 1988, further references ibid.). This marker sequence is well recognized by a special Ca^{+2}-dependent monoclonal antibody (Prickett et al., 1989, further references ibid., see also Chapter 2.2). This antibody is able to interact preferably with the marker sequence. Corresponding fusion proteins, therefore, can be identified, separated and/or purified under mild conditions by immunoaffinity chromatography in a one-step procedure applying this antibody. The elution is carried out in this special case by removing or chelating Ca^{2+} from the washing buffer and the peptide is subsequently detached from the protein by treatment with the protease enterokinase, which cleaves immediately

Table 3.11. Separation of Subcellular Particles and Organelles by Immunosorption

Source	First antibody	Second antibody	Adsorbent*)	Recovery[a] (referred to)	References
Plasma membranes					
Rat adipocytes	rabbit-anti-(rat erythrocyte) serum	donkey anti-rabbit globulin (IgG)	diazocellulose	≈ 35 % (5'-nucleotidase activity)	LUZIO et al., 1976
Rat liver or rat liver hepatocytes	rabbit-anti-(rat erythrocyte) serum	sheep anti-rabbit IgG	diazocellulose	≈ 40 % (5'-nucleotidase activity)	WESTWOOD et al., 1979
Rat liver	chicken or guinea pig anti-LAP ab [b]	-	*Staphylococcus aureus* cells [c]	> 70 %, 153 fold (LAP)	ROMAN and HUBBARD, 1984
Cultured rat hepatocytes (fao cells)	rabbit-anti-(5'-nucleotidase) serum against the plasma membrane	sheep anti-rabbit IgG	diazocellulose	40-60 %, 34 fold (5'-nucleotidase activity)	DEVANEY and HOWELL, 1985
Calf liver (membranes enriched in mannose-6-phosphate receptors)	rabbit anti-peptide ab	goat anti-rabbit IgG	**14**	50-60 %, 30-50 fold (receptors)	MESSNER et al., 1989
Neuronal components					
Rat brain mitochondrial fractions; cholinergic synaptosomes of of different origin	sheep anti-(Chol-1) serum	mouse anti-sheep IgG	cxellulose	24 %, 26-38 fold (choline acetyltransferase activity)	RICHARDSON et al., 1984
Rat brain; synaptic vesicles	mouse mab against synaptic junctional prrotein	protein A [d]	acrylamide beads	-	MATTEW et al., 1981
Endocytic pathway components					
Porcine brain; clathrin-coated vesicles	rabbit anti-clathrin ab	-	*Staphylococcus aureus* cells [c]	70-80 %	MERISKO et al., 1982
Porcine brain; clathrin-coated particles	two different mab [e]	goat anti-mouse ab	*Staphylococcus aureus* cells (^{125}I label)	13 and 25 %, respectively	PFEFFER and KELLY, 1985
Rat hepatocytes; endosome-derived vesicles	anti-(5'-nucleotidase) serum	sheep anti-rabbit IgG	diazocellulose	5 % (5'-nucleotidase activity)	LUZIO and STANLEY, 1983
Endoplasmatic reticulum					
Rat liver; whole and sonicated	rabbit anti-NADPH cytochrome c reductase Ig	-	rabbit ab bound to **1**	-	KAWAJIRI et al., 1977

Table 3.11. Continued from page 106

Source	First antibody	Second antibody	Adsorbent*)	Recovery[a] (referred to)	References
Golgi apparatus					
Rat liver; light Golgi fractions	rabbit anti-NADPH cytochrome c reductase ab	goat anti-rabbit IgG	polyacrylamide beads	60 % (NADPH cytochrome c reductase activity)	ITO and PALADE, 1978

*) numbewring of the adsorbents cf. Table 3.6.
[a] further investigations without cleavage of the adsorbent/particle complex, [b] in some cases crosslinked with glutaraldehyde and reduced with $NaBH_4$, [c] formalin-fixed, heat-inactivated, [d] first ab and protein A crosslinked by paraformaldehyde and glutaraldehyde, [e] elution: pellet was suspended in 2 % SDS/6 M urea, sonicated, boiled in a water bath and centrifuged.
LAP = leucine aminopeptidase; Chol-1 = Cholinergic antigen 1

after the Asp-Asp-Asp-Asp-Lys-sequence. This method is being developed by IMMUNEX as the so-called FLAG™ technique. Up to now it has been used successfully to generate various recombinant proteins from fusion products such as the interleukins IL-2, IL-3 (YANG et al., 1986) and IL-4, the granalocyte-macrophage colony stimulating factor, the colony stimulating factor-1 and the granulocyte stimulating factor (HOPP et al., 1988).

The identification, separation and/or purification as well as the cleavage of many other recombinant fusion proteins have been described in the literature. It is noteworthy that this technique has received increasing interest for industrial-scale preparation of various proteins (e.g. recombinant growth hormone) of practically importance.

Subcellular Materials

Immunoaffinity procedures for the fractionation of subcellular materials are generally more effective than the classical centrifugation techniques as well as more recent methods, including electrophoretic separation and polymer-phase partition systems, since they rely on biological differences (e.g. the expression of different antigenic determinants) in contrast to other techniques, all of which depend on differences in physical and/or physico-chemical parameters (size, shape, density, charge, hydrophobicity etc.). Furthermore, immunoaffinity procedures frequently offer the prospect of fast purification in high yields, even when only small amounts of sample material is available (e.g. tissue culture cells). Moreover, they have the advantage of being applicable in physiological salt solutions and they do not expose the sample material either to unusual media or to osmotic and electric shock.

Solid phase techniques for the immunoaffinity fractionation of antigen-bearing subcellular material (and also whole cells) can be subdivided into (a) direct and (b) indirect methods (Fig. 3.4.) (RICHARDSON and LUCIO, 1986).

In the case of direct immunoaffinity fractionation, the antigen-specific antibodies are themselves covalently bound to the solid phase, which is then used as the immunosorbent material (Fig. 3.4A.).

A feature of the indirect methods is that the subcellular materials are first incubated with an appropriate antibody (first antibody) and this complex is fractionated using a second antibody or bacterial immunoglobulin receptor bound to the solid phase (Fig. 3.4B.). Instead of bacterial immunoglobulin receptors, heat-inactivated *Staphylococcus aureus* bacteria may be used. In the latter case it is possible to stabilize the cells additionally by a crosslinking agent. The indirect techniques are frequently more effective and it is assumed that this is attributable to a spacer like

Table 3.12. Separation of Viruses by Immunosorbent Techniques

Virus (= V.)	**Source**	**Adsorbent**[*] (protein/gel)	**Elution medium**	**Recovery** (concentration)	**Comment**	**References**
Parvo V.	canine cell A-72	mouse mab bound to **1**	3 M NH_4SCN, pH 7.8	70-90 % related to the antigen (4 fold); 20 % related to infectious material (16 fold)	> 90 % of contaminating protein removed	RIMMEL-ZWAAN et al., 1987
Aleutian mink disease V.	tissue extracts (liver, spleen etc.) from mink infected with Aleutian virus	ab bound to **5**	a) 0.75 M NaCl; subsequently b) 0.2 M glycine in 0.75 M NaCl (pH 6.5-2.0)	n.g. [a]	two types of immunocomplexes proved	KENYON et al., 1973
Soybean mosaic V.	infected *glycine max. (L) Merr cv. Williams*	mab bound to **5** (7.2 mg/ 5.3 ml)	deionized destilled water	n.g.	method applicable for the purification of a wide variety of plant viruses	DIACO et al., 1986
Influenca V.; 3 different strains	infected calf kidney tissue cultures	disulfide-linked γ-globulin of rabbits [b] (cf. STEPHEN et al., 1966)	buffer: pH 11.3-11.5	depending on the run of the separation procedure	carried out as a) batch or b) column method	SWEET et al., 1974

[*] numbering of adsorbent material see Table 3.6., [a] n.g. = not given, [b] immunized with influenza virus from calf kidney tissue cultures.

behaviour of the two bridging molecules which diminish steric hindrance at immunosorption of the subcellular particle. Indirect immunosorption has also been used, therefore, for the chromatography of proteins and other single antigens. Examples of subcellular particles separated by immunosorption techniques are given in Table 3.11. Generally, further investigations (e.g. the determination of enzyme activities, electron microscopic recordings) may be performed directly on the sorbent/cell debris complex, so that a cleavage by any elution procedure is not necessary.

For the fractionation of subcellular materials (the same is valid for viruses and cells), moreover, special variants of direct and indirect methods of immunosorption are described in the literature (RICHARDSON and LUZIO, 1986) but it is not possible to deal with this matter in more detail in this short monograph.

Viruses and Cells

Besides methods using immobilized lectins (SHARON, 1979; KRISTIANSEN et al., 1979) immunosorption procedures have also gained considerably in importance for the separation of viruses and viable cells in the last few years. With the advent of monoclonal antibodies to numerous virus and cell surface antigens, several variants of such methods have been developed and supplied for the selection of fundamentally distinct virus

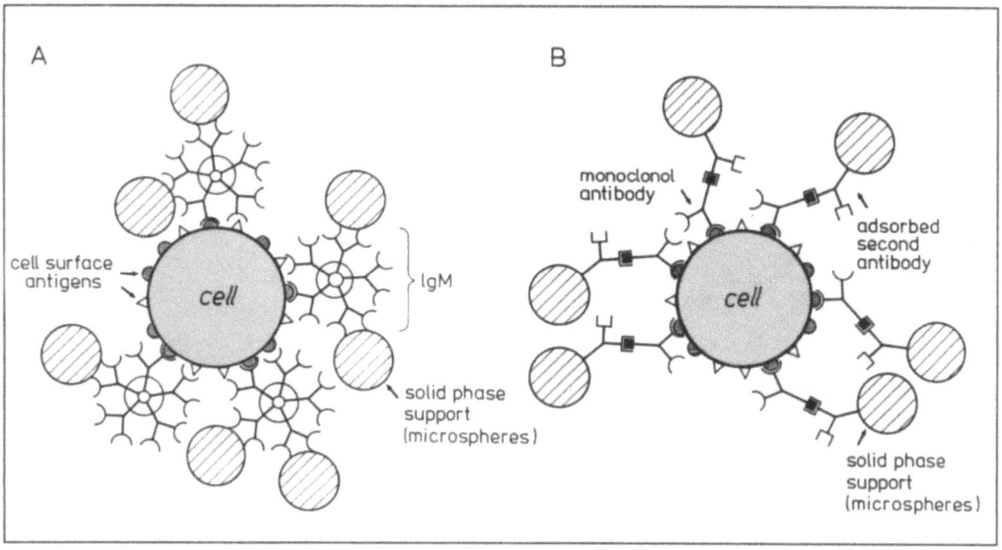

Fig. 3.5. Schematic representation of an antigen-bearing cell rosetted by microspheres via (A) immunoglobulin M; (B) a primary and a secondary antibody.

and cell populations. Besides their application in the field of research, they have also increased importance for analytical and medical purposes.

The concentration, separation and purification of viruses from different sources using immobilized virus protein specific antibodies to obtain effective vaccines or materials for fundamental investigations has been carried out successfully by numerous authors. Some selected examples described in the literature are given in Table 3.12..

Conventional methods for the separation of cells such as density gradient centrifugation, panning technique, rosetting with erythrocytes etc. are limited in their applicability. By utilization of immunological procedures essential progress in this field could be achieved.

A more or less specific immunoseparation of cells or cell subsets from suitable sample materials is frequently possible without considerable loss of their viability. The background of this specificity may be: (a) even the specificity of the immunocompetent cells themselves, (b) the affinity of an antibody for a cell surface-bound molecule, (c) the reactivity of an antibody for a haptenic determinant coupled to the cell surface or to a ligand binding to the cell surface (Basch et al., 1983). On this basis, the known immunological techniques practised for the separation of preferably lymphocyte populations can be subdivided into general variants (Table 3.13.) these being discussed in the following.

Table 3.13. Immunosorbent Techniques Used for Positive and Negative Selection of Cells

Procedure	Table	Figure
(A) Immunosorption of antigen (hapten) receptor-bearing cells by haptens or antigens [a)],	3.14.	3.6.
(B) Immunosorption of antigen-bearing cells by antibodies [a)],	3.15A.	3.5.
(C) Separation of antigen-bearing cells by antibodies via an interposed antigen or antibody conjugate [a)],	3.15B	3.9.
(D) Separation of antigen-bearing cells via cleavable or non-cleavable oligomeric antibody cross-linker [a)].	3.15A.	3.10.

[a)] bound to a solid phase matrix (beads, fibres, films, dishes, walls of tubes etc.).

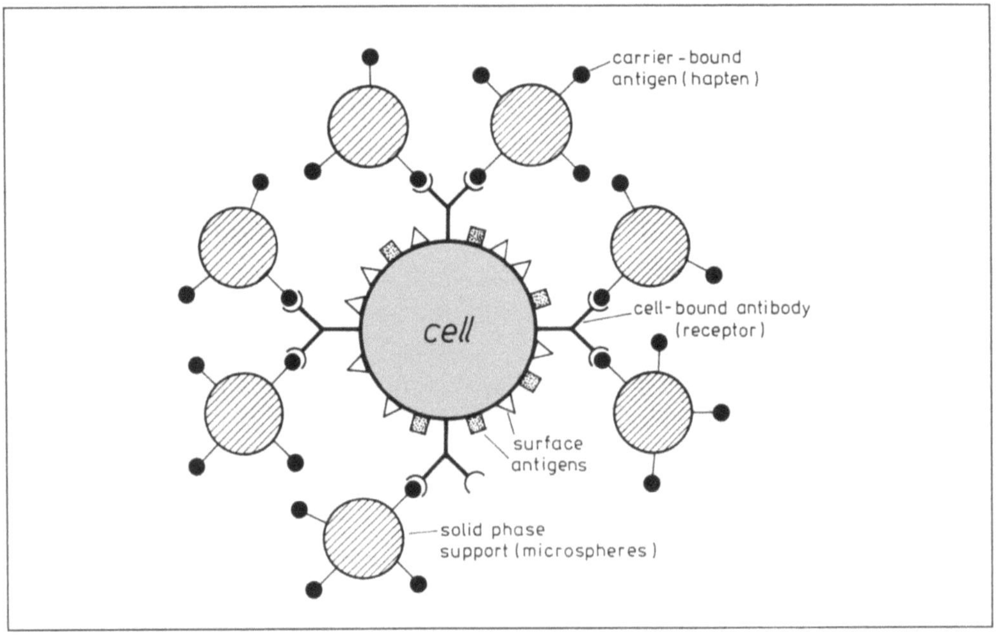

Fig. 3.6. Schematic representation of a receptor-bearing cell rosetted by microspheres.

In case B (Table 3.13.) one again has to distinguish between direct and indirect procedures (FUNDERUD et al., 1987), in which the definition given for the direct method used here corresponds widely to that given by RICHARDSON and LUZIO (1986) for the separation of subcellular particles (page 107 f.):

(a) In the case of direct procedures, the target cells are rosetted by the immunosorbent particles directly. In advance, however, these beads have to be coated with antibodies specific for certain antigens located on the surface of the cells to be separated (cf. Fig. 3.5.). Two different methods are preferably applied:

- monoclonal antibodies of the IgM type are bound to the beads (e.g. by adsorption). The pentameric structure of the IgM then allows a direct binding of the cells without a considerable yield-diminishing steric hindrance. A schematic representation of the so-formed immunocomplex is shown in Fig. 3.5A.
- Antibodies of the IgG type are bound to the beads via polyclonal second antibodies (e.g. sheep anti-mouse IgG) as it is presented in Fig. 3.5B. With this practice, steric hindrance can be likewise excluded, so that a selection of cells with acceptable yield is also possible.

(b) For indirect procedures, a crude suspension of mononuclear cells from blood or other origin has to be isolated beforehand (e.g. by density gradient centrifugation), and the target cells are sensitized with a primary antibody specific for any surface antigen on these cells. After this, the separation procedure is started analogously to the technique used for the indirect selection of subcellular particles (cf. Fig. 3.4.). Though the classification A-D given in Table 3.13. is rather schematic and overlapping cannot be avoided, it is used in the following, above all, from a practical point of view.

Furthermore, it has to be mentioned that none of these methods is universally applicable; in suitable separation procedures, however, excellent results can be obtained.

Table 3.14. Positive Selection of Antigen (Hapten) Receptor-Bearing Cells

Cell type, source	**Adsorbent**[*)] (protein/gel)	**Elution medium conditions**	**Comment**	**References**
Regional lymph node B cells of mice immunized against HSA, BSA or OA	HSA, BSA or OA adsorbed to glass or polymethacrylic beads	solutions of the free antigens (HSA BSA, OA), 4°C	adsorption of B cells inhibited by the free antigens	WIGZELL and ANDERSSON, 1969
IgG bearing B cells (spleen of mice)	rabbit anti-mouse F(ab) fragments bound to **13** (8 mg/g), effluent enriched in T cells	after adsorption the beads were solubilized by dextranase at room temperature	90 % of cells recovered were viable	SCHLOSSMAN and HUDSON, 1973
Spleen B cell populations of mice immunized against an azo-coupled lac-antigen	aminophenylglycoside coupled to **12**	PNP-β-lactoside, pH 7.2 (PBS), 4°C	adsorption of B cells is inhibited by PNP-β-lactoside	TRUFFA-BACHI and WOFSY, 1970
Spleen B cells of mice immunized against selected antigen (or hapten) conjugates	polystyrene tubes coated with rabbit anti-p-benzoate ab followed by the specific antigen or hapten-azobenzoate (antigen = KLH)	solution of the free antigen (or hapten) at neutral pH (1 mM p-nitrobenzoate)	generally applicable to the isolation of viable B cells bearing antigen (or hapten) receptors	CHOI et al., 1974
Spleen B cells of mice immunized against fluorescein-labeled antigens	anti-fluoresacein ab bound to **13**	solutions of the fluoresceinated antigens	fluoresceinated antigens: FL_5BSA, $FL_{15}HGG$, $FL_{3\text{-}5}SGG$, $FL_{2.5}TNP_8SGG$, FL-POL	SCOTT, 1976
Suppresor T cells of KLH-immunized mice (spleen)	KLH bound to **13**	cells (suspended in D'PBS+5 % heat-inactivated FCS) adsorbed at 37°C, eluted at 0-4°C (cf. Figure 3.7.)	to deplete B cells before the adsorption step the spleen cell suspension was passed through a column of mouse Ig bound to Sephadex G-200	OKUMURA et al., 1977

[*)] numbering of adsorbent material see Table 3.6.

Immunosorption of Antigen (Hapten) Receptor-bearing Cells

In the antigen-stimulated immunization of animals, lymphocytes bearing appropriate receptors on their surfaces increase. These may interact with the specific antigens or haptens respectively. To separate such receptor-bearing cells from sample solutions or suspensions (e.g. obtained from lymph nodes or spleens), the respective antigen or hapten bound to a solid phase matrix (e.g. beads) is used as the immunosorbent material (cf. BASCH et al., 1983). A schematic representation of cells rosetted by such beads is shown in Fig. 3.6. The elution of adsorbed cells is generally possible with the specific antibody or an excess of the appropriate free antigen or hapten. Furthermore, an application of EDTA (SINGER et al., 1978), temperature shifts (OKAMURA et al., 1977), matrix-degrading enzymes (SCHLOSSMAN and HUDSON, 1973), and others have been used successfully. Frequently, however, these methods seem to be more or less troublesome, and the recovery of viable cells is generally not so high. In the following, some examples for such procedures described in the literature are given (Table 3.14.). A diagram representing the elution of KLH-primed T cells from mice spleen by a simple temperature shift is shown in Fig. 3.7.

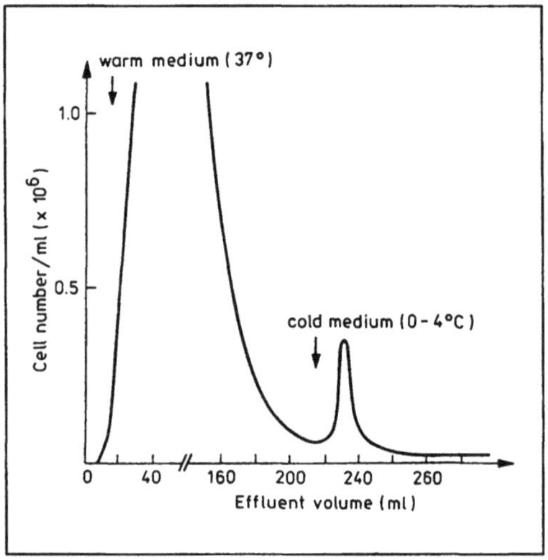

Fig. 3.7. Elution diagram of KLH-primed T cells from KLH-coated Sephadex G-200. A suspension of 5 x 10^8 spleen cells of mice were applied to a column at 37°C. After incubation for 30 minutes unbound cells were removed with warm medium (DULBECCO's PBS + 5% heat-inactivated FCS) followed by elution with cold medium. Normal and albumin-primed spleen cells did not provide the second peak under the same conditions (taken from OKAMURA et al., 1977).

Immunosorption of Antigen- or Hapten-bearing Cells

Further possibilities of isolating cells are provided by cell-surface bound antigens. For this purpose, antigen-specific poly- or monoclonal antibodies are bound to solid phase materials (e.g. microspheres) which then serve as the immunosorbent. A breakthrough in this field could be achieved with the advent of magnetizable beads as well as the development of suitable separation techniques (cf. FUNDERUD et al., 1987). The cells are surrounded (rosetted) by the beads as shown in Fig. 3.5. Fig. 3.8. represents an impressive scanning electron micrograph of mouse hepatocytes surrounded by such antibody-coated magnetizable microbeads.

The availability of highly specific monoclonal antibodies of relatively low affinity, offers new approaches to this problem for cells with relatively high antigen densities. The separation of cells with little antigen on their surface and a quantitative discrimination among cells differing in antigen density are beyond the capacity of most solid phase techniques in this field. Efforts to isolate adsorbed cells, in the case of positive selection by subsequent cleavage of the immunocomplexes formed, generally involve considerable difficulties. The procedures applied to dissociate antigen-

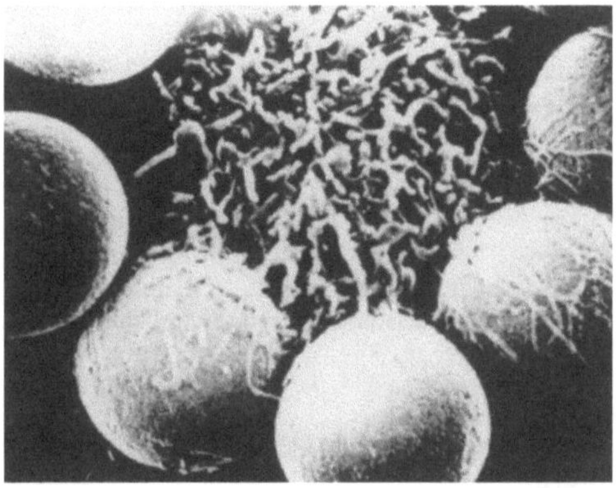

Fig. 3.8. Mouse hepatocyte isolated with immunomagnetic particles (Dynabeads) coated with monoclonal antibody against the cell surface marker H2 (S.E.M. x 14,500) (by courtesy of DANIELSEN, H. et al., Norwegian Cancer Hospital, Oslo).

antibody complexes themselves (p. 000), such as extremes of pH or chaotropic agents, are not suitable for the preparation of viable cells.

Frequently, however, removal of cells from the beads is not necessary since they also remain viable in this state and subsequent investigations (e.g. lymphocyte subset quantifications, HLA typing) are generally not appreciably affected. Separation of pure viable cells (predominantly lymphocytes) is in some cases successful through incubation of the immune complex for several hours in humidified CO_2 at 37°C. A dislodgement by gentle mechanical agitation is also possible. The degree of the detachment from the immunosorbent generally depends on the cell type and its avidity as well as on the specificity of the antibody. Unfortunately, at present these are the sole simple methods for this purpose. Further efficient and rapid procedures, e.g. cleavage of the complexes by addition of immunoglobulin or by chemical and enzymatic degradation respectively, of linker groups (cf. Procedure D in Table 3.13.) or of the sorbent material are under investigation.

In the Tables 3.15A. and 3.15B. are some examples of the positive (Table 3.15A.) and negative selection (Table 3.15B.) of antigen-bearing cells followed by a general protocol (Protocol 3.4.) demonstrating (a) the course of the isolation of pure viable CD8-positive T lymphocytes by antibody-coated immunomagnetic microspheres from whole blood, (b) their quantitation by cell counting and (c) the carrying out of HLA class I and HLA class II typing:

Protocol 3.4.: **Positive selection and direct quantitation of CD8-positive T lymphocytes from whole blood - the general course.**

(a) Positive selection.

In the following the direct positive selection and recovery of viable CD8-positive T cells as well as their quantification is described as a more general applicable example for such methods (taken from Funderud et al., 1987).

The procedure starts with the mixing of the sample solution containing the target cells with magnetizable microspheres (Dynabeads M-450) coated with adsorbed IgM antibodies specific for CD8 cell membrane antigen (which is a double chain 32 - 43 kD glycoprotein). The optimal bead:target cell ratio may be varied in the different systems but may be 3:1 for mononuclear cells isolated by density gradient centrifugation, 10:1 for buffy coat cells (without platelets) and 20:1 to 50:1 for whole blood. The bead-to-cell ratio, however, should be increased if a complete depletion is required (cf. below). During the cell separation and incubation procedure it is important to keep the cell suspension cold in each step (approximately 2 - 4 C) in order to prevent attachment of phagocytic cells to the beads.

After immunosorption the CD8-positive cells rosetted by the magnetizable beads are separated from the cell suspension by placing the test tube in an MPC for 2 - 3 minutes and the supernatant is removed by pipetting. Subsequently the cells are washed 4 - 5 times in PBS/FCS, again using an MPC, and are resuspended in the desired volume of an appropriate buffer (e.g. HBSS).

(b) Cell culture.

When a detachment of viable cells from the beads is desired, the bead-to-target cell ratio should be as low as possible in the preceding cell isolation step described above. This will increase both the recovery of the cells and will also facilitate their removal.

Usually, this procedure starts with resuspending the cells in an appropriate volume of cell culture medium, which is then transfered into a suitable vessel (for instance, into a cell culture flask) at a concentration of approximately 1 - 2 x 10^6 cells/ml, and incubated subsequently 10 - 15 hours at 37°C in humidified air with 5 % CO_2. The cultivated cells and the detached beads are resuspended by moderate pipetting using a narrow-bore Pasteur pipette (too vigorous pipetting may damage the cells). The detached beads and the remaining rosetted cells are then removed by an MPC. Pure and viable CD8-positive T cells can now be isolated from the supernatant for further studies. Generally, 70 % of CD8-positive cells will be recovered after incubation which are then washed 1-2 times in a cell culture medium before employing them for further studies.

Table 3.15A. Positive Selection of Antigen-bearing Cells for Analytical, Functional and Activation Studies

Cell type	Source	Adsorbent material[a)]	Comments	References
Various kinds of B lymphocytes	PBMC from heparinized blood; cells sensitized by the appropriate mab	**14** coated with rabbit anti-mouse IgG (2-4 beads/cell) are used in a rosetting step	indirect method; detachment of the particles frequently is possible in a humidified CO_2-containing incubator	Lea et al., 1986; Funderud et al., 1987
Lymphocyte subsets (CD4- and CD8-positive cells)	PBMC, T cells isolated by rosetting with AET-treated SRBC	**14** coated with ab of IgM type	indirect method; CD8-positive rosetted cells are used for further studies; the rosette-free fraction contains the CD4-positive cells	Gaudernack et al., 1986; Funderud et al., 1987; Leivestad et al., 1986, 1987
Lymphocyte subsets (CD2-, CD3-, CD4-, CD8-, CD19-, CD25-, CD37-, CD41b-, CD71-, CDw78-, ID5- and HKB1-positive cells)	25 µl samples of different origin (e.g. body fluids) from healthy and ill persons	**14** coated with goat anti-mouse IgG and the cell antigen specific mouse mab	indirect method; suitable for rapid phenotyping of cells (e.g. leukemia and other cancer cells); formation of rosettes may be inspected in a microscope or counted in a hemocytometer	Gaudernack and Lundin, 1989
Lymphocyte subsets (CD2-, CD4-, CD8-, CD19-positive cells)	500-1000 µl EDTA-anticoagulated blood	**14** directly coated with the specific mab's	nuclei of lysed cells are attained with acridine orange and counted in a hemocytometer; CD4- and CD8-positive cells serve as indicators for HIV infection; CD2-positive cell monitoring may be of interest in acute rejection of organ transplants	Brinchmann et al., 1988, 1989
Tac-(CD25)-positive lymphocytes	PBMC from defibrinated venous blood	**14** coated with sheep anti-mouse ab + tac mab as first ab	tac-positive cells are separated from the rosettes in humidified CO_2-containing incubator and used for T-cell cloning purposes	Lundin et al., 1989

Table 3.15A. Continued from page 114

Cell type	Source	Adsorbent material[a)]	Comments	References
Lymphocyte subsets [b)]	human and dog PBMC and BMNC	avidin linked to: a) CNBr-activated Sepharose 6MB, b) Biogel P-30 by the carbodiimide method, c) Biogel P-30 activated by glutaraldehyde	cells are incubated with mab's (Leu-4, Leu-5, 7.2 or DT2) and subsequently with biotinylated goat anti-mouse Ig, and passed through a gel-filled 3 ml column; adherent cells are dislodged by mechanical agitation (80-90 % of the cells were viable); regenerated gels of type a) and b) can be reused up to three times	Berenson et al., 1986
Lymphocyte subsets (CD3 and CD4-positive cells)	human PBMC and BMNC	glass beads coated with BSA-desferal and subsequently with a tetrameric ab complex consisting of: a) anti-CD3, anti-CD8 or anti-CD34 ab, b) mouse anti-desferal ab, c) $F(ab')_2$ rat anti-mouse IgG1	1-2 ml columns are filled with the hapten-modified glass beads; cells are removed by reduction with DTT and counted in a hemocytometer (in some cases the cells were removed by mechanical agitation); the method is more generally applicable	Thomas et al., 1989
Human erythrocytes		conjugate of anti-human red blood cell antibody and poly(ethylene glycol)	single step procedure in a model system of human erythrocytes and HL60 cells for the extraction of the red blood cells by affinity cell partitioning	Delgado et al., 1991; cf. Fisher and Sutherland, 1989

[a)] numbering of the adsorbent material see Table 3.6., [b)] cf. Figure 3.9.

Table 3.15B. Negative Selection of Antigen-bearing Cells

Target cells	Source	Adsorbent*)	Comments	References
T lymphocytes	human PBMC and BMNC	mab's to human T cell differentation antigens bound to CNBr-activated Sepharose 6MB	removing of viable cells by anti-leu-1 or anti-Leu-4 ab columns; 92.3-98.4 % T cells from PBMC with 43.5-47.5 % recovery of non-T cells; 98.3-99 % T cells from BMNC with recovery of ≈ 75 % non-T cells. Combining anti-Leu-1 and anti-Leu-4 mab's on the same column all detectable T cells may be removed; regeneration of the columns by mechanical agitation	Berenson et al., 1984
CD2- and CD3-positive T lymphocytes	human PBMC	**14** coated with rabbit anti-mouse Ig (5 μg/ml) and subsequently with anti-CD2 and anti-CD3 mab	PBMC suspension mixed with ab coated beads; rosetted cells separated with an MPC; the procedure leaves a maximum of 0.025 % SRBC rosette-forming cells and less than 0.02 % T cells	Vardtal et al., 1987
CD19-positive B lymphocytes	Rael Burkitt lymphoma cells	mice B cell mab (anti-CD19) chemically coupled to **14** (2.5-3.0 μg/mg)	cells admixed to human PBMC and separated with a MPC; after two consecutive cycles a depletion of (4-6)log10 was achieved	Kvalheim et al., 1987
Neoplastic B lineage derived cells [a)]	bone marrow of patients with multiple myeloma;	avidin-linked to CNBr-activated Sepharose 6MB	cells treated with mab and biotinylated goat anti-mouse Ig and then passed over the gel; linked cells dislodged by mechanical agitation; a mixture of mab's caused ≈ 3log10 of plasma removal	Lemoli et al., 1989
Leukemia CD10-positive B cells [a)]	^{111}In-oxine labeled Namalwa cells admixed to human BMNC	polypropylene floating beads (density: 0.91) incubated with: a) biotinylated BSA, b) avidin, c) biotinylated, CD10-positive murine ab	PBMC suspensions (2x10^7 cells/ml) contaminated with 0.5-5 % tumor cells incubated with floating beads; (3-4)log10 reduction of tumor load by an one-step treatment, 5log10 when the process is repeated	Hirn-Scavannec et al., 1988

Table 3.15B. Continued from page 116

Target cells	Source	Adsorbent*)	Comments	References
CD8-positive T-lymphocytes [b]	human PBMC	the tetramolecular ab complex consisting of anti-CD8, mouse anti-FITC mab and rat anti-mouse IgG1 is bound to glass beads (200-300 μm) coated with BSA-FITC conjugate	2×6^{10} PBMC's are passed over an 1 ml column at room temperature, retained cells are removed by agitating the beads	Thomas and Lansdorp, 1988

*) numbering of adsorbent material see Table 3.6., [a] cf. Figure 3.9., [b] cf. Figure 3.10.

(c) Direct quantitation of T cells (e.g. CD2-, CD4-, CD8- and CD19-positive cells) *from whole blood.*

For the direct quantitation described by Brinchmann et al. (1988, 1989) 0.5 ml cold EDTA blood is diluted with 1.0 ml cold PBS/FCS using an MPC for a minimum of 30 seconds between the single washing cycles again. Subsequently, the last washing buffer is removed completely and all the rosetted cells are flushed down from the side of the test tube with 25 μl of a cell lysing solution containing the detergent ZAPonin, thereby detaching the microspheres from the cells. PBS/BSA is added to make up a suitable volume and the cell nuclei are stained with a final concentration of 12.5 μg/ml acridine orange. Throughout these procedures the cells are kept at 2 - 8°C.

(d) Cell counting.

The stained cell nuclei and the free beads obtained in the preceding step are well mixed and counted in a Bürker hemocytometer using an immunofluorescence microscope both with fluorescent and white light to allow simultaneous identification of the lines in the hemocytometer and the cell nuclei. All the nuclei in the 8 Å squares (0.8 mm^3) are counted and the counts (C) are converted to a concentration of target cells in blood by the formula:

$$\frac{C \times VCN}{BV \times 0.8} \times 10^6 = \text{cells/l} \quad (3.1.)$$

where VCN represents the volume of the suspension of cell nuclei and BV denotes the volume of blood in the rosette suspension. If other types of hemocytometers are used, the calculation formula has to be adjusted accordingly in order to obtain correct counting results.

(e) HLA class I and HLA class II typing.

Paramagnetic, monodisperse microspheres coated with monoclonal antibodies of the IgM type specific for CD8-positive T cells or for the HLA class II ß-chain monomorphic epitope, permit both cell separation and the subsequent HLA class I (A, B, C) as well as HLA class II (DR, DP, DQ) typing. These procedures represent, in principle, a recent modification of microcytoxicity testing introduced by TERASAKI and MCCLELLAND (1964).

For HLA typing, the target cells are separated directly from peripheral anticoagulated blood (e.g. ACD blood) or from another source with an appropriate magnetizable immunosorbent. To avoid nonspecific attachment of phagocytic cells to the microspheres, the procedure is carried out at low temperatures (2 - 8°C). The rosetted cells are then purified by means of an MPC.

After sufficient washing and further treatment required for the HLA typing procedure (cf. VARTDAL et al., 1986) the assay can be read in an inverted microscope with ordinary light (one rosette is defined as a cell to which at least three beads adhere) (HANSEN and HANNESTAD, 1989), or an assessment may be achieved by staining with fluorescent substances, e.g. acridine orange and ethidium bromide. In this case a fluorescence microscope is applied. Dead cells have a red, viable cells a green colour. More detailed information on this topic is provided in the literature cited above.

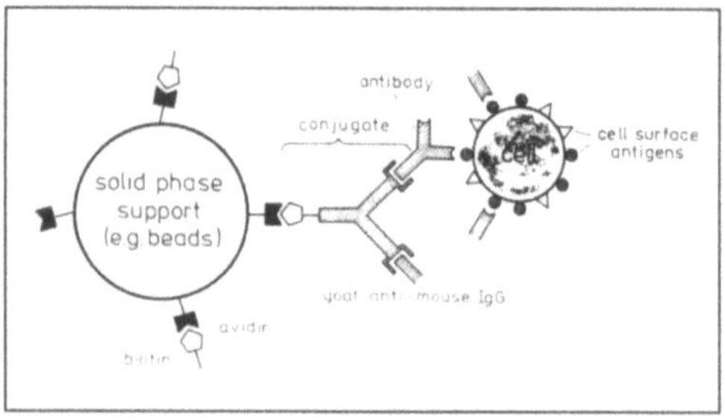

Fig. 3.9. Immunosorption of cells by avidin-coated beads via an interposed biotin-antibody conjugate - a schematic representation

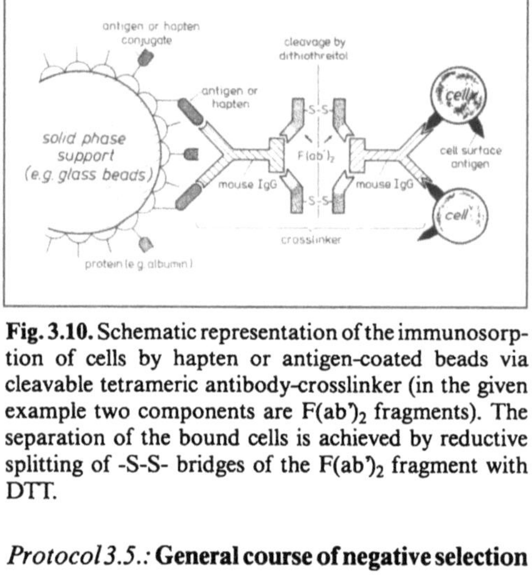

Fig. 3.10. Schematic representation of the immunosorption of cells by hapten or antigen-coated beads via cleavable tetrameric antibody-crosslinker (in the given example two components are $F(ab')_2$ fragments). The separation of the bound cells is achieved by reductive splitting of -S-S- bridges of the $F(ab')_2$ fragment with DTT.

Negative Selection of Cells

Negative selection is used for the depletion of cell suspensions (e.g. blood, PBMC, BMNC or other body fluids containing heterogeneous cell populations) from unwanted cell populations. This technique can be used (a) to study how removal of certain cell subsets may influence various functional parameters in cell culture experiments, (b) to deplete T cells from bone marrow grafts in order to avoid graft-versus-host disease in allogenic bone marrow transplantation (VARTDAL et al., 1987) or (c) to carry out tumor cell purging in autologous bone marrow transplantation in the treatment of neuroblastomas (TRELEAVEN et al., 1984). Compared with positive selection methods, the depletion of cells generally requires higher particle/cell ratios (approximately 10-20 beads/cell or more). Examples of cell depletion procedures described in the literature are given in Table 3.15B..

Protocol 3.5.: **General course of negative selection of CD4-positive T lymphocytes** (taken from Draft 10 - 220688, DYNAL AS, Norway).

The procedure starts with the isolation of cells from blood, buffy coat or some other material by density gradient centrifugation. After washing with PBS/FCS the cell pellet obtained by centrifugation is resuspended in a small volume of PBS. Magnetizable microspheres coated with anti-CD4 mab are added according to the expected number of target cells in the suspension and the sample is incubated for 30 minutes at 4°C under continuous tilting and rotation. Subsequently, the test tube is placed for 2 - 3 minutes in an MPC to collect rosetted cells and free beads followed by the transfer of the depleted supernatant into a clean culture flask for further studies. Generally, two consecutive incubations with magnetizable microspheres will give a depletion of more than three orders of magnitude.

Furthermore in Table 3.13. (C) examples for separation of antigen-bearing cells by antibodies via an interposed antigen or antibody conjugate as well as in (D) for separation of antigen-bearing cells via cleavable or non-cleavable oligomeric crosslinker are given. These two techniques were used successfully in depletion and positive selection procedures. Schematic representations demonstrating the structure of such immunocomplexes are shown in Fig. 3.9. and 3.10. References of some examples described in the literature are given in Tables 3.15A and 3.15B.

4. Techniques Based on Immunosorption

4.1. Immunoassays

4.1.1. General Considerations

Over the last four decades, tests based on the formation of hapten-antibody or antigen-antibody complexes respectively, and designated as immunoassays have become an essential analytical tool for both qualitative and quantitative determinations of analytes present in materials of different origin (human body fluids, foodstuffs, biotechnical preparations etc.).

The first immunoassay used successfully for the determination of insulin in human plasma was described by YALOW and BERSON in 1959. Since the development of this principle, not only increasingly more immunoassays for the determination of selected substances but also modified test procedures have been proposed, and it can be assumed that this trend is far from being finished. Therefore, it is impossible to provide an exhaustive treatment of this topic in the present monograph. Rather, the aim of this chapter is (1) to systematize the known procedures as far as practicable, (2) to treat several special procedures and (3) to list various selected immunoassays and their characteristic parameters. According to the present state-of-the-art, immunoassays can be classified from different points of view. Some possibilities are given in the following:

(a) Antigen-(hapten-)determining / antibody-determining assays.
(b) Tests for qualitative screening procedures / semiquantitative tests / quantitative assays.
(c) Subdivision on the basis of antigen (hapten) or antibody labels (markers) in use, which enable the indication of the test result (e.g. radiolabels, fluorescence, luminiscence and spin markers, numerous enzymes) providing the required analytical signal (cf. Table 4.1.).
(d) Solid phase tests (under consideration of the morphological and chemical structure of the solid phase material) / tests carried out in liquid phase (and, e.g., a subsequent precipitation of the immune complex formed) / tests carried out exclusively in liquid phase. Such methods are designated as homogeneous immunoassays whereas the two first-mentioned ones rest on the separation of bound and free labeled components and are designated as heterogeneous immunoassays.
(e) Direct / indirect assays.
(f) Assays with monoclonal / with polyclonal / with both monoclonal and polyclonal antibodies.
(g) Inhibition (competitive) assays / two-side binding (sandwich-) assays.
(h) Subdivision in variants: conventional assays / tests on the basis of bi- (and oligo-) specific monoclonal antibodies / application of antibody fragments / use of helper antibodies and others.

To treat this topic as completely as possible for the purpose of systematization the points (d), (g) and (h) shall be given priority here (whereas the other considerations will be dealt with as far as necessary).

4.1.2. Heterogeneous Immunoassays

These assays can be subdivided into competitive and two-side binding tests as illustrated in Fig.

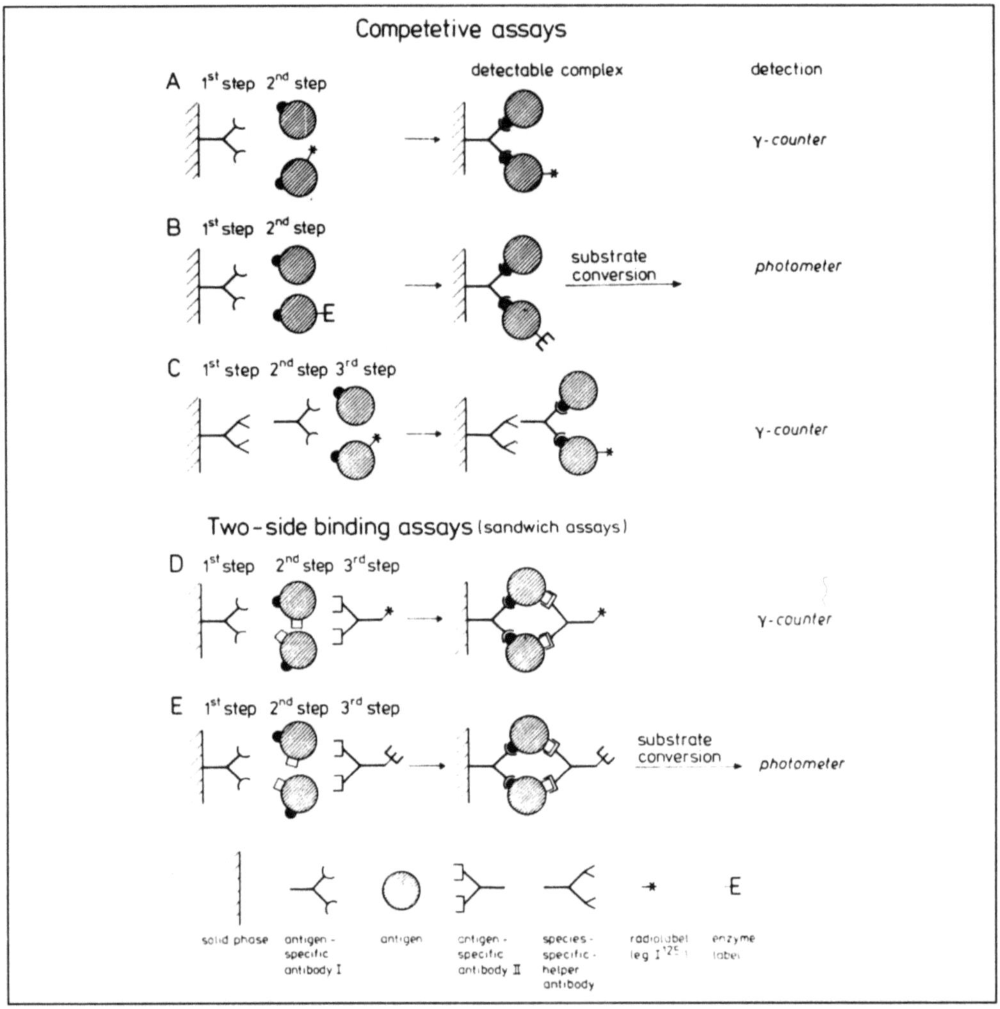

Fig. 4.1. Schematic representation of heterogeneous immunoassays (selected examples).
Competetive assays. Within a definite range, the antigen concentration in the sample correlates with the reciprocal of the intensity of the analytical signal obtained by γ-counting (e.g. for ^{125}I as marker) or β-counting (e.g. for ^{3}H as label) (a) and spectrophotometric determination at a suitable wavelength (b), respectively.
A) Radioimmunoassay (RIA) (a).
B) Enzymeimmunoassay (EIA) (also designated as ELISA = enzyme linked immnunosorbent assay) (b).
C) Radioimmunoassay using additionally a species specific (helper) antibody (a).
Two-site binding assays (sandwich-assays). Within a definite range, the antigen concentration in the sample correlates directly with the intensity of the analytical signal.
D) Immunoradiometric assay (IRMA) (a).
E) Immunoenzymometric assay (IEMA) (b).

Table 4.1. Heterogeneous Immunoassays and Principles of Signal Detection (cf. Schuurs et al., 1982)

Nature of particles	Kind of test	Analysis; detection, determination by:
Sensitized Particles [a]		
Latices (polystyrene[b], polyvinyltoluene, polymethacrylate etc.) [b,c]	agglutination (flocculation) tests; agglutination/ inhibition tests [d]	visual observation (e.g. slide tests, giving yes/no answers [e]; turbidimetry, nephelometry (Price et al., 1987); quasielectric light scattering (Looney, 1984); angular dissymmetry (Cannell et al., 1979); particle counting (Limit et al., 1979); spectrophotometry etc.
Gold sols		change of colour; sedimentation [f] (Geoghegan et al., 1980)
Colloidal organic dyes		(Gribnau et al., 1982)
Erythrocytes	rosette test	sedimentation pattern in round bottom tubes (Schuurs et al., 1982)
Immobibized reagents [g]		
Radionuclides	radioommunoassay (RIA)	β- or γ-counting e.g. ^{125}I, ^{131}I, ^{3}H, ^{75}Se, (Yalow and Berson, 1959)
Enzymes with high turnover numbers	enzyme immunoassay (EIA, cf. Tjissen, 1985)	spectrophotometry (cf. Saunders, 1979)
Other labels [h]		

[a] separation of any component during the implementation of the test procedure ist not required, [b] diameter of the particles $< 1\,\mu m$, [c] suitable for determination of bi- or polyvalent antigens (haptens) as well as of immunoglobulins; the required reactant can be passively adsorbed on the particles or is covalently bound, [d] the latex particles coated with the immunoglobulin, hapten or antigen (e.g. HCG) are agglutinated with a properly diluted hapten, antigen or antibody (e.g. anti-HCG serum); this agglutination can be inhibited by free antibody, hapten or antigen (HCG) present in the test sample (e.g. urine of a pregnant woman), [e] applied mainly for diagnosis of infection and autoimmune diseases, respectively, as well as for detection of hormones and drugs, [f] initial change of colour from deep red to purple and blue followed by sedimentation leaving a clear supernatant, [g] for bound/free separation (cf. Schuurs et al., 1982; Parker, 1990) generally, the label is not changed in its physical or chemical properties, [h] fluorescence markers in fluorescence immunoassays: FIA, (Aalberse, 1973); europium chelates in time resolved immunoassays (DELFIA™/Pharmacia), Hemmila et al., 1984; cf. Dimandis and Christopoulos, 1990; gold sol particles (SPIA); dye sol particles (DIA, Gribnau et al., 1982).

4.1A. to 4.1E. (more detailed information about this is given in the attached legend).

With the simplest of these test procedures, the antigen (or hapten) to be determined competes with the same but specifically labeled antigen (or hapten) added in a required concentration (which has to be known exactly) to the solution to be analyzed.

A particular immune test can be described according to these principles, e.g. the test presented in Fig. 1.18 (p. 20), which is suitable as a direct screening solid phase assay for antigen specific antibodies (e.g. performed as radioimmunoassay) using a polyclonal mouse Ig-specific catcher antibody and labeled antigen. Early antigen specific quantitative immune tests (e.g. the

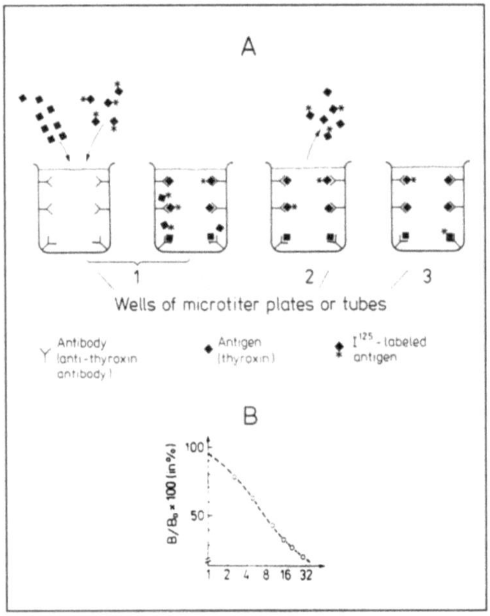

Fig. 4.2.
A) Schematic demonstration of a competetive radioimmunoassay (RIA) by the example of determination of thyroxin (T_4).
(1) Fixed volumes of the sample solution containing the ^{125}I-labeled hapten in the required concentration is pipetted into tubes covered on the inner walls with anti-thyroxin antibody.
(2) Unbound thyroxin is completely removed by repeated washing steps.
(3) The remaining surface-bound ^{125}I-labeled thyroxin is determined in a γ-counter.
B) The calibration curve obtained by six standards shows that the radioactivity measured by the γ-counter decreases when the hapten concentration in the sample increases.
Ordinate: Antibody-bound thyroxin conjugate in %; BO = amount of ^{125}I-labeled thyroxin necessary to saturate the surface-bound anti-thyroxin antibody completely; B = amount of the ^{125}I-labeled thyroxin bound in the presence of the analyte.
Abscissa: Thyroxin concentration in μg T_4 per dl (logarithmic).

first assay was developed by Yalow and Berson in 1959) were competitive liquid phase radioimmunoassays, using polyclonal antibodies and radiolabeled antigen (mostly ^{125}I as label). Before measurement in a γ-counter, therefore, the immunocomplex was precipitated by a suitable agent (e.g. a precipitating antibody).

In addition to the use of radionuclides as labels already referred to fluorescent substances, free radicals, numerous enzymes etc. (cf. Table 4.1.), which are anchored generally via covalent bonds on the antigen (or hapten) are also in use.

To carry out a simple heterogeneous immunoassay for the determination of antigen (or hapten), a fixed volume of the sample solution is pipetted, e.g., into suitable plastic tubes or into the wells of a microtiter plate covered with the complementary antibody followed by the addition of labeled antigen (or hapten) in the required concentration. This approach is represented schematically in Fig. 4.2A. by the example of determination of thyroxin in human serum with the aid of ^{125}I-labeled hapten. The test illustrated here is so constructed as to enable the analyte to compete directly with the labeled thyroxin for the surface-bound anti-thyroxin antibody. When the complex stability for both the unmodified and the labeled species do not differ considerably, the proportion of the bound molecules corresponds to that present in solution.

After removing both the unbound hapten and the unbound ^{125}I-conjugate by repeated washing steps, the amount of antibody-bound ^{125}I-labeled thyroxin is determined by measuring the radioactivity in a γ-counter. For a competitive test, as discussed here, in a definite range the hapten concentration in the sample correlates directly with the intensity of the analytical signal (number of counts) meaning that the value found will be the higher, the lower the concentration of the analyte in the sample to be analyzed.

To calculate its real concentration, a calibration curve is required in addition. This can be obtained by analyzing a sufficient number of standard solutions containing fixed amounts of both labeled and unlabeled hapten of different concentrations. As an example, in Fig. 4.2B., a calibration curve is shown for the determination of thyroxin by the competitive immunosorbent assay discussed above. This curve, moreover, demonstrates the high analytical sensitivity of such analytical procedures, but it should be noticed that linearity as a requirement for exact quantitation in immunosorbent assays is given only in a distinct range of the whole signal-analyte correlation.

In the following, a protocol (Protocol 4.1.) is given describing one possible run of a heterogeneous immunometric assay in a generalyzed form (see Fig. 4.1E.) which is particularly useful for the determination of protein antigens.

It is impossible to give a protocol which is optimized for all purposes. Therefore, for special cases reviews and monographs, for instance those by TIJSSEN (1985) or COLLINS (1988), should be consulted.

Protocol 4.1.: **Generalized procedure of an immunoenzymometric assay**

(1) Preparation of the immunosorbent

100 µl of a solution of purified antigen-specific (monoclonal) antibodies appropriately diluted with PBS is applied to wells of a microtiter plate, and the antibody is allowed to bind adsorptively to the plate at 4°C over night. For absorption, a 20 mM sodium bicarbonate buffer, pH 9.6, is recommended.

Residual absorption areas of the microtitre plate can be blocked with 0.1 % gelatin, 0.5 - 1 % skimmed milk powder, serum albumin or other inert protein (with respect to the antibody-antigen system to be used in the assay) in PBS. Then unbound material is removed thoroughly by washing with PBS (4 - 5 washes) or simply with cold running tap water (8 - 10 washes).

(2) Specific binding of the antigen

Antigen samples are definitely diluted with PBS containing 1 - 2 % bovine serum albumin (PBS/ BSA) which allows the omission of an additional blocking step of unsaturated binding sites at the plastic surface. In the same manner a dilution series of antigen solution is applied at least in duplicate to the wells of the immunosorbent plate prepared in step (1).

(3) Binding of an antigen-specific enzyme-labeled antibody

A second, antigen-specific monoclonal antibody recognizing an epitope different from that of the solid phase antibody and covalently labeled with horseradish peroxidase [a] is diluted appropriately with PBS/BSA. 100µl of this solution is applied to each well of the microtiter plate and incubated for one hour at room temperature in humid air. Unbound conjugate is then removed by thorough washing as described in step (1).

(4) Enzymatic indication

Each well of the plate is incubated with 100 µl of a solution containing a chromogenic substrate (e.g., 0.4 mg/ml of o-phenylene diamine (OPA) or 0.55 mg/ml diammonium 2,2'-azino-bis(3-ethylbenzthiazoline-6-sulfonate (ABTS) (PORSTMANN et al., 1981) and 0.5 µl/ml of 30 % H_2O_2 in a phosphate/citrate buffer, pH 5, made from 5.1 mg/ml of citric acid and 7.1 mg/ml $NaH_2PO_4{*}H_2O$) for 30 minutes at room temperature in the dark.

The enzymatic reaction is stopped with 100 µl of a stopper solution (e.g. 1 molar sulfuric acid), and the adsorbance is determined in a microplate reader at 492 nm.

Using this test principle, the antigen concentration correlates directly in a definite range linearly with the adsorbance at the selected wavelength. Thus the antigen concentration of a sample can be calculated from the standard curve using an internal program of the plate reader. To avoid deviations caused by inhomogeneities in coating of different plates it is recommended to run a set of standards on each plate.

For the sole discrimination between positive and negative samples the times of all incubation steps can be reduced to several minutes.

Although the protocol seems to be relatively simple, the development of an assay - and this is valid principially for most immunoassays - can be difficult since the best test combination of antibodies and optimal dilutions of both solid phase-bound and enzyme-labeled antibodies as well as the optimal incubation conditions have to be found empirically by more or less time-consuming test procedures.

[a] Other enzyme labels are also used, for instance alkaline phosphatase from calf intestine, ß-galactosidase or glucose oxidase (TIJSSEN, 1985).

Table 4.2A. Heterogeneous Immunoassays

Analyte	**Type of assay** (solid phase component)	**Label** (indication)	**Lower detection limit** (range)	**References**
hCG	agglutination (the label)	gold sol particles (visually) [a]	30 IU/l[b]	LEUWERING et al., 1980
hCG	sandwich (Indium-coated plastic strips)	without[c] or POD[d] (visually)	(1 μg/ml - 1 ng/ml)	GUPKA et al., 1991
Human placental lactogen	disperse(d) dye (the label)	colloidal organic dye particles (spectrophotometrically)	1-2 ng/ml (2-100 ng/nl) 0.25-1mIU/ml (visually, 4-1000 mIU/ml)	GRIBNAU et al., 1982
Anti-Rubella	"	"	2.5 IU/ml (3-50 IU/ml)	"
Testosterone	"	"	0.2-0.4 pmol/ml (0.5-5 pmol/ml)	"
Luteinizing hormone	competetive (Sephadex-particles)	^{125}I (γ-counting)	<1pg/ml	WIDE and PORATH, 1966
Human thyreotropin	competetive (plastic tubes)	glucose-oxidase (spectrophotometrically) [e]	1.5 μU/ml	TANSWELL et al., 1979
Testosterone	competetive (polystyrene microtiter strips)	Eu [f] (fluorimetrically)	15 fmol	BERTROFT et al., 1984
CEA	sandwich (polystyrene balls)	POD [g] (spectrophotometrically)	0.5 ng/ml	FAHTEH-MOGHADAM et al., 1979
HBsAg (adw subtype)	sandwich (balls of organic polymers, microtiter plates)	^{125}I (γ-counting) POD	1.4 ng/ml 1.9 ng/ml	GERLICH and STAMM, 1978
Myeloperoxidase	immunometric (polystyrene balls)	ABEN [h] + peroxide (by luminiscence [i]	(0-600 μg/l	JANDA et al., 1990
1,25-dihydroxy-vitamin D3 receptor	immunometric (Sepharose-particles)	^{125}I (γ-counting)	2-3 fmol (in crude extract)	SANDGREN et al., 1989

Table 4.2A. Continueed from page 124

Analyte	Type of assay (solid phase component)	Label (indication)	Lower detection limit (range)	References
Theophyllin	competetive (liposome flow injection immuno-assay) [j]	fluorescence derivative	3.9 x 10^{-8} M	LOCASIO-BROWN et al., 1990
IgE, IgA1 IgA2 and vitronectin	avidin-coated polyacrylamide beads + biotinylated anti-mouse IgGs [k]	H_2O_2 and o-phenylene diamine, per-oxidase (spectro-photomerically)	(0.25 - 2.0 ng/ml)	HAUN and WASI, 1990

[a] quantitation by means of a colorimeter is possible at 540 nm; [b] incubation time: 4h; [c] the test is based on the principle that adsorbed proteins turn the light brown surface to a darker brown; [d] development of precipitable colour by incubating with 3', 3'-diamino benzidine and H_2O_2; [e] + glucose, POD and ABTS; [f] time resolved fluorescence immunoassay (cf. HÄMMILÄ et al., 1984); [g] + orthophenylene diamine and H_2O_2; [h] 9-[N-(4-aminobutyl)N-ethyl]-amino benzo[f]phthalazine-1.4-(2H,3H) dione; [i] another possibility is given by spectrophotometric indication using both biotin and a streptavidine/alkaline phosphatase conjugate, [j] the antibody (anti-theophyllin) is bound on silica particles of a packed-bead column; liposomes containing a xanthine derivative and the fluorescence marker compete against theophyllin of the sample. Bound liposomes are disrupted by a glycopyranoside and the associated fluoressence is measured. The method is rapid and can be automated; the system is regenerable, [k] allows an increase of the ligand density on the matrix.

Recently a heterogenic immunoassay system based on the dry reagent technique and self-contained fluorometric ELISA, respectively, was developed by Polaroid Corporation (U.S.A.) and Behringwerke AG (Germany) under the trademark OPUS™ Immunoassay System.
The system utilizes known formats of immunoassays combined with (i) a new dry thin film multilayer technique (e.g. for low molecular weight compounds, such as valproic acid, carbamazepine and gentamycine), or (ii) self-contained test modules which house all the reagents needed for the respective test (e.g. for determination of high molecular weight substances, such as antibodies, hCG or CEA) (PBDS Scientific Posters, 1990). In both variants a fluorescent dye (e.g. rhodamine) serves as label.
The specific and precise quantitative determination of an analyte can be carried out over a wide range of molecular concentrations in a total assay time between 6 and 20 minutes. No pretreatment or dilution of sample (e.g. 10 μl serum in case of the film technique) is required. An adapted multitask microprocessor controls all functions, data processing included.
It can be assumed that the OPUS™ will offer a broad menu of tests, including thyroid markers, therapeutic drug monitoring, hormones, tumor markers and germs of infectious diseases.
Selected examples of heterogeneous immunoassays are given in Table 4.2A.

4.1.3. Homogeneous Immunoassays

The first homogeneous test was described by RUBINSTEIN et al. in 1972 using lysozyme as a marker. Contrary to heterogeneous assays, these procedures do not require any solid phase-bound component. All substances included in the test procedure (e.g. the substance to be analyzed, the conjugate used, the antigen or (hapten)) are solved at least in the initial phase. In principle, however, a separation step is not necessary, so that this approach provides excellent possibilities for automation.

Table 4.2B. Homogeneous Immunoassays [a] (selected examples)

Analyte	**Type of immunoassay**	**Label** (indication)	**Lower detection limit** (range)	**References**
Ovalbumin	fluorescence polarization	FITC bound ovalbumin [b]	(nmole range)	DANDLIKER and FEIGEN, 1961
Human IgM	fluorescence polarization	Lucifer Yellow [c]	0.8 μg/ml	URIOS and CITTANOWA, 1990
Morphin	enzyme	lysozyme bound to morphine [d]	< 1 x 10^{-9}M	RUBINSTEIN et al., 1972
Vitamin B12	recombinant protein-based (CEDIA™)	polypeptides forming an enzyme with	(0-2000 pg/ml)	KHANNA and WORTHY, 1990
Folate	"	β-galacto-sidase ac-	(0-20 ng/ml)	"
Digoxin	"	tivity (colorime-trically) [e]	(0-4 ng/ml)	HENDERSON et al., 1986
Drugs (opiates, barbiturates, amphetamine etc.) [f]	enzyme (EMIT™)	malate dehydroge-nase; glucose-6-phosphate dehy-drogenase [g]	(0.5 - 1.5 mg/l on average	LEUTE and ORTH, 1978; OELLERICH, 1979

[a] nephelometric and turbidimetric systems disregarded; [b] and combined with rabbit anti-fluorescein ovalbumin; fluorescence polarization decreases when anti-ovalbumin is added; [c] bound to (anti-μ chain human IgM)-Fab fragments; [d] dislodgement of the lysozyme-morphine conjugate from anti-morphine antibodies by morphine under increase of the enzyme activity; [e] using chromogenic and fluorogenic substrates with high extinction coefficients; [f] semiquantitative; [g] glucose-6-phosphate dehydrogenase from *Leuconostoc mesenteroides* (since this enzyme is NAD-dependent contrary to the enzyme from erythrocytes).

As labels for these tests are used, e.g. single electron containing (spin immunoassay, LEUTE et al., 1972) and fluorescent substances (e.g. fluorescence polarization assay, DANDLIKER et al., 1961; URIOS and CITTANOVA, 1990), β-galactosidase forming polypeptides (HENDERSON et al., 1986) - these test systems are commercially available as CEDIA™ - and, in a qualified sense, bacteriophages too (HAIMOVICH et al., 1970a, 1970b) as well as various selected enzymes.

The essential property of homogeneous assays consists of a change of the characteristic signal of an applied marker when an antibody is bound to the labeled antigen (or hapten) (cf. Fig. 4.3.).

At present, enzymes (e.g. malate dehydrogenase and glucose-6-phosphate dehydrogenase as well as NAD^+ as substrate) are favoured as labels in commercially available assays (e.g. in the so-called EMITS™ distributed by SYVA; EMIT = enzyme multiplied immune technique) which will be discussed in more detail in the following.

When suitable enzymes are used as markers, their activity is modulated (most frequently inhibited) at formation of the antigen (or hapten) complex. The inhibition (e.g. by hapten) can be explained as follows (cf. Fig. 4.3B.): it has to be assumed that the hapten molecule is arranged in the direct neighborhood of the catalytic center when it is bound covalently to the marker enzyme. An antibody directed against this hapten covers the active center and prevents an access of the substrate. For this reason the application of homogeneous enzyme immunoassays is largely limited to the determination of low molecular

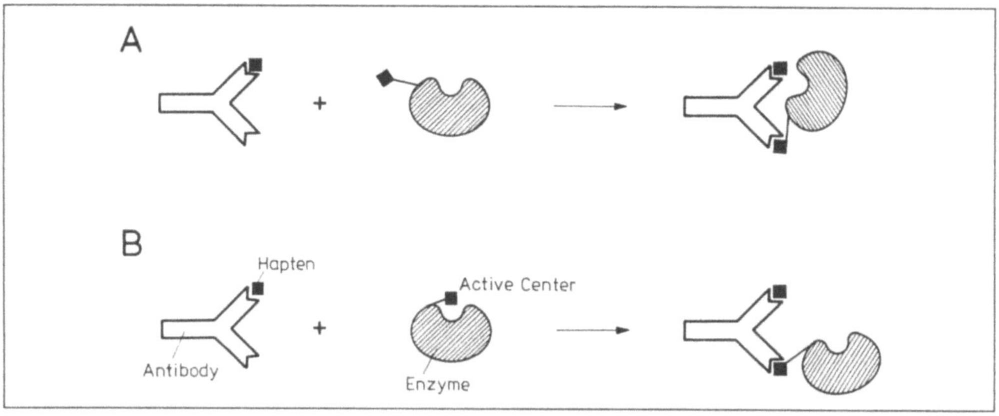

Fig. 4.3. Illustration of enzyme inhibition and activation, respectively, in homogeneous enzyme immunoassays. A) The active center of the marker enzyme is masked by the hapten component. By binding of the antibody it is accessible for substrates.
(B) Vice versa, it is also possible that the active center of an enzyme is accessible for substrates in the unbound state and that it can be masked by the antibody after binding the conjugate.

weight substances (haptens). In case of high molecular weight substances (antigens), the active center of the enzyme used as label is either not or only insufficiently modulated for sensitive indication.
Contrary to an inhibition, however, an activation of hapten-bound enzymes has also been observed. A simplified illustration of this behavior is given in Fig. 4.3A.
Homogeneous enzyme immunoassays are excellently suited to the screening and monitoring of drugs and their metabolites formed under in vivo conditions, and they are increasingly utilized in this field (Chang, 1979; Oellerich, 1979).
Adjacent to this part of the chapter, a selection of some representative homogeneous immunoassays described in the literature is provided in Table 4.2B.

4.1.4. Amplification of Immunoassays

A general enzyme amplification system was developed by Stanley et al. (1985) (cf. Johannsson et al., 1985, Self, 1985, Stanley et al., 1988) which can be used to increase both the speed and the sensitivity of enzyme immunoassays. In this method, the enzyme label is used to catalyze the dephosphorylation of $NADP^+$. The NAD^+ so formed then catalytically activates an NAD^+ specific redox cycle, yielding an intensely coloured formazan dye (Fig. 4.4.). This step requires the enzymes diaphorase and alcohol dehydrogenase. The application of this detection method has made possible an assay for thyroid-stimulating hormone (TSH) (Fig. 4.5.) and a progesterone assay which takes only 15 minutes to complete.
Another version of the enzyme amplified principle uses $K_4[Fe(CN)_6]$ instead of the tetrazolium salt, which effects the transfer of electrons from the $NAD^+/NADH$ cycle to a platinum electrode and the analytical value is recorded amperometrically (Stanley et al., 1988; cf. Cardosi et al., 1989). The application of this assay for determination of prosthatic acid phosphatase provided sensities comparable to the optical method.
Amplified enzyme immunoassays of the principle represented in Fig. 4.4. are commercially offered at present by Novo BioLabs Ltd. as NovoClone^{TM} (AELIA^{TM}) for the determination of numerous substances (e.g. TSH, prostata alkaline phosphatase, luteinising hormone, follicle stimulating hormone etc.).

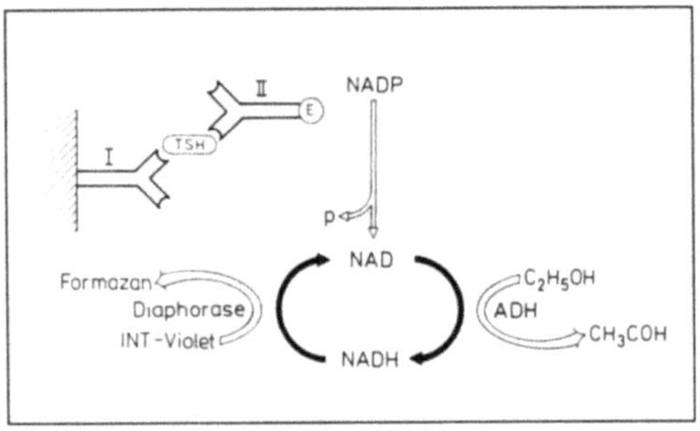

Fig. 4.4. Representation of an amplified enzyme-linked immunoassay for TSH.
I and II are mouse monoclonal antibodies specific for TSH. I is immobilized on wells of a polystyrene microtiter plate and has bound to the appropriate antigen. A second antibody II, labeled with alkaline phosphatase completes the "sandwich". The formed NAD is reduced by alcohol dehydrogenase (ADH) and ethanol. The hydrogen of NADH is transfered by diaphorase to the coloured substrate INT.
P, phosphate; INT, p-iodonitrotetrazolium violet (2-[4-iodophenyl]-3-[4-nitrophenyl]-5-phenyltetrazolium chloride). (Taken from Stanley et al., 1985).

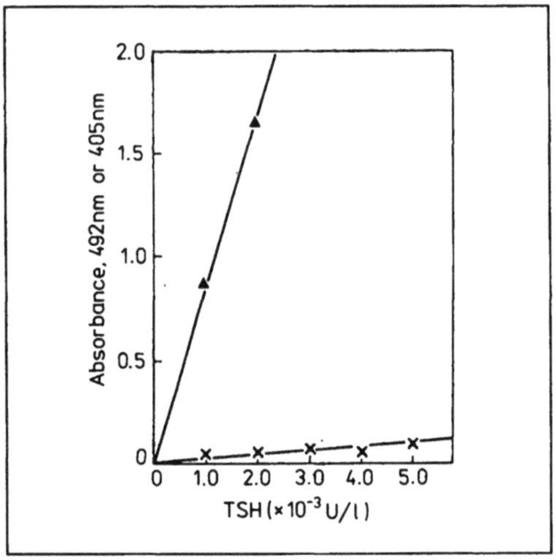

Fig. 4.5. Comparison of conventional and enzyme-amplified assay methods in an ELISA for TSH.
The adsorbance of the liquid in the wells over the reagent blank was measured at 492 nm for the enzyme-amplified system (▲) and at 405 nm for the conventional assay (x). Each point represents an average of 6 readings.
The sensitivities (defined as that concentration of TSH which corresponds to an adsorbance of the replicates of the zero standard) were as follows. Conventional method, 7 x 10^{-4} IU/l; amplified method, 1 x 10^{-5} IU/l. The 70-fold increase in sensitivity made possible by enzyme amplification provides an assay enabling precise measurements to be made of TSH levels that are in the normal adult range (Roddis et al., 1985). (Taken from Stanley at al., 1985).

4.2. Immunoblotting and Immunodot Techniques

Blotting is the process of transfering electrophoretically separated macromolecules from gels (e.g. agarose, polyacrylamide) to the surface of an immobilizing matrix (e.g. nitrocellulose (NC), polyvinylidenfluoride (PVDF), nylon membranes or chemically activated paper); reviews concerning support materials and techniques are given, for instance, by Bjerrum and Heegard, 1988, Stott, 1989, Garfin and Bers, 1989, Hunger et al., 1990) with the aim of their sensitive analytical detection.
The idea for this approach arose from the technique developed by Southern (1975) for analyzing DNA fragments. Adequate procedures for the transfer of RNA and proteins became known as Northern blotting (Bonner and Laskey, 1974; Reed and Mann, 1985; Li et al., 1987) or Western blotting (Towbin and Gordon, 1984), respectively. All these methods are highly sensitive analytical tools and suitable for the detection and characterization of even the smallest amounts of target molecules. The protein detection procedures (Western blotting) comprise three main groups:

- Total protein staining of membranes e.g. by dyes such as Coomassie brillant blue R-250, Fast green FCF and Ponceau C (Gershoni and Palade, 1983; Hancock and Tsang, 1983; Towbin and Gordon, 1984; Bers and Garfin, 1985), colloidal gold (Rohringer and Holden, 1985) or using a (strept)avidin-enzyme system after biotinylation of whole the blot (Dunn and Patel, 1988) providing a visual image of the complete protein pattern which is required for the identification of specific antigen detected in a complete protein mixture

- Protein blotting standards providing a reference for determining the molecular weights of interest, identified by suitable probes. Protein standards, moreover, are also useful for monitoring transfer efficiency and serve as controls to ensure proper location of transfer bands in repetitive screening applications.
- Immunological blotting detection abbreviated to immunoblotting (an extensive review of immunoblotting of proteins was given by BJERRUM and HEEGARD, 1988; cf. also STOTT, 1989; HOLTZHAUER, 1988): The term immunoblotting means that the protein transfered by the Western blot technique is detected via specific antibodies as probes in a one- or two-step procedure. This is possible because on the membrane surface the proteins are easily accessible to a broad variety of macromolecules inclusively immunoglobulins, whereas inside a gel the matrix generally inhibits the penetration of such probes.

Dot blotting (dot immunobinding): is a variant of Western blotting in which antigens are detected in samples spotted directly onto a membrane without prior separation (cf. Protocol 4.2.).

Three different techniques for protein transfer from gels on to membranes are in use today:

(a) Blotting by simple diffusion (transfer time 36 - 48 h): for this reason membranes may be placed on each site of the gel immersed in a suitable transfer buffer (BOWEN et al., 1980; LEE et al., 1982).

(b) A second method designated as capillary blotting (transfer time about 2 h; STOTT, 1989) rests on the flow of the solvent from the gel through the membrane induced by capillary attraction. For this purpose, the membrane is placed on top of the gel followed by chromatography paper and a pile of paper towels on the top of the membrane (SMITH and SUMMERS, 1980; REINHART and MALAMUD, 1982). Transfer is aided by placing a source of buffer in the form of wet chromatography paper under the gel (cf. SOUTHERN, 1975).

Methods (a) and (b) work best with agarose gels which have very large pores that do not hinder the movement of high molecular weight proteins (SCHIBECI et al., 1986).

(c) Electrotransfer (Western blot) (TOWBIN et al., 1979; BITTNER et al., 1980) normally prefered for polyacrylamide gels and which is the technique most frequently applied today (transfer time about 2 h; cf. STOTT, 1989). In each of these ways, replica blots are obtained on the membrane.

A variant of electroblotting of proteins is the so-called semi-dry transfer described by KYHSE-ANDERSEN (1984), which now is preferred because it is faster and easier to manipulate than procedures following TOWBIN's protocol.

For the semi-dry blotting the wet transfer membrane, on which the electrophoresis gel is positioned, is placed between several sheets of filter paper, soaked with buffer. This stack is than put between two carbon electrodes as described in Protocol 4.3. As a consequence of the tight structure mostly only 0.8 milliamps per cm^2 (constant current) are needed, resulting in a voltage lower than 20 V. The low power consumption of the transfer system affords no further cooling. In spite of the low voltage applied inside the transfer unit a field strength of more than 10 V/cm will be achieved which guarantees high transfer speed as well as high transfer yield.

Recently, ZENG et al. (1990) described an enhancement in transfer efficiency onto nitrocellulose or polyvinylidene difluoride (PVDF) membranes when the electrophoresis gel was soaked in a buffer containing up to 30% polyethylene glycol (PEG 2000) prior to semi-dry transfer.

Analogous to ELISA or dot blot procedures, after finishing a transfer it is first necessary to block (quench) unbound membrane sides to prevent nonspecific binding of the used probes in the subsequent detection step. The blocking agent(s) and blocking conditions will largely depend on the type of the membrane and the sensitivity of the system under investigation. A general protocol (Protocol 4.2.) demonstrating both the run of dot immunobinding and immunoblotting of electrotransfered proteins is given in the following:

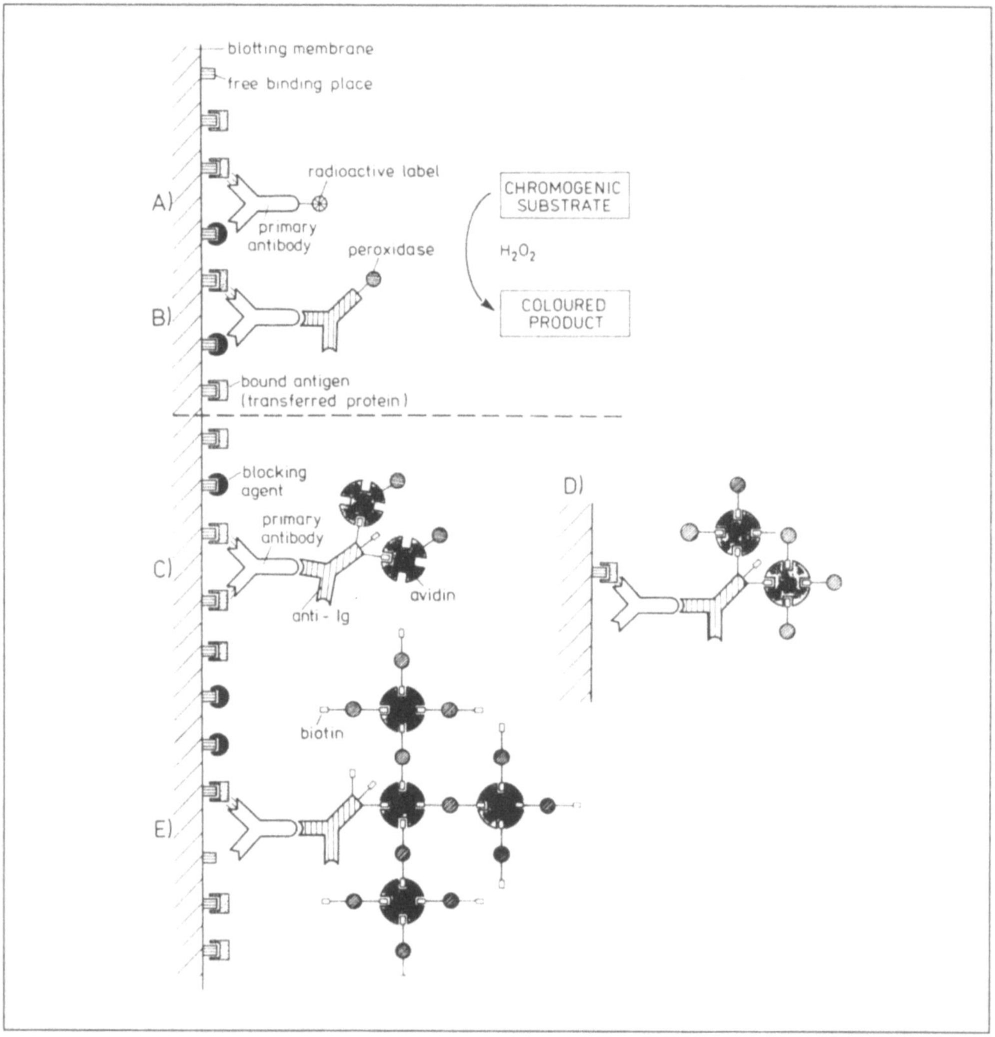

Fig. 4.6. Schematic representation of immunodetection of proteins transferred on a blotting membrane
A) Detection by binding a radioactively labeled specific antibody;
B) Detection by binding a specific antibody followed by a peroxidase-labeled anti-Ig. After adding the chromogenic substrate the membrane is stained on places where the protein is bound.
C) - E) Enhancement of sensitivity by application of the avidin/biotin system.
C) The secondary antibody is labeled with biotin and interacts with enzyme-avidin conjugate(s);
D) further enhancement of sensitivity is attained when unmodified avidin is added after binding the secondary biotin-labeled antibody followed by an enzyme-biotin conjugate;
E) finally considerable amplification is possible when the enzyme conjugate contains two or more biotin molecules.

Protocol 4.2.[a]: **Determination of proteins by dot immunobinding and immunoblotting**

1. Application of antigen

1.1. Dots:

0.5 - 1.0 μl of antigen-containing sample solution is given on to 3 x 3 mm squares of nitrocellulose membranes. After drying at 45°C within 15 minutes they are agitated for 5 minutes in TBS (pH 7.3) and subsequently given in the wells of a microtiter plate.

1.2. Blots:

Proteins are separated by gel electrophoresis according to LAEMMLI (1970) and electrotransfered onto nitrocellulose sheets. These are dried and subsequently cut in strips which are given onto glass tubes or grooves.

2. Detection of antigen (cf. Fig. 4.6B.)

- block unspecific binding places of nitrocellulose surface with a solution of 5 % skimmed milk powder (other substances as, for instance, gelatin, serum albumin or polyvinyl pyrrolidone may also be used in lower concentrations) in TBS + 0.05 % Tween 20 for 10 minutes under agitation at room temperature (0.05 - 1.0 ml/dot or 0.5 -1.0 ml/ blotted strip);
- remove the blocking solution;
- add the antibody-containing solution(s) in volume(s) nearly identical to that (those) used in the blocking step and incubate overnight at 4°C (3 hours at room temperature are also sufficient);
- rinse twice with PBS + 0.05 % Tween 20;
- add secondary antibody (anti-rabbit or anti-sheep/goat peroxidase conjugate) in suitable dilution with the blocking solution (in most cases between 1:1,000 - 1:5,000) and incubate for 90 - 120 minutes under agitation at room temperature;
- rinse five times with TBS and suck off;
- stain the dot/blots by addition of TBS containing 0.06 ml/ml of a freshly prepared solution of 4-chloro-1-naphthol (3 mg in 1 ml methanol; store it dry and in the dark for up to two weeks only) and 0.001 ml/ml 30 % H_2O_2.
- from this solution give 0.1 ml per dot or 0.05 - 1.0 ml on blotted strips, respectively. The staining is generally finished within 30 minutes;
- finally rinse with water and dry the sheets or strips.

[a] We thank Dr. J. STAHL for providing the protocol.

KYHSE-ANDERSEN described in his paper the application of this transfer method for simultaneous electrotransfer of up to six gels in one stack. In the following the transfer protocol for only one gel is given.

Protocol 4.3.: **Semi-dry blotting of proteins from polyacrylamide gels**

(modified KYHSE-ANDERSEN protocol according to HOLTZHAUER (1988), pp. 54-57)

This protocol is given for the transfer from SDS-polyacrylamide gels (LAEMMLI system). When proteins were separated in other systems, the transfer buffers should be adapted to the buffer constituents of the separating system.

- Cut thick filter paper in the dimension of the electrophoresis gel to be blotted.
- Soak it in 0.3 M Tris base and put it on a flat carbon electrode (anode).
- Wet a further filter paper and the tansfer membrane (nitrocellulose, PVDF or the like) in 25 mM Tris base.
- Put the second filter paper, the membrane and the gel onto the first filter sheet.
- Cover this stack with a third filter paper, soaked in a buffer containing 0.3 M Tris base, 0.5 % ε-aminocaproic acid, 0.05 % SDS.
- Remove air blubles between the different layers by gentle pressure. Close the transfer stack with the second carbon electrode (cathode).
- Electrotransfer is performed for 1 h at room temperatur with a current densitiy 0.8 mA/cm^2.
- Originally, KYHSE-ANDERSEN described a buffer system containing 20 % methanol. It should be tested for the distinct problem to be solved whether the precence or absence of methanol improves sensitivity, transfer efficiency and/or transfer time.

A transfer system, different to that of KHYSE-ANDERSEN only in the use of boric acid instead of ε-aminocaproic acid, was described by HIRANO

Table 4.3. Proteins Detected by Immunoblotting (selected examples)

Antigenic protein(s)	Gel	Membrane	Transfer buffer	Blocking agent	Primary antibody	Second overlay	References
Human serum proteins	a)	b)	c)	4% BSA in TBS	rabbit ab against human serum proteins	anti-rabbit swine ab (HRP-conjugate)	Kyse-Anderson, 1984
Non-histone chromatine proteins from mouse plasma cytoma Adj PC5	a) + urea	b)	Tris/glycine, pH 8.8	10% sheep serum	rabbit anti-serum, 3% BSA	^{125}I-labeled anti-Ig or HRP-conjugated Ig, stained with o-dianisidine/H_2O_2	Stott, et al., 1985
Rat brain subcellular fractions	a)	b)	0.7% acetic acid	10% FCS in TBS pH 7.4	ConA	HRP in blocking solution, stained with 4-chloro-1-naphthol/H_2O_2	Hawkes, 1983
SV40 specific proteins	a)	diazo-phenyl-thioether paper	Na-borate pH 9.2	10% ethanolamine 0.25% gelatin pH 9	rabbit antisera	^{125}I-labeled protein A[d]	Reiser and Wardale, 1981
SV40 viral polypeptides	a)	b)	Tris/HCL, pH 8.3, glycine + 20% methanol	0.25% gelatin in Tris/HCl, pH 7.4	rabbit antiserum	^{125}I-labeled protein A[d]	Lin and Katsamatsu, 1983
Glycoproteins [e]	a)	b)	tris/glycine + 20% methanol	3% gelatin in PBS	ConA	HRP, stained with 4-chloro-1-naphthol/H_2O_2	Faye and Chrispeels, 1985
Bovine brain homogenates	a)	b) or f)	a) Tris/glycine, pH 8.3 (with or without methanol) or b) Tris/boric acid	for b): 2% BSA or 1% Hb; for f): 10% BSA	rabbit anti-protein I (synapsin)	^{125}I-labeled protein A[d]	Gershoni and Palade, 1982

Table 4.3. Continued from page 132

Antigenic protein(s)	Gel	Membrane	Transfer buffer	Blocking agent	Primary antibody	Second overlay	References
BLV proteins	[a] + urea	cyanuric chloride activated paper	2 % acetic acid	1 % gelatin	ab against complete BLV protein, protein p24 and protein p15	^{125}I-labeled protein A	Hunger et al., 1986
Human parotid saliva proteins	PAA	[b]	e.g. Tris/HCl [g]	3 % BSA, pH 7.5	antiserum against a partially purified bacterial aggregating factor found in parotid saliva	HRP-conjugated goat anti-rabbit IgA, IgG, IgM, stained with o-dianisidine/H_2O_2	Reinhart and Malamud, 1982
Actin binding high molecular weight proteins from HeLa cells	[a]	[b]	Tris, pH 7.3	BSA pH 7.3	goat anti-serum	rhodamin conjugated rabbit antigoat IgG	Weihing, 1983
Chicken intestinal calbindin D_{28K}	[a]	[b]	[c]	3 % BSA, pH 7.4	specific ab	alkaline phosphatase conjugated ab, nitro-blue tetrazolium salt + BCIP[h]	Ono and Tuan, 1990
Human milk galactosyltransferase; pig kidney glucosidase II	[a]	[b]	0.7 % acetic acid	0.5 % BSA, pH 7.4	specific ab	protein A gold, subsequently silver staining	Brada and Roth, 1984

[a] SDS-PAA, [b] nitrocellulose, [c] a) 0.3 M Tris, pH 7.4, b) 25 mM Tris, pH 10.4, c) 25 mM Tris, pH 9.4, 40 mM 6-amino-n-hexanoic acid; each with 20 % methanol, [d] detected by autoradiography, [e] phaseolin, phytohemagglutinin, jackbean α-mannosidase, glycosylated ConA precursor, [f] nylon, [g] non electrophoretic transfer, [h] 5-bromo-4-chloro-3-indolylphosphate

(1989). This system should be used when amino acids interfer with the following steps, for instance in amino acid analysis.

- The individual protein bands on the membrane were visualized as described in Protocol 4.2, Part 2.

It is noteworthy that Coomassie-stained gels can also be transfered after a 2 x 15 min equilibration in the Tris-SDS-ε-aminocaproic acid buffer of the gel stored in aqueous methanol-acetic acid solution.

- Immunochemical detection of antigens is performed after blocking as described in Protocol 4.2, point 2. An enhancement in sensitivity is possible if 4,4'-diaminobenzidine or the non-carcinogenic 4,4-diamino diphenylether is used as substrate of peroxidase in the presence of 0.1 mg/ml $CuSO_4$ and 0.05 mg/ml $NiSO_4$.

- An importent increase in sensitivity is achieved by chemoluminiscence detection. The Western blot is performed as usual, but instead of a colour-forming substrate a substance is used which emits light when cleaved by the indicator enzyme. The light is registrated by a contact copy onto a X-ray film.

Substrates for alkaline phosphatase are AMPPD (3-(2'-spiroadamantane)-4-methoxy-4-(3"-phosphoryloxy)phenyl-1,2-dioxethane, Boehringer Mannheim, Germany) and the ECL reagents (Enhanced Chemiluminiscent, Amersham, GB) for peroxidase.

Some examples of usual membranes, transfer buffers, blocking (quenching) agents, primary antibodies and detectable secondary overlays are included in Table 4.3. Further detailed information is given in the review articles by GERSHONI and PALADE (1983), TOWBIN and GORDON (1984), BERS and GARFIN (1985) as well as STOTT (1989). For the detection of any transfered protein use direct probing with an antigen-specific labeled antibody (primary antibody) as schematically represented in Fig. 4.6A. Lectin conjugates for the detection of glycoproteins, labeled DNA or RNA for nucleic acid binding proteins and hormones as probes for the corresponding receptors are also used as primary layers.

If this primary probe has not been labeled, a secondary labeled probe is applied. For this purpose conjugates of anti-immunoglobulins and bacterial Ig-receptors (protein A, protein G) or colloidal gold conjugates obtained by mixing antibodies, protein A or protein G, respectively, with colloidal gold spheres (15 - 20 nm in diameter) (SUREK and LATZKO, 1984; HSU, 1984; BRADA and ROTH, 1984) may be employed.

Early systems used reagents conjugated with ^{125}I and the target protein was determined by autoradiography. The multiple drawbacks (e.g. short lifetime of the conjugate, protracted washing steps), however, have encouraged an increasing use of other nonradioactive labels as enzymes (e.g. colour reactions of alkaline phosphatase, horseradish peroxidase (cf. Fig. 4.6B.)), fluorochromes (e.g. fluorescein (TOWBIN et al., 1979; MIRANDE et al., 1982, rhodamine (WEIHING, 1983)), chemiluminiscence (peroxidase-catalyzed oxidation of luminol (LEONG et al., 1986) or enzymatic dephosphorylation of luciferin-O-phosphate (HAUBER and GEIGER, 1987), for review see KRICKA et al., 1988) or colloidal gold spheres. Some advantages and disadvantages of selected detection reagents are given in Table 4.4.

A sensitive detection of membrane-bound proteins is also made possible by exploiting the avidin/biotin system (in which streptavidin is preferably applied because it is more rarely adsorbed unspecifically than egg white avidin; cf. also Chapter 2.5.). This system may be used in three different variants (cf. Fig. 4.6C. and 4.6D.).

I. In the first, the primary antibody interacting with the transfered protein is overlayed with the biotinylated anti-Ig followed by a labeled avidin (in which horseradish peroxidase may be used as label; cf. Fig. 4.6C.).

II. An enhanced detection effect is achieved when a second, biotinylated anti-Ig is overlayed with avidin followed by the biotinylated enzyme (Fig. 4.6D.).

III. In the most sensitive variant (Fig. 4.6E.) a complex of avidin and biotinylated enzyme is allowed to bind biotinylated anti-Ig. Various detection kits basing on avidin-biotin interaction are available commercially (e.g. systems offered by

Table 4.4. Comparsion of Several Detection Reagents [a)]

Detectable component:	HRP	Alkaline phosphatase	Colloidal gold
Sensitivity [pg]	250-500	10-50	100-200 1-25 [b)]
Stability of stored blot	poor	poor	good
Total assay time [h]	3	3-24	5-24
Costs	low	medium	high

[a)] according to WALKER (1988), [b)] the gold stained membrane is incubated 10 - 15 minutes in a silver/lactate solution whereby the gold spheres are overlayed by metallic silver.

AMERSHAM, BIO-RAD, PIERCE, VECTOR LABORATORIES).

Frequently a quantitation of the amount of antigen present in a transfered band is desirable. When the probe is radiolabeled for example, this is possible by scanning the autoradiograph in a transmission densiometer or manually with a planimeter or by cutting out the band and counting. A linear correlationship between the image density and antigen concentration could be obtained in this way for some substances (HOWE and HERSHEY, 1981; VAESSEN et al., 1981; BATTEIGER et al., 1982).

Coloured bands on transfer membranes can be quantified by reflectance densitometry (GUENGERICH et al., 1982; RORDORF et al., 1983) or by rendering the membrane transparent (e.g. by soaking in an organic solvent such as toluene or xylene) and scanning with a transmission densitometer (NAKAMURA et al., 1985; STOTT et al., 1985; PALFREYMAN et al., 1988). But in all cases, it should be mentioned that this linearity exists only in a distinct range of protein amaount and varies with the protein species. For exact determination of protein quantities by radioactive as well as by photometric methods dose-response curves have to be constructed for each antigen (problems of data processing are discussed for instance by TJISSEN (1985), pp. 385-421).

4.3. Immunosorbents for Therapeutical Application - Immunosorbent Reactors

The removal of pathogenic substances (drugs, toxins, other undesirable low and high molecular weight substances) from the circulation by immunosorption is a technique with promising clinical significance. For this purpose, extracorporeal reactors filled with immobilized antibodies specific for the substance to be removed have been developed in the last few years. At first these were applied in animal experiments and, thereafter, increasingly too for selected therapeutic purposes in human medicine.

Such devices that remove preferentially low-density lipoprotein (LDL) from plasma have been used successfully in some hospitals to treat patients with severe hypercholesterolemia (STOFFEL et al., 1981; PARKER and STUDEBAKER, 1988; cf.: SAAL et al., 1986; GORDON et al., 1990). One of the principal techniques for performing this procedure uses immunoadsorption columns containing monospecific polyclonal sheep antibodies to human LDL covalently linked to Sepharose CL-4B by the CNBr-method (STOFFEL and DEMANT, 1981; PARKER and STUDEBAKER, 1988).

The efficiency of this method is demonstrated in Table 4.5. which summarizes the results of four plasma separator-anti-LDL-Sepharose immunoadsorption experiments in pigs (STOFFEL and DEMAND, 1981). With increasing volumes of blood passing through the shunt, there was a progressive decrease in the plasma LDL concentration.

LDL-pheresis in man proved to be both safe and effective as a procedure for selective lowering of the plasma LDL cholesterol levels. In longer treatments under in vivo conditions up to 93 % of the LDL could be removed by two columns each filled with 400 ml of the gel to achieve posttreatment levels as low as 12 mg/dl. The degree of LDL-lowering is limited only by the amount removed at each procedure and the frequency of the treatment. Both of these variables are under the control of the investigator (PARKER and STUDEBAKER, 1988).

Table 4.5. LDL Removal in vivo by Plasma Separation-anti-LDL-Sepharose Immunoadsorption

Exp.	Duration [min]	Blood volume passing [ml/min]	LDL removed [mg]	Initial plasma LDL remaining [a] [%]
1	105	60	660	36
2	150	110	670	33
3	145	230	1560	27
4	230	220	1830	16

[a] Initial concentration ranged from 1.5 to 1.8 mg LDL per ml of plasma (taken from STOFFEL and DEMAND, 1981)

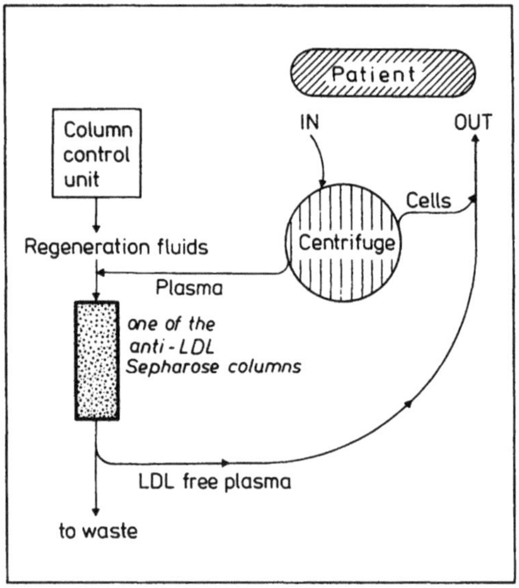

Fig. 4.7. Representation of the LDL-pheresis system (taken from PARKER and STUDEBAKER, 1988; for detailed information see ibid.)

A schematic representation of such a practically applied LDL-apherese system is shown in Fig. 4.7. The components have to accomplish four separate tasks under sterile and endotoxin-free conditions: (i) plasma separation: plasma separators are required because solid supports such as foreign materials can change several reactive components of the blood (e.g. clotting platelets); (ii) immunosorption as the essential step: 2 to 3 immunoadsorption columns, each capable of binding 10-12 g of LDL, are committed to the exclusive use of each patient; (iii) preservation and regeneration of the immunosorbent: NaN_3 is used for preservation, acid glycine, pH 2.9, for regeneration of the columns and saline as well as phosphate-buffered saline, pH 7.4, for washing steps; (iv) flow control units for blood, plasma and regeneration units.

One of the most essential problems to be solved, however, is the prevention of adsorbent leakage leading to impurties of plasma and blood respectively followed by immune reactions of the patient.

Beyond this, extracorporeal reactors have also been applied for the removal of various other plasma proteins by immunoadsorption. Columns with immobilized A or B blood group substances are used in the therapy of patients with existing antibodies to these substances prior to bone marrow transplation (BENSINGER et al., 1981).

Immobilized protein A is used in extracorporeal reactors to remove IgG or circulating immune complexes in patients with systemic lupus erythematosus (TERMAN et al., 1979) and cancer (TERMAN et al., 1981), respectively, as well as inhibitors to clotting proteins (NILSSON et al., 1981).

A possible procedure for the selective extracorporeal removal of anti-acetylcholine receptor antibodies appearing in patients with Myasthenia gravis (an organ-specific autoimmune disease) by protein A-Sepharose columns from plasma was evaluated by SOMMER and LANGVAD (1989). A full-scale in vitro experiment (a 4 litre volume of myasthenic plasma in a reservoir alternatingly recirculated over two columns filled with 100 ml gel) demonstrated the adsorption of 43% of the circulating anti-acetylcholine receptor antibodies within 70 minutes.

SATO et al. (1989) described a therapeutic immunosorption system that can remove IgE effectively and specifically from the plasma of patients with allergy or other hyper-IgE syndromes. As the immunosorbent, immunopurified anti-IgE antibodies immobilized on controlled pore glass beads (50 nm pore sizes) were used for this purpose. Such methods subjected to in vitro and clinical tests worked sufficiently in a wide range of IgE concentrations.

An example of the removal of drugs by an extracorporeal reactor, the immunoadsorption of digoxin from the circulation using immobilized monoclonal antibodies was recently described by BRIZGYS et al. (1989)

All these results so far obtained demonstrate impressively that the principle of immunoadsorption is more widely applicable and could provide new possibilities in medical therapy. To what extent this assumption is true will have to be proved by future investigations.

4.4. Immunosensors

Immunosensors are analytical devices based primarily on the immune complex formation (cf. Chapter 1.2.4.). In contrast to enzyme sensors relying on catalytic principles they are still in an experimental stage. Therefore, the introduction of marketable systems can be expected only in the next few years.

Table 4.6. Classification of Immunosensors *)

Sensors with electrochemical detection

1. amperometric devices, 2. potentiometric devices,
3. immunofield effect transistors,
4. immunoreactors with electrochemical detection.

Non-electrode sensors

5. immunoreactors with thermometric detection,
6. optical immunosensors (optrodes),
7. piezoelectric systems.

*) It is possible: (a) to cover the active surface of a transducer (electrodes, transistors, piezoelectric quartz crystals, reflecting layers etc.) directly with the immune component able to recognize the analyte, or (b) to bind this component at first on a suitable support (e.g. particles, membranes) followed by its (indirect) combination with the transducer.

Classification of immunosensors can be made under various aspects. In the following, selected examples illustrating the general principle of such devices will be discussed in the order shown in Table 4.6. (a comprehensive coverage of this matter was recently given by SCHELLER and SCHUBERT (1989).

4.4.1. Immunosensors with Electrochemical Detection

1. Amperometric devices: A membrane immunosensor for the determination of insulin and albumin, respectively, was described by MATTIASSON and NILSSON already in 1977. This sensor was designed as a flow-through cell and consists of a pO_2-electrode which is combined with a nylon net covered with covalently bound rabbit anti-human serum albumin or guinea pig anti-porcine insulin antibodies.

The cycle starts with 0.1 M potassium phosphate buffer, pH 7.0, followed by the addition of a mixture of the antigen to be assayed and the enzyme-labeled antigen molecules (insulin-catalase or albumin-glucoseoxidase conjugate, respectively). After a wash in 0.1 M phosphate buffer, pH 7.0, being in 1 M NaCl for 1 minute, the sensor is ready for assay. The amount of enzyme trapped in the immunoreaction is determined by introducing a pulse of a suitable substrate solution (H_2O_2 or glucose, respectively) followed by buffer until the system is in equilibrium again. A 3 minutes pulse of 0.2 M glycine/HCl buffer, pH 2.2, is used to split the antigen-antibody complex. After 1 minute washing with buffer, the system is ready for another assay.

A further typical example described by AIZAWA et al. (1980) concerns the determination of AFP. For this reason, rabbit anti-AFP is immobilized on a cellulose triacetate membrane via 1,8-diamino-4-aminomethyloctane and glutaraldehyde. This antibody-covered membrane is combined with a Clark-type oxygen electrode and applied for determination of the analyte in the presence of known concentrations of an AFP/catalase conjugate. After (competitive) binding of

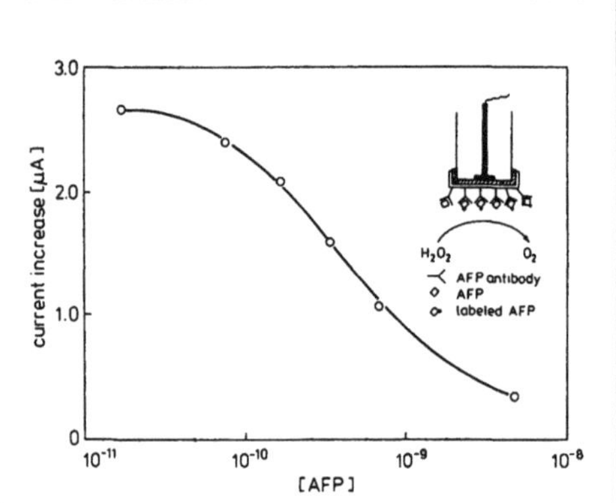

Fig. 4.8. Schematic representation of an amperometric immunosensor and calibration curve for determination of α-fetoprotein (AFP) by a competitive assay.
The sensor containing an anti-AFP covered membrane is brought in contact with a sample solution containing AFP and 650 "catalase units" of labeled AFP and is allowed to stand at 37°C for 2 h. After washing with 0.05 M phosphate buffer, pH 7 (the pH range 6.0 - 7.5 was found to be the optimum for the immunochemical reaction), the activity of the membrane-bound catalase is assayed by placing the sensor in phosphate buffer. When the output current of the sensor becomes constant, 100 μl of 3 % H_2O_2 is injected, and the increase in current is measured after a steady state has been achieved (taken from AIZAWA et al., 1980).

the free and catalase-labeled AFP, H_2O_2 was added as substrate and the sensor was tested for its catalase activity (cf. Fig. 4.8.). AFP can be determined by this sensor in a range of 10^{-11} - 10^{-8} g/ml as is shown in Fig. 4.8. (Standard deviation: 15 % at an AFP concentration of 10^{-9} g/ml; n = 25).

A further principle of an electrode-supported competitive enzyme immunoassay for the determination of factor VIII-antigen using alkaline phosphatase as marker enzyme was described by RENNEBERG et al. (1983). After the addition of native and labeled phosphatase, the bound phosphatase activity was determined by a glucoseoxidase containing biosensor. For this reason, glucose-6-phosphate is added and the H_2O_2 formed from liberated glucose by reaction with O_2 is measured. This approach still allows determinations of 1.56 x 10^{-2} U/ml factor VIII-antigen in plasma (lower detection limit) and, therefore, is quite comparable in its sensitivity to spectrophotometric methods.

An amperometric principle for the determination of serum insulin using a H_2O_2-sensitive electrode was described by KAKU et al. (1989). A microporous polypropylene membrane was partially hydrophilized by vapour/plasma treatment and activated with octamethylene diamine and glutaric aldehyde followed by binding of protein A. After addition of anti-insulin IgG this device was found to be suitable for the determination of insulin between 1 and 10^4 μU/ml in serum by the competitive method in the presence of glucoseoxidase-labeled insulin.

2. Potentiometric devices: Direct potentiometric immunosensors are based on changes of the potential or the dielectric constant near the surface of an electrode caused by adsorption of charged biomolecules and the resulting variation of the electrochemical double layer. Both membrane electrodes with immobilized antibodies and electrodes directly covered with antibodies or antigens have been described in the literature.

A simple potentiometric sensor-supported enzyme immonoassay based on the principle of a competitive immunoassay was developed by MEYERHOFF and RECHNITZ already in 1979 for the determination of BSA (lower detection limit 10 ng/ml) and cAMP (lower detection limit about 10 nmol/l). The enzyme urease was used as marker, and the enzyme activity was determined by means of a NH_3-sensitive electrode.

Ionic selective electrodes for the determination of antibodies against cortisol, digoxin, dinitrophenol and serum albumin were described by KEATING and RECHNITZ (1983, 1984) as well as by SOLSKY and RECHNITZ (1981). Further types of potentiometric immunosensors have been tested successfully by MEYERHOFF and RECHNITZ (1979) and ALEXANDER and MALTRA (1982).

Recently, catalytic antibodies for molecular recognition were introduced as a new class in potentiometric biosensors relying on selective catalysis by the antibody to generate acidic products which change the pH at the surface of an underlying pH electrode. BLACKBURN et al. (1990) described such a prototype biosensor in which a micro-pH electrode is modified with a catalytic antibody (induced in mice by phenylphosphonate coupled to KLH) that catalyzes the hydrolysis of phenylacetate, producing hydrogen ions that can be monitored by the electrode. The reversible response was linear with the log of substrate concentration over a range of 20 - 500 μM.

Generally, potentiometric immunosensors need a longer time for adjustment of the equilibrium and are less sensitive than the comparable immunoassays.

3. Immuno-field effect transistors (immuno-FET's): Immuno-FET's are obtained when the gate of an ion-selective field effect transistor (ISFET) is combined with an isolating membrane covered with an antibody or an antigen. On this basis, for example, immuno-FET's sensitive for anti-albumin and anti-syphilis antibodies have been developed (BERGVELD et al., 1987). Investigations in this field, however, have not yet gone beyond the experimental level.

4. Immunoreactors with electrochemical detection: The combination of an immunoassay with an electrochemical or thermometric probe allows the application of reactors (e.g. a column) as an analytical device.

Contrary to "real" immunosensors, where the detector and the biologically active layer are combined directly, reactor immunosensors are flow-through systems with a detector being arranged behind the chemically anchored, biologically active molecules. Reactor immunosensors are generally sensitive and allow rapid determinations; they can be regenerated and used repeatedly ($\approx$ 500 times). Despite the high technical expense of their process control, they are the most suitable ones at present.

An immunoreactor with electrochemical detection based on a two-side binding test (sandwich-ELISA) was described by DEALWIS and WILSON in 1985.

For the determination of anti-IgGs, as part of the flow-through system a minireactor was filled with bovine IgG immobilized on Reactigel-6X (PIERCE). At a flow rate of 0.5 ml/min, samples of mouse monoclonal anti-bovine IgG and GOD-labeled goat anti-mouse IgG (GOD-conjugate) were added at intervals of two minutes. The enzymatic activity of GOD correlating with the concentration of anti-IgG in the sample was then ascertained by three successive injections of glucose, and the H_2O_2 formed was measured amperometrically. After each determination the bound antibody and the conjugate were eluted with an acidic buffer, pH 2, and after equilibration with the measuring buffer the reactor was ready for further use. This method was suitable for the determination of IgG concentrations between the femtomol to the picomol range, with a coefficient of variation amounting to 3 %. At higher antibody concentrations it was possible to work with a minimal incubation time of 6 seconds. The reactor could be used for three months or at least for about 500 determinations.

An improved reactor immunosensor for the determination of theophyllin and insulin respectively, was described by LEE and MEYERHOFF (1988). The native and the enzyme labeled antigens at first compete with a non-fixed primary antibody followed by injection of this complex into the reactor chamber which contains an excess of a bound secondary antibody. After washing, the substrate of the enzyme is added and the signal registered. With this method, theophyllin can be measured between 0.025 - 0.25 μM and insulin between 1 - 250 μg/l.

4.4.2. Non-electrode Sensors

5. Immunoreactors with thermometric detection: Another group of immunoreactors based on heterogeneous immunoassays (ELISA's) uses the principle of calorimetric measurement (designated the TELISA-method; cf. BIRNBAUM et al., 1986). Antibodies are bound covalently to a solid phase support (e.g. Sepharose CL-4B particles) and filled in the reactor chamber of a flow-through device. After binding of the native and enzyme-labeled antigen to the respective antibody and washing, the activity of the bound enzyme is determined with the aid of a thermistor.

Table 4.7. Thermometric Enzyme Immunotests Using Antibodies Covalently Bound on Sepharose CL-4B

Substance	Immobilized antibody	Label	Detection range	Required time	Life-time of the reactor
Gentamycin	anti-gentamycin ab	catalase POD	0.01-0.9 μg/ml	9-12 min	8 days [a]
HSA	anti-HSA ab	catalase	10^{-13} - 10^{-8} mol/l		15-20 determinations [a]
Proinsulin	anti-insulin ab	POD	0.1-50 μg/l	13 min	14-21 days [b]

[a] Borrebeack et al., 1978, [b] Birnbaum et al., 1986.

Enzyme immunoreactors with thermometric indication have been described, e.g. for the analytical determination of gentamycin and HSA (Borrebeack et al., 1978) as well as for proinsulin (Birnbaum et al., 1986). Catalase and peroxidase respectively have been used as marker enzymes. By rinsing with low pH buffer (0.2 M glycine/HCl, pH 2.2) the immune complexes were split off and the matrix was ready for the next use. Some parameters of interest concerning the discussed method are given in Table 4.7.

Since the specificity of an assay method depends on the type of antibodies immobilized, the TELISA method is also widely applicable to many other substances of interest, provided that the required antibodies are available.

6. Optical immunosensors (optrodes): Antigen-antibody reactions on surfaces modify certain optical properties on these surfaces. Such optical parameters include light adsorption, reflection, refraction, scattering etc., which may vary as a result of immune complex formation. Therefore, repeated attempts have been made to use these effects as a basis for analytical test systems (cf. GBF Monographs, Vol. 13; 1989). Furthermore, methods have also been described which utilize shifts of fluorescence signals for analytical purposes (Place et al., 1985).

A simple optical method based on a substrate with a high refractive index (e.g. silicon) and the reflection of light was described by Arwin and Lindström (1985). For the application, silicon wafers (10 x 5 x 0.3 mm) were covered with dichloromethylsilane followed by treatment with a solution of HSA. Subsequently, these pieces were incubated in serum containing anti-HSA of different dilutions. Silicon has a high refractive index of $n \approx 4$, which provides an optical contrast to organic layers which normally have $n \approx 1.5$. These differences were used by the authors to study changes of surface dependent properties of anti-HSA adsorption with the aid of an ellipsometer (cf. Stenberg and Nygren, 1982). It was shown that this method provides a linear correlation of the reflectance change between 5-50 μg anti-HSA/ml serum.

Recently, Robinson et al. (1990) described an immunosensor named FCFD (fluorescence capillary fill device ; cf. Badley et al., 1987) which is based on the fluorescence of labeled antibodies and can be carried out in the capillary interspace of two parallel glass plates as a sandwich or a competitive assay respectively.

A sandwich assay format using two monoclonal antibodies against different epitopes was used to monitor HCG (Deacon et al., 1990) or Rubella antibodies in serum (Parry et al., 1990). The first antibody was covalently immobilized to the base-plate wave guide. The second was conjugated to a fluorophore (e.g. FITC) and microdosed onto the top plate of the FCFD. On addition of the sample, the labeled antigen dissolves and the resulting immune complex forms the base plate. Due to the very small capillary gap, the FCFD is able to produce equilibrium data within 3 to 15 minutes, depending on the analyte, assay format and antibody affinity.

As FCFD is illuminated with light of the fluorophore excitation wavelength, both bound and free (excess) fluorophore is excited. The signal is measured at the FCFD end face. Light emitted from the end face within the range of angles which are bounded by the critical angle result from fluorophore within the evanescent region only (i.e. the bound fluorophore in the assay). Measurements in this range are largely independent of excess solution fluorescence.

Another recent optical technique for quantitative analysis of molecular interactions in real time and without the need for labels or purification steps is being developed for commercial purposes by Amersham International and Pharmacia Biosensor AB. Both systems employ surface plasmon resonance (SPR) as the basic principle (cf. Scheller and Schubert, 1989).

SPR is a phenomenon which occurs between incoming photons and the electrons in the surface of a thin metal film mounted on a glass support. At a specific angle of incident plane-polarized light, energy is transfered to the electrons causing the reflected light to disappear. This angle of "non-reflectance", the resonance angle, changes proportionally to the change of mass concentration caused, e.g. by binding of substances to, or dissociation from, the surface of the chip.

The sensing interface of the BIAcore™ device (BIA = biospecific interaction analysis) as developed by Pharmacia is an exchangeable sensor chip consisting of a glass support coated with a gold film. Additionally, a layer of carboxylated dextran is covalently bound to the surface. This layer increases the effective surface area and eliminates non-specific binding.

By immobilizing a biospecific ligand within the dextran layer specific interactions can be analyzed directly in complex samples without prior purification. For immobilization of the ligand, the carboxyl groups on the surface are activated by N-hydroxy-succinimide and N-ethyl-N'-(dimethylaminopropyl) carbodiimide. Unreacted groups are deactivated after binding of the ligand by ethanolamine/HCl. The SPR resonance is measured in resonance units (RU); for most proteins 1,000 RU (1 kRU) corresponds to a surface concentration of approximately 1 ng/mm^2. Determinations of specific proteins in serum down to 20 ng/ml and macromolecular association constants from 10^7 M^{-1} up to $4 * 10^{11}$ M^{-1} are documented examples. An average analysis takes approximately 5 to 10 minutes. Moreover, the technique does not require molecular labels such as isotopes or spectroscopic markers.

BIAcore™ has been applied for concentration measurements of theophyllin (PAN 202) and β_2-microglobulin in the clinically important concentration range of 20 to 1,000 ng/ml (PAN 201). For determination of β_2-microglobulin in serum samples anti-β_2-microglobulin was covalently bound to the sensor chip. The sample containing the analyte is injected over the immobilized antibody followed by addition of polyclonal anti-β_2-microglobulin to improve the sensitivity. The sensor chip is regenerated with 10 mM HCl before the next use.

Further application of this principle is described for characterization of monoclonal antibody epitope specificity (PAN 101), for epitope mapping of HIV-1 p24 by peptide inhibition of antibody binding (PAN 102), for assessment of antigen-antibody interaction constants (PAN 301) and others.

7. Piezoelectric systems and surface acoustic wave devices: Piezoelectric crystals can oscillate at a very specific resonant frequency when placed in an appropriate circuit. The frequency of this resonant (generally 9 or 14 MHz) is changed by adding mass to the surface of the crystal. The total frequency change Δ F is proportional to the amount of adsorbed substance (Δ mass) according to the basic equation of Sauerbrey (cf. Farnell (1976):

$\Delta F = -k * \Delta \text{ mass}$

Selectivity of a piezoelectric immunosensor is developed by the coating, and sensitivity is a characteristic of the crystal (Guilbault, 1990). Advances in piezoelectric methodology in the last few years have also allowed dynamic measurements of minute mass changes ($< 10^{-9}$ g/cm^2) on surfaces, thin films and on electrode interfaces in liquid media (Ward and Buttry, 1990).

Using this principle, a procedure for the determination of human IgG between 10^{-6} - 10^{-2} mg/ml (10^{-11} - 10^{-7} mol/l) by means of protein A immobilized on a quartz crystal via 3-aminopropyl-triethoxysilane has been developed by Muramatsu et al. (1987). This technique has also been applied for the determination of microorganisms (Muramatsu et al., 1986; cf. Karube, 1988). For this reason, Candida sp. antibodies were immobilized (also via 3-aminopropyl-triethoxysilane) on the sensor covered with palladium. During the immunobinding of pathogenic Candida albicans the resonant frequency is lowered and correlates in the range 0.5 - 1.4 kHz with a concentration of 10^6 to 5 x 10^8 cells. A disadvantage, however, is the measuring time of ≈ 1 h and that the crystals have to be dried before every detection.

In a similar fashion, surface acoustic wave (SAW) detectors can be used. The operation principle of such transducers is as follows (Wholtjen and Dessy, 1979): an acoustic wave confined to the surface of some substrate material is generated and allowed to propagate. If matter is present on the same surface, then the wave and the matter will interact in such a way as to alter the properties of the wave (e.g. amplitude, phase, harmonic content etc.). The measurement of changes in the surface wave characteristics is a sensitive indicator of the properties of the material present on the surface of the device. The convenient generation of SAW requires a substrate material which is piezoelectric. Applying a time varying electric field to the piezoelectric material will cause a synchronous deformation of the substrate with a coincident generation of an acoustic wave in the material. The oscillation of a crystal, in this case, is at a higher frequency (several hundred MHz instead of 9 - 14 MHz), and corresponding sensors should be more sensitive than piezoelectric devices.

A SAW immunosensor for the determination of human IgG and type A influenza virus has been developed by Roederer and Bastiaans (1983). The measurements were carried out against an antibody-free reference crystal directly in the liquid. The detection time was reduced to 20 seconds. A regeneration of the sensor was attained by high ionic strength solutions. Disadvantages here are that this method is exclusively applicable to high molecular compounds and that the results may be falsified by unspecific effects.

A SAW method for monitoring anti-immunoglobulins has been described by Davis and Leary (1989). The AT-cut crystal with a fundamental resonant frequency of 10 MHz used was directly coated on one side with protein A. Upon exposure to solutions containing rabbit or human IgG, the resonant frequency decreases due to the binding of IgG to protein A. Subsequent addition of sheep anti-human IgG to the now immobilized human IgG caused a specific 3-fold further decrease in resonant frequency (change of ≈ 1 Hz for each 10 ng of added Ig). Decreasing the pH to 3 released the bound IgG but not the protein A and permitted re-use of the sensor for further determination.

Despite these successful applications of the SWA technique, it has not yet been possible to go beyond the experimental level (cf. Ward and Buttry, 1990).

References

Aalberse, R.C.(1973): Quantitative fluoroimmunoassay. Clin. Chem. **48**, 109-111

Abe, C., Saito, H., Tomioka, H., Fukasawa, Y. (1989): Production of a monoclonal antibody specific for *Mycobacterium avium* and immunological activity of the affinity-purified antigen. Infect. Immunity **57**, 1095-1099

Agris, P.F., Armstrong, S.A., Guenther, R.H. (1989): Biomacromolecular liquid chromatography yesterday and today: Advancements in the separation and study of nucleic acids and their related proteins. J. Liquid Chromatogr. **12**, 1347-1366

Aguet, M., Merlin, G. (1987): Purification of human γ-interferon receptors by sequential affinity chromatography on immobilized monoclonal antireceptor antibodies and human γ-interferon. J. exp. Med. **165**, 988-999

Ahn, I.S., Choi, C.Y. (1989 a): Development of chromatographic downstream processing for the purification of monoclonal antibodies from ascites fluid. Part I. Tandem use of hydroxylapatite chromatography and gel permeation chromatography. Sanop. Misaengmul. Hakhoechi **17**, 19-23

Ahn, I.S., Choi, C.Y. (1989 b): Development of chromatographic downstream processing for the purification of monoclonal antibodies from ascites fluid. Part II. Use of single hydroxylapatite chromatography step. Sanop. Misaengmul. Hakhoechi **17**, 269-272

Aithal, H.N., Knigge, K.M., Kartha, S., Czyzewski, E.A, Tobak, F.G. (1988): An alternate method utilizing small quantities of ligand for affinity purification of monospecific antibodies. J. Immunol. Meth. **112**, 63-70

Aizawa, M., Morioka, A., Suzuki, S. (1980): An enzyme immunosensor for the electrochemical determination of the tumorantigen α-fetoprotein. Anal. Chem. Acta **115**, 61-67

Åkerström, B., Björck, L. (1986): A physicochemical study of protein G, a molecule with unique immunglobulin G-binding properties. J. Biol. Chem. **261**, 10240-10244

Åkerström, B., Brodin, T., Reis, K., Björck, L. (1985): Protein G: A powerful tool for binding and detection of monoclonal and polyclonal antibodies. J. Immunol. **135**, 2589-2592

Alexander, P.W., Maltra, C. (1982): Enzyme-linked immunoassay of human immunoglobulin G with the fluoride-ion-selective electrode. Anal. Chem. **54**, 68-71

Ali, M.A., Jacob, T.M. (1984): Specificity and purification of antibodies to adenylic acid. J. Appl. Biochem. **6**, 126-134

Altshuler, G.L., Dziewulsky, D.M., Sowek, J.A., Belfort, G. (1986): Continuous hybridoma growth and monoclonal antibody production in hollow fiber reactors-separators. Biotechnol. Bioengng. **28**, 646-658

Andersen, K.K., Benyamin, Y., Douzon, P., Balny, C. (1975): The effects of organic solvents and temperature on the desorption of yeast 3-phosphoglycerate kinase from immunosorbent. J. Immunol. Meth. **25**, 375-381

Anderson, B.G., Gruenberg, M.L. (1987): Optimization techniques for the production of monoclonal antibodies utilizing hollow-fiber technology. In: Seaver, S.S. (ed.) The Commercial Production of Monoclonal Antibodies, Marcel Dekker Inc., New York-Basel, pp. 175-195

Annunziato, E., Marciani, D.J. (1987): Efficient purification of mouse monoclonal antibodies from ascites fluid by medium-performance anion exchange chromatography. Gene Anal. Technol. **4**, 1-4

Arwin, H., Lindström, I. (1985): A reflectance method for quantification of immunological reactions on surfaces. Anal. Biochem. **145**, 106-112

Aston, R., Cooper, L., Holder, A., Ivanyi, J., Preece, M. (1985): Monoclonal antibodies to human growth hormone can distinguish between pituitary and genetically engineering forms. Mol. Immunol. **22**, 271-277

Aucouturier, P., Pineau, N., Brugier, J.-C., Mihaesco, E., Duarte, F., Skvaril, F., Preud'homme, J.-L. (1989): Jacalin: A new laboratory tool in immunochemistry and cellular immunology. J. Clin. Lab. Anal. **3**, 244-251

Awdeh, Z.L., Williamson, R., Askonas, B.A. (1970): One-cell-one immunoglobulin. Origin of limited heterogeneity of myeloma proteins. Biochem. J. **116**, 241-248

Axen, R., Ernback, S. (1971): Chemical fixation of enzymes to cyanogen halide activated polysaccharide carriers. Eur. J. Biochem. **18**, 351-360

Babashak, J.V., Phillips, T.M. (1988): Use of avidin-coated glass beads as a support for high-performance immuno-affinity chromatography. J. Chromatogr. **444**, 21-28

Backer, M.P., Metzger, L.S., Slaber, P.L., Nevitt, K.L., Boder, G.B. (1988): Large-scale production of monoclonal antibodies in suspension culture. Biotechnol. Bioengng. **32**, 993-1000

Badley, R.A., Drake, R.A.L., Shanks, I.A., Smith, A.M., Stephenson, P.R. (1987): Optical biosensors for immunoassays: the fluorescence capillary fill device. Phil. Trans. Roy. Soc. London B, **316**, 143-160

Baeseler, M., Boeden, H.-F., Koelsch, R., Lasch, J. (1991): Cellulose beads: A weak leaking affinity support. J. Chromat. (in press)

Baldwin, S.W. Bier, J.R., Schafer, C.A., Schlender, K.K., Reimann, E.M. (1989): Immunoaffinity purification of glycogen synthase: Phosphopeptide mapping of glycogen synthase isolated from skeletal muscle. Adv. Prot. Protease **5**, 507-516

Ball, G.D. (1985): Clarification and sterilisation. In: Animal Cell Biotechnology, Academic Press Inc., London, Vol. 2, pp. 87-127

Bankert, R.B., Des Soye, D., Powers, L. (1980): Antigen-promoted cell fusion: Antigen-coated myeloma cells fuse with antigen-reactive spleen cells. Transplant. Proc. **12**, 443-446

Bartholomew, R., Beider, D., David, G. (1983): Immunoaffinity chromatography with monoclonal antibodies. In: Peters, H. (ed.) Proteides of the Biological Fluids, Vol. 30, Pergamon Press, Oxford, pp. 667-670.

Basch, R.S., Berman, J.W., Lakow, E. (1983): Cell separation using positive immunoselective techniques. J. Immunol. Meth. **16**, 269-280

Baskir, J.N., Hatton, T.A., Suter, U.W. (1989): Protein partitioning in two-phase aqueous polymer systems. Biotechnol. Bioengng. **34**, 541-548

Batteiger, B., Newhall, W.J., Jones, R.B. (1982): The use of Tween 20 as a blocking agent in the immunological detection of proteins transferred to nitrocellulose. J. Immunol. Meth. **55**, 297-307

Bayer, E.A., Wilcheck, M. (1978): The avidin-biotin complex as tool in molecular biology. TIBS **3**, 257-259

Bayer, E.A., Wilchek, M., Skutelsky, E. (1976): Affinity cytochemistry: The localization of lectin and antibody receptors on erythrocytes via the avidin-biotin complex. FEBS Lett. **68**, 240-244

Bazin, H., Cormont, F., De Clercq, L. (1984 b): Rat monoclonal antibodies: II. A rapid and efficient method of purification from ascitic fluid or serum. J. Immunol. Meth. **71**, 9-16

Bazin, H., Cormont, F., De Clerq, L. (1986): Purification of rat monoclonal antibodies. Meth. Enzymol. **121**, 638-652

Bazin, H., Malache, J.-M. (1986): Rat (and mouse) monoclonal antibodies. V. A simple automated technique of antigen purification by immunoaffinity chromatography. J. Immunol. Meth. **88**, 19-24

Bazin, H., Xhurdebise, L.-M., Burtonboy, G., Lebacq, A.M., De Clercq, L., Cormont, F. (1984 a): Rat monoclonal antibodies: I. Rapid purification from *in vitro* culture supernatants. J. Immunol. Meth. **66**, 261-270

Belew, M., Juntti, N., Larsson, A., Porath, J. (1987): A one-step purification method for monoclonal antibodies based on salt-promoted adsorption chromatography on a thiophilic adsorbent. J. Immunol. Meth. **102**, 173-182

Bensinger, W.I., Baker, D.A., Buckner, C.D., Clift, R.A., Thomas, E.D. (1981): Immunoadsorption for removal of A and B blood group antibodies. New Engl. J. Med. **304**, 160-162

Berenson, R.J., Bensinger, W.I., Kalamasz, D. (1986): Positive selection of viable cell populations using avidin-biotin immunoadsorption. J. Immunol. Meth. **91**, 11-19

Berenson, R.J., Levitt, L.J., Levy, R., Miller, R.A. (1984): Cellular immunoadsorption using monoclonal antibodies: Selective removal of T cells from peripheral blood and bone marrow. Transplantation **38**, 136-143

Bergmann, K.-Ch., Wieser, R. (1978): Einsatz der Laser-Nephelometrie zur quantitativen Bestimmung von IgA, IgM, IgG und anderer Serumproteine. Dt. Gesundh.-Wesen **33/18**, 855-857

Bergveld, P., Van Der Schoot, B.H., Schasfoort, R.B.M. (1987): in "GBF Monographs", Vol. 10, VCH Verlagsgesellschaft, Weinheim, pp. 165-171

Bernardi, G. (1971): Chromatography of proteins on hydroxyapatite. Meth. Enzymol., **22**, 325-339

Bernardi, G. (1973): Chromatography of proteins on hydroxyapatite. Meth. Enzymol., **27**, 471-479

Bernardi, G., Giro, M.G., Gaillord, G. (1972), Chromatography of polypeptides and proteins on hydroxyapatite columns: Some new developments. Biochim. Biophys. Acta **278**, 409-420

Bernardi, G., Kawasaki, T. (1968): Chromatography of polypeptides and proteins on hydroxyapatite columns. Biochim. Biophys. Acta **160**, 301-311

Bers, G., Garfin, D.(1985): Protein and nucleic acid blotting and immunobiochemical detection. BioTechniques **3**, 276-288

Bertroft, E., Eskola, J.U., Näntö, V., Lövgren, T. (1984): Competetive solid phase immunoassay of testosterone using time-resolved fluorescence. FEBS Lett. **173**, 213-216

Bhatia, S.K., Shriver-Lage, L.C., Prior, K.J., Georger, J.H., Calvert, J.M., Bredehorst, R., Ligler, F.S. (1989): Use of thiol-terminal silanes and heterobifunktional crosslinkers for immobilization of antibodies on silica surfaces. Anal. Biochem. **178**, 408-413.

Bier, O. (1986): Fundamentals of Immunology. Springer-Verlag, Berlin

Birch, J.R., Lambert, K., Boraston, R., Thompson, P.W., Boss, M.A. (1985): Large scale production of monoclonal antibodies. Presented at BIOTECH '85

U.S.A., World Biotech. Rep., Online Publications 2, pp. 179-188

Birch, J.R., Lambert, K., Boraston, R., Thompson, P.W., Garland, S., Kenney, A.C. (1987): The industrial production of monoclonal antibodies in cell culture. NATO ASI Ser., Ser. A **128**, 97-109

Bird, R.E., Hardman, K.D., Jacobson, J.W., Johnson, S., Kaufman, B.M., Lee, S.-M., Lee, T., Pope, S.H., Riordan, G.S., Whitlow, M. (1988): Single-chain antigen-binding proteins. Science **242**, 423-426

Birnbaum, S., Bülow, L., Hardy, K., Danielson, B., Mosbach, K. (1986): Automated thermometric enzyme immunoassay of human proinsulin produced by Escherichia coli. Anal. Biochem. **158**, 12-19,

Bittner, M., Kupferer, P., Morris, C.F. (1980): Electrophoretic transfer of proteins and nucleic acids from slab gels to diazobenzyloxymethylcellulose or nitrocellulose sheets. Anal. Biochem. **102**, 459-471

Bjerrum, O.J., Heegard (eds.) (1988): CRC Handbook of immunoblotting, Vol. I, Technical Descriptions, Vol. II, Experimental and Chemical Applications, CRC Press Inc., Boca Raton, Forida

Blackburn, G.F., Talley, D.B., Booth, P.M., Durfor, C.N., Martin, M.T., Napper, A.D., Rees, A.R. (1990): Potentiometric biosensor employing catalytic antibodies as the molecular recognition element. Anal. Chem. **62**, 2211-2216

Blackburn, G.M., Kang, A.S., Kingsbury, G.A., Burton, D.R. (1989): Catalytic antibodies. Biochem. J. **262**, 381-390

Blackburn, S. (1986): CRC Handbook of chromatography: Peptides, Vol. 1, CRC Press, Boca Raton, pp. 298-322

Bloom, J.W., Wong, M.F., Mitra, G. (1989): Detection and reduction of protein A contamination in immobilized protein A purified monoclonal antibodies. J. Immunol. Meth. **117**, 83-89

Björck, L., Kronvall, G. (1984): Purification and some properties of Streptococcal protein G, a novel IgG-binding reagent. J. Immunol. **133**, 969-974

Boeden, H.-F., Büttner, W., Rupprich, Ch., Büttner, D., Heinrich, S., Becker, M., Holtzhauer, M. (1991a): Acylation of hydroxyl groups in polymers with carbonic acid derivatives in the presence of tertiary amines. Makromol. Chem. (submitted)

Boeden, H.-F., Pommerening, K., Becker, M., Rupprich, Ch., Holtzhauer, M., Loth, F., Müller, R., Bertram, D. (1991b): Bead cellulose derivatives as supports for immobilization and chromatographic purification of proteins. J. Chromatogr. **552**, 389-414

Bonner, M., Laskey, L.A. (1974): A film detection method for tritium-labelled protein and nucleic acids in polyacrylamide gels. Eur. J. Biochem. **46**, 83-88

Borrebaeck, C., Börjeson, J., Mattiasson, B. (1978): Thermometric enzyme linked immunosorbent assay in continuous flow system: Optimization and evaluation using human serum albumin as model system. Clin. Chim. Acta **86**, 267-278

Borrebaeck, C.A.K., Danielsson, L., Möller, S.A. (1988): Human monoclonal antibodies produced by primary in vitro immunization of peripheral blood lymphocytes. Proc. Natl. Acad. Sci. U.S.A. **85**, 3995-3999

Boss, M. (1986): Large scale production of monoclonal antibodies. Pract. Biotechnol., Febr. 1986, 7-9

Böttcher, I., Hämmerling, G., Kapp, J.F. (1978): Continuous production of mouse IgE antibodies with known allergenic specificity by a hybrid cell line. Nature **275**, 761-762

Bouzerna, N., Hammadi, H., Richard, C., Formstecher, P., Dautrevaux, M. (1988): Improvement in the purification of an anti-steroid antiserum resistant to conventional immunoadsorption chromatography. J. Immunol. Meth. **112**, 251-259

Bowen, B., Steinberg, J., Laemmli, U.K., Weintraub, H. (1980): The detection of DNA-binding proteins by protein blotting. Nucl. Acids Res. **8**, 1-20

Boyle, M.D.P., Reis, K.J. (1987): Bacterial Fc receptors. BioTechnology **5**, 697-702

Brada, D., Roth, J. (1984): "Golden Blot"-detection of polyclonal and monoclonal antibodies bound to antigens on nitrocellulose by protein A - gold complexes. Anal. Biochem. **142**, 79-83

Brinchman, J.E. Leivestad, T., Vartdal, F. (1989): Quantitation of lymphocyte subsets based on positive immunomagnetic selection of cells directly from blood. J. Immunogenet. **16**, 177-183

Brinchmann, J.E., Vartdal, F., Gaudernack, G., Markusson, G., Funderud, S., Ugelstad, J., Thorsby, E. (1988): Direct immunomagnetic quantitation of lymphocyte subsets in blood. Clin. Exp. Immunol. **71**, 182-186

Brizgys, M.V., Pincus, S., Siebert, C.J., Rollins, E. (1989): Removal of digoxin from circulation using immobilized monoclonal antibodies. J. Pharm. Sci. **78**, 393-398

Brodeur, B.R., Tsang, P., Larose, Y. (1984): Parameters affecting ascites tumour formation in mice and monoclonal antibody production. J. Immunol. Meth. **71**, 265-272

Brodeur, B.R., Tsang, P.S. (1986): High yield monoclonal antibody production in ascites. J. Immunol. Meth. **86**, 219-241

Brooks, T.L., Stevens, A. (1985): Techniques for purifying monoclonal antibodies. American Laboratory, Oct. **85**, 54-64

Bruck, C., Drebin, J.A., Glineur, C., Portetelle, D. (1986): Purification of mouse monoclonal antibodies from ascitic fluid by DEAE Affi-Gel Blue chromatography. Meth. Enzymol., **121**, 587-596

Bruck, C., Portetelle, D., Glineur, C., Bollen, A. (1982): One-step purification of mouse monoclonal antibodies from ascites fluid by DEAE-Affi-Gel Blue chromatography. J. Immunol. Meth. **53**, 313-320

Bruera, M.R., Sevlever, D., Gatti, C.A. (1983): Measurement of binding constants for divalent antibody-immobilized antigen interaction by antigen-Sepharose 4B chromatography. Immunol. Commun. **12**, 529-538

Bukovsky, J., Kennett, R.H. (1987): Simple and rapid purification of monoclonal antibodies from cell culture supernatants and ascites fluids by hydroxylapatite chromatography on analytical and preparative scales. Hybridoma **6**, 219-228

Burchiel, S.W. (1986): Purification and analysis of monoclonal antibodies by high-performance liquid chromatography. Meth. Enzymol. **121**, 596-622

Burchiel, S.W., Billman, J.R., Alber, T.R. (1984): Rapid and efficient purification of mouse monoclonal antibodies from ascites fluid using high-performance liquid chromatography. J. Immunol. Meth. **69**, 33-42

Burchiel, S.W., Rhodes, B.A. (1983): Radioimmunoimaging and Radioimmunotherapy, Elsevier, New York

Büttner, W., Becker, M., Rupprich, Ch., Boeden, H.-F., Henklein, P., Loth, F., Dautzenberg, H. (1989): A novel carbonochloridate for activation of supports containing hydroxyl groups. Biotechnol. Bioengng. **33**, 26-31

Cannell et al. (1979): Immunoassay by light scattering intensity anisotropy measurements. U.S. Patent 4.174.952

Cardosi, M.F., Birch, S.W., Stanley, C.J., Johannsson, A., Turner, A.F.P. (1989): An electrochemical immunoassay for prosthatic phosphatase incorporating enzyme amplification, Internat. Biotechnol. Lab., June 1989, pp. 8, 10, 12-17

Carlsson, M.A., Hedin, A., Inganäs, M., Härfast, B., Blomberg, F. (1985): Purification of *in vitro* produced mouse monoclonal antibodies. A two-step procedure utilizing cation exchange chromatography and gel filtration. J. Immunol. Meth. **79**, 89-98

Carr, D.D.J., Decosta, B., Jacobson, A.E., Bost, K.L. Rice, K.C., Blalock, J.E. (1987): Immunoaffinity-purified opiate receptor specifically binds S-class opiate receptor ligand cis-(+)-3-methylfentanylisothiocyanate. FEBS Lett. **224**, 272-276

Carty, P., O'Kennedey, R. (1988): Use of high-performance liquid chromatography for the purification of antibodies and antibody conjugates and the study of antibody-antigen interactions. J. Chromatogr. **442**, 279-288

Chandler, J.P. (1987): Factors influencing monoclonal antibody production in mouse ascites fluid. In: Seaver, S.S. (ed.) The Commercial Production of Monoclonal Antibodies, Marcel Dekker Inc., New York-Basel, pp. 75-92

Chang, J.Y. (1979): Der homogene Immunoassay - neueste Entwicklungen und Aspekte. In: Vogt, W. (ed.) "Praktische Anwendung des Enzymimmunoassays in klinischer Chemie und Serologie", Georg Thieme Verlag Stuttgart, pp. 1-9

Chanutin, A., Curnish, R.R. (1960): The precipitation of plasma proteins by short chain fatty acids. Arch. Biochim. Biophys. **89**, 218-220

Chard, T. (1980): Ammonium sulfate and polyethylene glycol as reagents to separate antigen from antigen-antibody complexes. Meth. Enzymol. **70**, 280-291

Chase, H.A. (1984): Scale-up of immunoaffinity separation processes. J. Biotechnol. **1**, 67-80

Chen, F.-M., Naeve, G.S., Epstein, A.L. (1988): Comparison of Mono Q, Superose-6 and ABx fast protein liquid chromatography for purification of IgM monoclonal antibodies. J. Chromatogr. **444**, 153-164

Chernajowsky, Y., Mori, Y, Chen, L., Marks, Z., Novick, D., Rubenstein, M., Revel, M. (1984): Efficient constitutive production of human fibroblast interferon by hamster cells transformed with the interferon ß1 gene fused to an SV40 early promoter. DNA 3, 297-308

Chersi, A., Ruocco, E., Muratti, E. (1989): Preparation and properties of gel-peptide immunosorbents. J. Immunol. Meth. **122**, 285-289

Chhatwal, G.S., Blobel, H. (1987): Isolation and properties of a novel IgG-binding protein from Streptococci of serological group U. Med. Microbiol. Immunol. **176**, 1-12

Ching, C.B., Uddin, M.S., Hidajat, K. (1989): Diffusional kinetics of monoclonal antibody, transferrin and bovine serum albumin on Sephacryl S-200 HR gel. Chem. Engng. J. **42**, B47-B52

Choi, T.K., Sleight, D.R., Nisonoff, A. (1974): General method for isolation and recovery of B cells bearing specific receptors. J. Exp. Med. **139**, 761-766

Clausen, J. (1988) Immunochemical techniques for the identification and estimation of macromolecules. In: Burdon, R.H., van Knippenberg, P.H. (eds.) Laboratory Techniques in Biochemistry and Molecular Biology, Vol. 1 pt. 3), 3rd ed., Elsevier Sci. Publ., Amsterdam

Clements, G.B. (1975): Selection of biochemically variant in some cases mutant, mammalian cells in culture. Adv. Cancer Res. **21**, 273-290

Clements, P.R., Brooks, D.A., Mccourt, P.A.G., Hopwood, J.J. (1989): Immunopurification and characterization of human α-L-iduronidase with the use of monoclonal antibodies. Biochem. J. **259**, 199-208

Clezardin, P., Hunter, N.R., McGregor, I.R., McGregor, J.L., Pepper, D.S., Dawes, J. (1986): Tandem purification of mouse IgM monoclonal antibodies produced in vitro using anion-exchange and gel fast protein liquid chromatography. J. Chromatogr. **358**, 209-216

Clezardin, P.J., McGregor, J.L., Manach, M., Boukerche, H., Dechavanne, M. (1985): One-step procedure for the rapid isolation of mouse monoclonal antibodies and their antigen binding fragments by fast protein liquid chromatography on a Mono Q anion exchange column. J. Chromatogr. **319**, 67-77

Clonis, Y.D. (1989) High-performance affinity chromatography (HPAC). In: Oliver, R.W.A. (ed.) HPLC of Macromolecules - a Practical Approach, IRL Press, Oxford, pp. 157-182

Cobbold, S.P., Waldman, H. (1984): Therapeutic potential of monovalent monoclonal antibodies. Nature **308**, 460-462

Collawn, J.F., Wallace, C.J.A., Proudfoot, E.A.I., Paterson, Y. (1988): Monoclonal antibodies as probes of conformational changes in protein-engineered cytochrome c. J. Biol. Chem. **263**, 8625-8634

Collins, W.P. (ed.) (1988): Complementary Immunoassays. J. Wiley & Sons, Chichester

Commission of the European Committees (1988): Guidelines on the production and quality control of monoclonal antibodies of murine origin for use in man. TIBTECH, **6**, 5-8

Cormont, F., Monouvriez P., De Clercq, L., Bazin, H. (1986): The use of rat monoclonal antibodies to characterize, quantify, and purify polyclonal or monoclonal mouse IgM. Meth. Enzymol. **121**, 622-631

Crane, L.J. (1987): Purification of monoclonal antibodies by high-performance ion-exchange chromatography. In: Schook, L.B. (ed.) Monoclonal Antibody Production Techniques and Applications, Marcel Dekker, Inc., New York-Basel, pp. 139-171

Cripps, A.W., Neoh, S.H., Smart, I.J. (1983): Isolation of human IgA and IgM from normal serum using polyethylene glycol precipitation and affinity chromatography. J. Immunol. Meth. **57**, 197-204

Dahlberg, E., Snochowski, M., Gustafsson, J.-A. (1980): Removal of hydrophobic compounds from biological fluids by a simple method. Anal. Biochem. **106**, 380-388

Dakour, J., Lundblad, A., Zopf, D. (1987): Separation of blood A-active oligosaccharides by high-pressure liquid affinity chromatography using a monoclonal antibody bound to concanavalin A silica. Anal. Biochem. **161**, 140-143

Dandliker, W.B., Feigen, G.A. (1961): Quantitation of the antigen-antibody reaction by polarization of fluorescence. Biochem. Biophys. Res. Comm. **5**, 299-304

Danielsson, A., Ljunglöf, A., Lindblom, H. (1988): One-step purification of monoclonal IgG antibodies from mouse ascites. J. Immunol. Meth. **115**, 79-88

Davidson, III, R.L. (1988): Monoclonal Antibodies, Technical Insights, Inc., Englewood-Fort Lee, Emerging Industries, No 2

Davies, D.H., Sheriff, S., Padian, E.A. (1988): Antibody- antigen complexes. J. Biol. Chem. **263**, 10541-10544

Davis, G.C., Hein, M.B., Chapman D.A. (1986): Evaluation of immunosorbents for the analysis of small molecules. Isolation and purification of cytokinins. J. Chromatogr. **366**, 171-189

Davis, K.A., Leary, T.R. (1989): Continuous liquid-phase piezoelectric biosensor for kinetic immunoassays. Anal. Chem. **61**, 1227-1230

Dawson, R.M.C., Elliot, D.C., Elliot, W.H., Jones, K.M. (1986) Data for Biochemical Research, 3rd ed., Clarendon Press, Oxford

Day, E.D., Hashim, G.A. (1984): Affinity purification of two populations of antibodies against format determinants of synthetic myelin basic protein peptide S82 from S82-AH- and S82-CH-Sepharose 4B columns. Neurochemical Research **9**, 1453-1465

De Rie, M.A., Zeijlemaker, W.P., Von Dem Borne, A.E.G.K., Out, T.A. (1987): Evaluation of a method of production and purification of monoclonal antibodies for clinical applications. J. Immunol. Meth. **102**, 187-194

Deacon, J.K., Stops, J.E., Thomson, A., Roberts, P.R., Whiteley, S.C., Attridge, J.W., Love, C.A., Robinson, G.A., Davidson, G.P. (1990): An assay for human chorionic gonadotropin using the fluorescence capillary fill immunosensor. Abstr. 1st World Congress on Biosensors, 2.-4. May, Singapure, p. 57-58

DeAlwis, W.U., Wilson, G.S. (1985): Rapid sub-picomole electrochemical enzyme immunoassay for immunoglobulin G. Anal. Chem. **57**, 2754-2756

Dean, P.D.G., Johnson, W.S., Middle, F.A. (eds.) (1985): Affinity Chromatography - a Practical Approach, IRL, Press, Oxford

Dedianous, S., Kopeyan, C., Bahraouni, E.M., Rochat, H. (1987): Purification of contracture-inducing insect toxins from buthinae scorpion venoms by immunoaffinity and high-pressure liquid chromatography. Toxicon **25**, 731-741

Deisenhofer, J. (1981): Crystallographic refinement and atomic models of a human Fc fragment and its complex with fragment B of protein A from *Staphylococcus aureus* at 2.9 and 2.8 Å resolution. Biochem. **20**, 2361-2370

Delacroix, D., Vaerman, J.-P. (1979): Simple purification of goat IgG1 and IgG2 subclasses by chromatography on protein A-Sepharose at various pH. Mol. Immunol. **16**, 837-840

Delgado, C., Anderson, R.J., Francis, G.E., Fisher, D. (1991) Separation of cell mixtures by immunoaffinity cell partitioning: Strategies for low abundance cells. Anal. Biochem. **192**, 322-328

DeLisi, C., Hethcote, H.W. (1982): A theory of column chromatography for sequential reactions in heterogenous nonequilibrium systems: Application to antigen-antibody reactions. In: Gribnau, T.C.J., Visser, J., Nivard, R.J.F. (eds.) Affinity Chromatography and Related Techniques. Elsevier Sci. Publ., Amsterdam, pp. 63-78

Demignot, S., Garnett, M.C., Baldwin, R.W. (1989): Mouse IgG2b monoclonal antibody fragmentation. Preparation and purification of Fab/c fragments. J. Immunol. Meth. **121**, 209-217

Deschamps, J.R., Hildreth, J.E.K., Derr, D., August, J.T. (1985): A high performance liquid chromatographic procedure for the purification of mouse monoclonal antibodies. Anal. Biochem. **147**, 451-454

Devaney, E., Howell, K.E. (1985): Immuno-isolation of a plasma membrane fraction of the fao. EMBO J. **4**, 3123-3130

Diaco, R., Hill, J.H., Durand, D.P. (1986): Purification of soybean mosaic virus by affinity chromatography using monoclonal antibodies. J. Gener. Virol. **67**, 345-351

Diaz, A.J.M., Kohnert, K.D., Keilacker, H., Ziegler, B., Ziegler, M. (1989): Purification of mouse monoclonal antibodies by chromatography on Sepharose 6B. Allerg. Immunol. **35**, 173-179

Dimandis, E.P., Christopoulos, T.K. (1990): Europium chelate labels in time-resolved fluorescence immunossays and DNA hybridization assays, Anal. Chem. **62**, No.22 (Report, 7 p.)

Dimandis, E.P., Christopoulos, T.K. (1991): The biotin-(strept)avidin system: Principles and application in biotechnology. Clin. Chem. **37**, 625-636

Drechou, A., Perez-Gonzales, N., Biou, B., Rouzeau, J.D., Feger, J., Durand, G. (1989): One-step purification of rat plasma α1-acid glycoprotein by antibody affinity chromatography: Application to normal and inflamed rat sera. J. Chromatogr. **489**, 273-282

Dubin, P.L. (Ed.) (1988): Aqueous Size-Exclusion Chromatography. J. Chromatogr. Library, Vol. 40, Elsevier, Amsterdam

Duerksen, P.J., Wilkinson, K.D. (1987): Immobilization of proteins via arginine residues. Anal. Biochem. **160**, 444-454

Duerksen-Hughes, P.J., Williamson, M.M., Wilkinson, K.D. (1989): Affinity chromatography using protein immobilized via arginine residues: Purification of ubiquitin carboxyl-terminal hydrolases. Biochem. **28**, 8530-8536

Duffy, S.A., Moellering, B.J., Prior, G.M., Doyle, K.R., Prior, C.P. (1989): Recovery of therapeutic grade antibodies: Protein A and ion-exchange. BioPharm. **2**, 34-45

Duncan, J.K., Chen, A.J.C., Siebert, C.J. (1987): Performance evaluation of non-porous versus porous ion-exchange packings in the separation of proteins by high-performance liquid chromatography. J. Chromatogr. **397**, 3-12

Dunn, M.J., Patel, K. (1988): Detection of protein blots using the avidin-biotin system. In: Walker, J.M. (ed.) Methods in Molecular Biology, vol. 3, Humana Press, Clifton, pp. 419-426

Durley, R.C., Sharp, C.R., Maki, S.I., Brenner, M.L., Carnes, M.G. (1989): Immunoaffinity techniques applied to the purification of gibberellins from plant extracts. Plant Physiol. **90**, 445-481

Egen, N.B., Bliss, M., Mayersohn, M., Owens, S.M., Arnold, L., Bier, M. (1988): Isolation of monoclonal antibodies to phenycyclidine from ascites fluid by preparative isoelectric focusing in the Rotofor. Anal. Biochem. **172**, 488-494

Ehle, H., Gödicke, C., Horn, A. (1989): A new graphical method for determining the affinity constants of monoclonal antibodies to enzymes. J. Immunol. Meth. **117**, 17-23

Ehrnström, R., Gustavsson, B. (1988): Purification and analysis of monoclonal antibodies from mouse ascites fluid. Internat. Biotech. Lab., June '88, 40-45

Eliasson, M., Andersson, R., Olsson, A., Wigzell, H., Uhlen, M. (1989): Differential IgG-binding characteristics of Staphylococcal Protein A, Streptococcal Protein G, and a chimeric Protein AG. J. Immunol. **142**, 575-581

Endo, Y., Miyai, K., Hata, N., Ichihara, K. (1985): Fractionation of polyclonal antibody by isoelectric focusing: Separation of high-affinity rabbit donotype anti-thyroxine antibody. Anal. Biochem. **144**, 41-46

Engelhardt, J. (1986): HPLC of proteins and peptides. In: Engelhardt, H. (ed.) Practice of High-Performance Liquid Chromatography, Springer Verlag, Berlin, pp. 409-425

Eppert, G. (1988): Einführung in die schnelle Flüssigchromatographie, 2. Aufl., Akademie Verlag, Berlin

Eshar, Z., Ofarim, M., Waks, T. (1980): Generation of hybridomas secreting murine reaging antibodies of anti-DNP specificity. J. Immunol. **124**, 775-780

Eveleigh, J.W. (1982): Practical considerations in the use of immunosorbents and associated instrumentation. In: Gribnau, T.C.J., Visser, J., Nivard (eds.) Affinity Chromatography and Related Techniques. Elsevier Sci. Publ., Amsterdam, pp. 293-303

Ey, P.L., Prowse, S.J., Jenkins, C.P. (1978): Isolation of pure IgG1, IgG2a and IgG2b immunoglobulins from mouse serum using protein A-Sepharose. Immunochemistry **15**, 429-436

Farnell, G.W. (1976): SAW propagation in piezoelectric solids. Wave electron **2**, 1-24

Fateh-Moghadam, A. Neumeier, D., Pape, S. (1979): Vergleichende enzymimmunologische Untersuchungen zur Bestimmung von carcinoembryonalem Antigen (CEA) im Plasma. In: Vogt, W. (ed.) Praktische Anwendung des Enzymimunoassays in klinischer Chemie und Serologie, Georg Thieme Verlag Stuttgart, pp. 59-65

FAYE, L., CHRISPEELS, M.J. (1985): Characterization of N-linked oligosaccharides by affinoblotting with concanavalin A-peroxidase and treatment of the blots with glycosidases. Anal. Biochem. **149**, 218-224

FAZEKAS DE ST.GROTH, S. (1979): The quality of antibodies and cellular receptors. In: LEVKOVITS, I., PERNIS, B. (eds.) Immunological Methods, Vol. 1, Academic Press, New York, pp. 1-42

FISHER, D., SUTHERLAND, I.A. (Eds.) (1989): Separation Using Aqueous Systems: Application in Cell Biology and Biotechnology. Plenum Press, New York

FLEMINGER, G., HADAS, E., WOLF, T., SOLOMON, B. (1990): Oriented immobilization of periodate-oxidized monoclonal antibodies on amino and hydrazide derivatives of Eupergit C. Appl. Biochem. Biotechnol. **23**, 123-137

Food and Drug Administration (1987): Points to consider in the manufacture and testing of monoclonal antibody products for human use. Memorandum from the Director, Dr. Thomas HOFFMAN, Chairman, Hybridoma Committee, Office of Biologics, Research and Review, Center for Drugs and Biologics, Food and Drug Administration, Bethesda, U.S.A

FORMSTECHER, P., HAMMADI, H., BOUZERNA, N., DAUTREVAUX, M. (1986): Rapid purification of antisteroid antibodies by high-performance liquid affinity chromatography. J. Chromatogr. **369**, 379-390

FRANEK, F. (1986): Purification of IgG monoclonal antibodies from ascitic fluid based on Rivanol precipitation. Meth. Enzymol. **121**, 631-638

FRANKS, F. (1975): The hydrophobic interaction, In: FRANKS, F. (ed.) Water - a Comprehensive Treatise, Vol. 4, Plenum Press, New York, pp. 1-94

FRASER, C.M., VENTER, J.C. (1982): The size of the mammalian lung β2-adrenergic receptor as determined by target size analysis and immunoaffinity chromatography. Biochem. Biophys. Res. Commun. **109**, 21-29

FREDRIKSSON, U.-B., FÅGERSTAM, L.G., COLE, A.W.G., LUNDGREN, T. (1986): Protein A-Sepharose CL-4B affinity purification of IgG monoclonal antibodies from mouse ascites. Presented at the 6th Int. Congr. Immunol., Toronto, 1986

FRIGUET, B., CHAFFOTTE, A.F., DJAVADI-OHANIANCE, L., GOLDBERG, M.E. (1985): Measurements of the true affinity constant in solution of antigen-antibody complexes by enzyme-linked immunosorbent assay. J. Immunol. Meth. **77**, 305-319

FÜGLISTALLER, P. (1989): Comparison of immunoglobulin binding capacities and ligand leakage using eight different protein A affinity chromatography matrices. J. Immunol. Meth. **124**, 171-177

FUNDERUD, S., NUSTAD, K., LEA, T., VARTDAL, F., GAUDERNACK, G., STENSTAD, P., UGELSTAD, J. (1987): Fractionation of lymphocytes by immunomagnetic beads: In: KLAUS, G.G.B. (ed.) Lymphocytes - A Practical Approach, IRL Press, Oxford, Washington, pp. 55-65,

GALLO, P., OLSSON, O., SIDEN, Å. (1986): Small column chromatofocusing of cerebrospinal fluid and serum immunoglobulin. J. Chromatogr. **375**, 277-283

GARCIA, L.A., ORDONEZ, G.A. (1976): The use of pluronic polyols in the precipitation of plasma derivatives. Transfusion **16**, 32-41

GARCIA-GONZALES, M., BETTINGER, S., OH, S., OLIVER, P., KADOUCHE, J., POULETTI, P. (1988): Purification of murine IgG3 and IgM monoclonal antibodies by euglobulin precipitation. J. Immunol. Meth. **111**, 17-23

GARFIN, D.E., BERS, G. (1989): Basic aspects of protein blotting. In: BALDO, B.A., TOVEY, E.R., LEONARDS, S. (eds.) Protein Blotting, S.Karger, Basel, pp. 5-42

GARVEY, J.S., CREMER, N.R., SUSSDORF, D.H. (1977): A laboratory text for instruction and research. In: Meth. in Immunology, Addison Wesley, Reading, Mass., pp. 223-226

GAUDERNACK, G., LEIVESTAD, T., UGELSTAD, J., THORSBY, E. (1986): Isolation of pure functionally active $CD8^+$ T cells. Positive selection with monoclonal antibodies directly conjugated to monosized magnetic microspheres. J. Immunol. Meth. **90**, 179-187

GAUDERNACK, G., LUNDIN, K.E.A. (1989): Rapid immunomagnetic phenotyping of cells. J. Immunogenet. **16**, 169-175

GBF Monographs, Vol. 13 (1989): Biosensors. Application in Medicine, Environmental Protection and Process Control (SCHMID, R.D., SCHELLER, F., eds.), VCH Verlagsgesellschaft, Weinheim

GEMSKI, M.J., DOCTOR, B.P., GENTRY, J.K., PLUSKAL, M.J., STRICKLER, M.P. (1985): Single-step purification of monoclonal antibodies from murine ascites and tissue culture fluids by anion exchange high performance liquid chromatography. BioTechniques **3**, 378-384

GEOGHEGAN, W.D., AMBEGAONKAR, S., CALVANICO, N.J. (1980): Passive gold agglutination. An alternative to passive hemagglutination. J. Immunol. Meth. **34**, 11-21

GERLICH, W., STAMM, B. (1978): Erfahrungen mit einem Enzymimmunoassay zum Nachweis von Hepatitis B surface antigen. In: VOGT, W. (ed.) Enzymimmunoassay, Grundlagen und praktische Anwendung, Georg Thieme Verlag Stuttgart, pp. 61-65

GERSHONI, J.M., PALADE, G.E. (1982): Electrophoretic transfer of proteins from sodium dodecylsulfate polyacrylamide gels to a positively charged membrane filter. Anal. Biochem. **124**, 396-405

GERSHONI, J.M., PALADE, G.E. (1983): Protein blotting: Principles and applications. Anal. Biochem. **131**, 1-15

Gilbert, M. T. (1987): High performance liquid chromatography, Wright, Bristol

Girard, R., Goichot, J. (1981): Preparation of monospecific anti-Salmonella lipopolysaccharide antibodies by affinity chromatography. Ann. Immunol. (Inst. Pasteur) **132 C**, 211-217

Glassy, M.C., Tharakan, J.P., Chau, P.C. (1988): Serum-free media in hybridoma culture and monoclonal antibody production. Biotechnol. Bioengng. **32**, 1015-1028

Glöckner, G. (1988) Polymer characterization by liquid chromatography. J. Chromatogr. Library Vol. 34, Elsevier Sci. Publ., Amsterdam

Goding, J.W. (1978): Use of Staphylococcal protein A as an immunological reagent. J. Immunol. Meth. **20**, 241-253

Goding, J.W. (1986): Monoclonal Antibodies, Principle and Practice, Academic Press Inc., London, 2nd Edition, pp. 108-125

Goldring, O., Gray, B., Graham, D., West, I., Pepper, D. (1988): Parameters affecting monoclonal antibody purification using protein A affinity chromatography. DECHEMA Biotechnol. Conf., Vol. 2, pp. 253-259

Goldstein, G. (1985): A randomised clinical trial of OKT 3 monoclonal antibody for acute rejection of cadaveric renal transplants. New Engl. J. Med. **313**, 337-342

Goldstein, L. (1976): Methods for the immobilization of enzymes. In: Fasman, C.D. (ed.) CRC Handbook of Biochemistry and Molecular Biology, 3rd ed., Proteins Vol. II, Cleveland, pp. 722-741

Gooding, K.M., Regnier, F.E. (eds.) (1990): HPLC of Biological Macromolecules. Marcel Dekker Inc., New York

Goodman, T., Lefrancois, l. (1988): Expression of the γ-δ T-cell receptor on intraepithelial lymphocytes, Nature **333**, 855-858

Gorbunoff, M.J. (1984 a): The interaction of proteins with hydroxyapatite. I. Role of protein charge and structure. Anal. Biochem. **136**, 425-432

Gorbunoff, M.J. (1984 b): The interaction of proteins with hydroxyapatite. II. Role of acidic and basic groups. Anal. Biochem. **136**, 433-439

Gorbunoff, M.J., Timasheff, S. (1984): The interaction of proteins with hydroxyapatite. Part III. Mechanism. Anal. Biochem. **136**, 440-445

Gordon, B.R., Sloan, B.J., Parker, T.S., Saal, S.D., Levine, D.M., Rubin, A.L. (199O): Humoral immune response following extracorporeal immunoadsorption therapy of patients with hypercholesterolemia, Transfusion **30**, 327-332

Gratecos, D., Astier, M., Semeriva, M. (1987): A new approach to monoclonal antibody production. In vitro immunization with antigens on nitrocellulose using Drosophila myosin heavy chain as an example. J. Immunol. Meth. **103**, 169-178

Green, N.M., Toms, E.J. (1970): Purification and crystallization of avidin. Biochem. J. **118**, 67-70

Green, N.M. (1975): Avidin. Adv. Protein Chem. **29**, 85-133

Gretch, D.R., Suter, M., Stinsky, M.F. (1987): The use of biotinylated monoclonal antibodies and streptavidin affinity chromatography to isolate herpes virus hydrophobic proteins and glycoproteins. Anal. Biochem. **163**, 270-273

Gribnau, T., Roeles, F., Biezen, J.V.D., Leuvering, J., Schuurs, A.(1982): The application of colloidal dye particles as label in immunoassays. In: Gribnau, T.C.J., Visser, J., Nivard, R.J.F. (eds.) Affinity Chromatography and Related Techniques, Elsevier Sci. Publ., Amsterdam, pp. 411-424

Gribnau, T.C.J. (1977): Coupling of effector-molecules to solid supports. Development and application of a new method for affinity chromatography and enzyme/hormone-immobilization. PhD thesis. Univ. Nijmegen

Griswold, W.R., Nelson, D.P. (1984): A rapid method for the determination of antibody affinity. Immunol. Lett. **7**, 229-232

Griswold, W.R., Nelson, D.P. (1985): Calculation of monoclonal antibody affinity constants directly from antibody dilution curves. Immunol. Lett. **9**, 15-18

Groopmann, J.D., Donahue, P.R., Zhu, J., Chen, J., Wogan, G.N. (1985): Detection of metabolites and nucleic acids in urine by affinity chromatography, Proc. Natl. Acad. Sci. U.S.A. **82**, 6492-6496

Guengerich, F.P., Wang, P., Davidson, N.K. (1982): Estimation of isoenzymes of microsomal cytochrome P-450 in rats, rabbits and humans using immunochemical staining coupled with sodium dodecyl sulphate polyacrylamide gel electrophoresis. Biochem. **21**, 1698-1706

Guesdon, J.L., Ternynck, T., Avrameas, S. (1979): The use of avidin-biotin interaction in immunoenzymatic techniques. J. Histochem. Cytochem. **27**, 1131-1139,

Guilbault, G.G. (1990): Piezoelectric immunosensors. Abstr. 1st World Congress of Biosensors, May, 2nd-4th, Singapure, p. 38-40

Guilbert, L.J., Iscove, N.N. (1976): Partial replacement of serum by selenite, transferrin, albumin and lecithin in haemopoietic cell culture. Nature **263**, 594-595

Gupka, S.K., Talwar, G.P., Rose, N.R. and Burek, C.L. (1991): Preliminary studies on the indium slide immunoassay for estimation of human chorionic gonadotropin antibody. Proc. Soc. Exp. Biol. Med. **196**, 106-109

Habeeb, A.F.S.A., (1981): A novel preparation of immunosorbents. Controlled coupling of proteins to Sepharose-gelatin by heterobifunctional reagent. Biochem. Biophys. Acta **673**, 527-538

Hage, D.S., Walters, R.R., Hethocote H.W. (1986): Split-peak affinity chromatographic studies of the immobilization-dependent adsorption kinetics of protein A. Anal. Chem. **58**, 274-279

Haimovich, J., Hurwitz, E., Novik, N., Sela, A. (1970b): Use of protein bacteriophage conjugates for detection and quantitation of proteins. Biochim. Biophys. Acta **207**, 125-129

Haimovich, J., Hurwitz, E., Novik, N., Sela, M. (1970a): Preparation of protein-bacteriophage conjugates and their use in detection of anti-protein antibodies. Biochim. Biophys. Acta **207**, 115-124

Hall, R., Hydr, J.E., Goman, M., Simons, D.L., Hope, I.A., Mackay, M., Scaife, J. (1984): Major surface antigens of a malaria parasite cloned and expressed in bacteria. Nature **311**, 379-382

Hamiliton, R.G., Roebber, M., Reimer, C.B., Rodkey, L.S. (1987): Quality control of murine monoclonal antibodies using isoelectric focusing affinity immunoblot analysis. Hybridoma **6**, 205-217

Hancock, K., Tsang, V.C.W. (1983): India ink staining on nitrocellulose paper. Anal. Biochem. **133**, 157-162

Hansen, T., Hannestad, K. (1989): HLA typing by rosetting with immunomagnetic beads coated with specific antibodies. J. Immunogenet. **16**, 137-139

Harlow, E., Lane, D.P. (1988): Antibodies. A Laboratory Manual. Cold Spring Harbor Laboratory, pp. 551-552

Harshman, J.S. (1989): Purification of murine IgM monoclonal antibodies by hydroxylapatite chromatography. J. Tissue Culture Meth. **12**, 115-117

Hassl, A., Aspock, H. (1988): Purification of egg yolk immunoglobulins: A two-step procedure using hydrophobic interaction chromatography and gel filtration. J. Immunol. Meth. **110**, 225-228

Hauber, R., Geiger, R.A. (1987): A new, very sensitive, bioluminiscnce-enhanced detection system for protein blotting. J. Clin. Chem. Biochem. **25**, 511-514

Haun, M., Wasi, S. (1990): Biotinylated antibodies bound to streptavidin beads: A versatile solid matrix for immunoassays. Anal. Biochem. **191**, 337-342

Hawkes, R. (1983): Identification of concanavalin A-binding proteins after sodium dodecyl sulphate gel electrophoresis and protein blotting. Anal. Biochem. **123**, 143-146

Hayashi, T., Sakamoto, S., Shikanabe, M., Wada, I., Yoshida, H. (1989): HPLC analysis of human epidermal growth factor using immunoaffinity precolumn. I. Optimization of immunoaffinity column. Chromatogr. **27**, 569-573

Hearn, M.T., Davies, J.R. (1990): Evaluation of factors which affect column performance with immobilized antibodies. Model studies with a lysozyme-antilysozyme system. J. Chromatogr. **512**, 23-39

Heifetz, A.H., Braatz, J.A., Wolfe, R.A., Barry, R.M., Miller, D.A., Solomon, B.A. (1989): Monoclonal antibody production in hollow fiber bioreactors using serum-free medium. BioTechniques **7**, 192-197

Heisz, O. (1987): Hochleistungs-Flüssigkeits-Chromatographie. A. Hüthig Verl., Heidelberg

Hemmilä, I., Dakubu, S., Muukula, V.-M., Siitari, H., Löwgren, T. (1984): Europium as label in time-resolved immunofluorometric assays. Anal. Biochem. **137**, 335-343

Henderson, D.R., Friedman, S.B., Harries, J.D., Manning, W.B., Zoccoli, M.A.(1986): CEDIA™, a new homogeneous immunoassay system, Clin. Chem. **32** 1637-1641

Heney, G., Orr, G.A. (1981): The purification of avidin and its derivatives on 2-iminobiotin-6-aminohexyl-Sepharose 4B. Anal. Biochem. **114**, 92-96,

Heyningen, van, V., Brock, D.J.H., Heyningen, van, S. (1983): A simple method for ranking the affinities of monoclonal antibodies. J. Immunol. Meth. **62**, 147-153

Hiatt, A., Cafferkey, R., Bowdish, K. (1989): Production of antibodies in transgenic plants. Nature 342, 76-78

Hill, C.R., Birch, J.R., Benton, C. (1986): Affinity chromatography using monoclonal antibodies. Spec. Publ. Soc. Gen. Microbiol. **18**, 175-190

Hinman, C., Green, C.L., Denno, D., Rauch, J.C., Hudson, R.A. (1985): Affinity chromatographic purification of antibody subsets depends on the mode of cross-linking of antigen to the affinity matrix. Mol. Immunol. **22**, 681-688

Hirn-Scavennec, J., Brailly, H., Maraninchi, D., Mannoni, P., Mawas, C., Delaage, M. (1988): Elimination of leukemia cells from human bone marrow using floating beads. Transplantation **46**, 558-563

Hirano, H. (1989): Microsequence analysis of winged scan seed proteins electroblotted from two-dimensional gel. J. Protein Chem. **8**, 115-130

Hirata, H., Kambe, T., Kagawa, Y. (1984): A purified alanine carrier composed of a single polypeptide from thermophilic bacterium PS3 driven by either proton or sodium ion gradient. J. Biol. Chem. **259**, 10653-10655

Hjelm, H., Hjelm, K., Sjöquist, J. (1972): Protein A from Staphylococcus aureus. Its isolation by affinity chromatography and its use as an immunosorbent for isolation of immunoglobulins. FEBS Lett. **28**, 73-76

Hjerten, S. (1959): Calcium phosphate chromatography of normal human serum and of electrophoretically isolated proteins. Biochim. Biophys. Acta **31**, 216-235

Hochuli, E. (1990): Affinity purification of human interferon synthesized in bacteria. In: Briand, Y., Doinel, C., Faure, A. (eds.) Technologies de Purification des Proteins, Vol. 4, Clermon-Ferrant, pp. 155-158

HOFFMAN, W.L., O'SHANNESSY, D.J. (1988): Site-specific immobilization of antibodies by their oligosaccharide moities to new hydrazide derivatized solid supports. J. Immunol. Meth. **112**, 113-120

HOLTZHAUER, M. (1988): Biochemische Labormethoden: Arbeitsvorschriften und Tabellen, Heidelberger Taschenbücher, Vol. 249, Springer Verlag Heidelberg

HOPP, T.P., PRIKETT, K.S., PRICE, V.L., LIBBY, R.T., MARCH, C.J., CERRETTI, D.P., URDAL, D.L., CONLON, P.J. (1988): A short polypeptide marker sequence useful for recombinant protein identification and purification. Bio/Technology **6**, 1204-1210

HOREJSI, J., SMETANA, R. (1956): The isolation of gamma globulin from blood-serum by Rivanol. Acta Med. Scand. **155**, 65-70

HOUTEN, W.H. (1987): A survey of enzyme coupling techniques. Meth. Enzymol. **135**, 30-65

HOWE, J.G., HERSHEY, J.W.B. (1981): A sensitive immunoblotting method for measuring protein synthesis initiation factor levels in lysates of *Escherichia coli*. J. Biol. Chem. **256**, 12836-12839

HRKAL, Z., REJNKOVA, J., STOCKBAUER, P., RYBAK, M., BENES, M.J. (1989): Isolation of monoclonal antibodies from mouse ascites fluids by chromatography on "Blue" DEAE cellulose. Cesk. Farm. **38**, 276-278

HSIUNG, L.-M. BARCLEY, A.N., BRANDON, M.R., SIM, E., PORTER, R.R. (1982): Purification of human C3b inactivator by monoclonal antibody affinity chromatography. Biochem. J. **203**, 293-298

HSU, J.H. (1984): Immunogold for detection of antigen on nitrocellulose paper. Anal. Biochem. **142**, 221-225

HSU, S.M., RAINE, L., FANGHER, H. (1981): The use of avidin-biotin-peroxidase complex (ABC) in immunoperoxidase techniques. Comparison between ABC and unlabeled antibody (PAP) procedures. J. Histochem. Cytochem. **29**, 577-580,

HUDSON, L., HAY, F.C. (1989): Practical Immunology, Blackwell Sci. Publ., Oxford, 3nd Edition

HUMBERT, P., NIROOMAND, F., FISCHER, G., MAYER, B., KOESLING, D., HINSCH, K-D., GAUSEPOHL, H., FRANK, R., SCHULTZ, G., BÖHME, E. (1990): Purification of soluble guanylyl cyclase from bovine lung by a new immunoaffinity chromatographic method. Eur. J. Biochem., **190**, 273-278

HUNGER, H.-D., BERENDT, G., BRETER, H., COUTELLE, C. (1990): Flächige Trägermaterialien in der Molekularbiologie. GIT Labor-Medizin, 438-444 (Teil 1), 531-540 (Teil 2), 622-636 (Teil 3)

HUNGER, H.-D., COUTELLE, C., BERENDT, G., FLACHMEIER, C., ROSENTHAL, A., SPEER, A, SZARGAN, R., FRANKE, P., STAHL, J., CUONG, N.V., BARCHAND, G. (1986): CCA paper: A new two-dimensional cyanuric chloride-activated matrix for universal application in molecular biology. Anal. Biochem. **156**, 286-299

HUR, S.-J., TODA, H., YAMADA, M. (1989): Isolation and characterization of an unprocessed extracellular myeloperoxidase in HL-60 cell cultures. J. Biol. Chem. **264**, 8542-8548

HWANG, H.H., HEALEY, M.C., JOHNSTON, A.V. (1988): Purification of ascitic fluid-derived monoclonal antibodies by anion exchange and size-exclusion high-performance liquid chromatography. J. Chromatogr. **430**, 329-339

IDEYAMA, S., NAKAGAWA, S., ARAKAWA, M., SUGINO, H., KAKINUMA, A. (1986): Purification and characterization of IgE produced by human myeloma cell line U 266. Mol. Immunol. **23**, 159-167

IINO, S. (1988): Separation and purification of monoclonal antibody by hydroxyapatite packed column. Bio. Ind. **5**, 903-909

INGANÄS, M. (1981): Comparison of mechanisms of interaction between protein A from *Staphylococcus aureus* and human monoclonal IgG, IgA and IgM in relation to the classical Fcγ and the alternative F(ab')$_2$ protein A interactions. Scand. J. Immunol. **13**, 343-352

ITO, A., PALADE, G.E. (1978): Presence of NADPH-cytochrome P-450 reductase in rat liver Golgi membranes. J. Cell. Biol. **79**, 590-597

JACOBSON, C., FRICH, J.R., STEENSGAARD, J. (1982): Determination of affinity of monoclonal antibodies against human IgG. J. Immunol. Meth. **50**, 77-88

JAMES, R.W., PROUDFOOT, A., POMETTA, D. (1989): Immunoaffinity fractionation of high-density lipoprotein subclasses 2 and 3 using anti-apolipoprotein A-I and A-II immunosorbent gels. Biochim. Biophys. Acta **1002**, 292-301

JANDA, I, JAENSCH, H. BRAUN, J., WOOD, W.G. (1990): A comparison of four immunometric assays for myeloperoxidase using luminiscent and colorimetric signal detection. J. Clin. Chem. Clin. Biochem. **28**, 475-480

JANSON, J.-C. (1984): Large-scale affinity purification - state of the art and future prospects. Trends in Biotechnol. **2**, 31-38

JATON, J.-C., BRAMDT, D.C., VASSALLI, P. (1979): The isolation and characterization of immunoglobulins, antibodies, and their constituent polypeptide chains. In: LEFKOVITS, I., PERNIS, B. (eds.) Immunological Methods, Vol. 1, Academic Press, New York, pp. 44-68

JEFFREY, A.M., ZOPF, D.A., GINSBURG, V. (1975): Affinity chromatography of carbohydrate-specific immunoglobulins: Coupling of oligosaccharides to Sepharose. Biochem. Biophys. Res. Commun. **62**, 608-613

JOHANNSON, H., OESTLING, M., SOFER, G., WHALSTROEM, H., LOW, D. (1988) Chromatographic equipment for large-scale protein and peptide purification. In: MIZRAKI, A. (ed.) Downstream Processes: Equipment and Techniques. A.R. Liss Inc., New York, pp. 128-157

JOHANNSSON, A., STANLEY, C.J., SELF, C.H. (1985): A fast highly sensitive colorimetric enzyme immunoassay system demonstrating benefits of enzyme amplification in clinical chemistry, Clin. Chim. Acta **148**, 119-124

JOHNSON, E., MIRIBEL, M., ARNAUD, P., TSANG, K.Y. (1987): Purification of IgM monoclonal antibody from murine ascitic fluid by a two step column chromatography procedure. Immunol. Lett. **14**, 159-165

JOHNSTON, A., HEARN, M.T.W. (1990): High-performance liquid chromatography of amino acids, peptides and proteins. CIII. Mass transfer resitances in ion-exhange and dye-affinity chromatography of proteins. J. Chromatogr. **512**, 101-114

JOHNSTONE, A., THORPE, R. (1982): Immunochemistry in Practice, Blackwell Scientific Publ., Oxford, pp. 27-31

JONSDOTTIR, J., SKOOG, B. EKRE, H.-P.T., PAVLU, B., PERLMAN, P. (1986): Purification of pituitary and biosynthetic human growth hormone using monoclonal antibody immunoadsorbent. Mol. Cell Endocrinol. **46**, 131-135

JOSIC, D., HOFMANN, W., HABERMANN, R., SCHULZE, J.-D., REUTTER, W. (1988): Isolation of immunoglobulins and their use in immunoaffinity HPLC. J. Clin. Chem. Clin. Biochem. **26**, 559-568

JUAREZ-SALINAS, H., BIGBEE, W.L., LAMOTTE, G.B., OTT, G.S. (1986): New procedures for the analysis and purification of IgG murine MAbs. Amer. Biotech. Lab. March/April '86, 38-43

JUAREZ-SALINAS, H., ENGELHORN, S.C., BIGBEE, W.L., LOWRY, M.A., STANKER, L.H. (1984): Ultrapurification of monoclonal antibodies by high performance hydroxyapatite (HPHT) chromatography. BioTechniques **5**, 164-169

JUAREZ-SALINAS, H., OTT, G.S., CHEN, J.-C., BROOKS, T.L., STANKER, L.H. (1986 a): Separation of IgG idiotypes by high-performance hydroxylapatite chromatography. Meth. Enzymol., **121**, 615-622

JUNGBAUER, A., TAUER, CH., REITER, M., PURTSCHER, M., WENISCH, E., STEINDL, F., BUCHACHER, A., KATINGER, H. (1989): Comparison of protein A, protein G and copolymerized hydroxyapatite for the purification of human monoclonal antibodies. J. Chromatogr. **476**, 257-268

JUNGBAUER, A., TAUER, CH., WENISCH, E., UHL, K., BRUNNER, J., PURTSCHER, M., STEINDL, F., BUCHACHER, A. (1990): Isolation of isoproteins from monoclonal antibodies and recombinant proteins by chromatofocusing. J. Chromatogr. **512**, 157-163

JUNGBAUER, A., UNTERLUGGAUER, F., STEINDL, F., RÜKER, F., KATINGER, H. (1987): Combination of mass ion-exchange media and high performance cation exchange chromatography for the purification of high purity monoclonal antibodies. J. Chromatogr. **397**, 313-320

JUNGBAUER, A., UNTERLUGGAUER, F., UHL, K., BUCHACHER, A., STEINDL, F., PETTAUER, D., WENISCH, E. (1988): Scale-up of monoclonal antibody purification using radial streaming ion exchange chromatography. Biotechnol. Bioengng. **32**, 326-333

JUNGBAUER, A., WENISCH, E. (1989): High performance liquid chromatography and related methods in purification of monoclonal antibodies. In: MIZRAKI, A. (ed.) Monoclonal Antibodies: Production and Application, Alan R. Liss Inc., New York, pp. 161-192

KADISH, J.L., WENC, K.M. (1983): Contamination of polyethylene glycol with aldehydes: Implications for hybridoma fusion. Hybridoma **2**, 87-89

KAISER, G., MICHEEL, B. (1991): Immunoaffinity purification of human α-fetoprotein using monoclonal antibodies. Biomed. Biochim. Acta **50**, 1033-1039

KAKU, I., NAKANISHI, S., HORIGUCHI, K. (1989): Enzyme immunoelectrode for insulin incorporating a membrane partially treated with water-vapour plasma. Anal. Chim. Acta **22**, 283-292

KARAWAJEW, L., BEHRSING, O., KAISER, G., MICHEEL, B. (1988): Production and ELISA application of bispecific monoclonal antibodies against fluorescein isothiocyanate (FITC) and horseradish peroxidase (HRP). J. Immunol. Meth. **111**, 95-99

KARAWAJEW, L., MICHEEL, B., BEHRSING, O., GAESTEL, M. (1987): Bispecific antibody-producing hybrid-hybridomas selected by a fluorescence activated cell sorter. J. Immunol. Meth. **96**, 265-270

KARLSEN, A., LERNMARK, A., KOFOD, H., DYRBERG, T. (1990): A novel affinity purification method to isolate peptide specific antibodies. J. Immunol. Meth. **128**, 151-157

KARSTEN, U., STOLLEY, P., WALTHER, I., PAPSDORF, G., WEBER, S., CONRAD, K., PASTERNAK, L., KOPP, J. (1988): Direct comparison of electric field-mediated and PEG-mediated cell fusion for the generation of antibody producing hybridomas. Hybridoma **7**, 627-633

KARUBE, I. (1988): Novel immunosensor systems. Biotec., Vol. 2, Gustav Fischer Verlag, Stuttgart, pp. 37-47

KATAOKA, K., SAKURAI, Y., TSURATA, T. (1987): Affinity selection of cells on solid-phase matrices with immobilized proteins. In: BRASH, J.L., HORBETT, T.A. (eds.) Proteins at Interfaces, ACS Symposium Series No. 343, pp. 603-614

KATO, Y., NAKAMURA, K., HASHIMOTO, T. (1982): Evaluation of conventional and medium-performance ion exchangers for the preparation of proteins. J Chromatogr. **253**, 219-225

KATO, Y., NAKAMURA, K., HASHIMOTO, T. (1984): New high performance cation exchangers for the separation of proteins. J. Chromatogr. **294**, 207-212

KAWAJIRI, K., ITO, A., OMURA, T. (1977): Subfractionation of rat liver microsomes by immunoprecipitation and immunoadsorption methods. J. Biochem. **81**, 779-789

Kawasaki, T., Takahashi, S., Ikeda, K. (1985): Hydroxyapatite high-performance liquid chromatography: Column performance for proteins. Eur. J. Biochem. **152**, 361-371

Keating, M.Y.G, Rechnitz, G.A. (1984): Potentiometric digoxin antibody measurements with antigen ionophore-based membrane electrodes. Anal. Chem. **56**, 801-806

Keating, M.Y.G., Rechnitz, G.A. (1983): Cortisol (hydrocortisone) antibody electrode. Analyst **108**, 766-768

Keenan, M.J. (1988): Purification of rabbit anti-DBP antibodies and porcine DBP using immunoadsorption chromatography. Biochem. Arch. **4**, 239-245

Kennedy, J.F., Phillips, G.O., Wedloc, D.J., Williams, P.A. (eds.) (1985): Cellulose and its Derivatives. E. Horwood Ltd, Chichester

Kenney, A., Goulding, L., Hill, C. (1988): The design, preparation, and use of immunopurification reagents. In: Walker, J.M. (ed.) Methods in Molecular Biology, Vol. 3, Humana Press, Clifton, pp. 99-110

Kenney, A.C. (1986): A process for separating animal cells from a liquid culture. U.S. Patent 4,589,987

Kenney, A.C. (1989): Large-scale purification of monoclonal antibodies. In: Mizraki, A. (ed.) Monoclonal Antibodies: Production and Application, Alan R. Liss Inc., New York, pp. 143-160

Kenney, A.C., Chase, H.A. (1987): Automated production scale affinity purification of monoclonal antibodies. J. Chem. Tech. Biotechnol. **39**, 173-182

Kenny, P.A., McCaskill, A.C., Boyle, W. (1981): Enrichment and expansion of specific antibody-forming cells by adoptive transfer and clustering, and their use in hybridoma production. AJEBAC **59**, part 4, 427-437

Kenyon, A.J., Gander, E.J., Lopez, C., Good, R.A. (1973): Isolation of Aleutian Mink disease virus by affinity chromatography, Science **179**, 187-189

Keynes, M. (1988): Rapid purification of mouse monoclonal antibodies from ascites by fast protein liquid chromatography. Chromatography Int., April 1988, 14-21

Khanna, P.L., Worthy, T.E.(1990): A recombinant protein-based homogeneous immunoassay. Eur. Clin. Lab., June, 31-35

Khurana, A.L., Butts, E.T., Ho, C.-T. (1989): Analysis of mouse, monkey and baboon sera IgGs by HPL-affinity chromatography. J. Liquid Chromatogr. **12**, 3019-3031

Kim, W.B., Kim, B.M., Choi, E.C, Kim, B.K. (1990): Immunoaffinity purification of hepatitis B surface antigen using anti-idiotype as a specific eluent. J. Immunol. Meth. **126**, 119-124

Kints, J.P., Manouvriez, P., Bazin, H. (1989): Rat monoclonal antibodies. VII. Enhancement of ascites production and yield of monoclonal antibodies in rats following pretreatment with pristane and Freunds adjuvant. J. Immunol. Meth. **119**, 241-245

Kitagawa, Y., Sasaki, T. (1987): Specific purification of monoclonal anti-DNA antibodies from culture medium using a DNA-coupled Sepharose 4B affinity column. J. Immunol. Meth. **96**, 7-10

Klausner, A. (1986): Taking aim at cancer with monoclonal antibodies. BioTechnology **4**, 194-195

Köhler, G., Milstein, C. (1975): Continuous cultures of fused cells secreting antibody of predefined specificity. Nature **256**, 495-497

Komisar, J.L., Fuhrman, J.A., Cebra, J.J. (1982): IgA producing hybridomas are readily derived from gut-associated lymphoid tissue. J. Immunol. **128**, 2376-2378

Kondo, A., Kishimura, M., Katoh, S., Sada, E. (1989): Improvement of proteolytic resistance of immunoadsorbents by chemical modification with polyethylene glycol. Biotechnol. Bioengng. **34**, 532-540

Kondo, A., Takamatsu, H., Katoh, S., Sada, E. (1990): Adsorption equilibrium in immunoaffinity chromatography with antibodies to synthetic peptides. Biotechnol. Bioengng. **35**, 146-151

Kondoh, H., Kobayashi, K., Hagiwara, K. (1987): A simple procedure for the isolation of human secretory IgA of IgA1 and IgA2 subclass by a jackfruit lectin, jacalin, affinity chromatography. Mol. Immunol. **24**, 1219-1222

Kovar, J. (1986 a): Hybridoma cultivation in defined serum-free media: Growth supporting substances, II. Insulin, other hormones and growth factors. Folia biol. **32**, 304-310

Kovar, J. (1986 b): Hybridoma cultivation in defined serum- free media: Growth supporting substances, III. Ethanolamine, vitamins and other low molecular weight nutrients. Folia biol. **32**, 369-376

Kovar, J., Franek, F. (1985): Hybridoma cultivation in defined serum-free media: Growth supporting substances, I. Transferrin. Folia biol. **31**, 167-175

Kovar, J., Franek, F. (1987): Iron compounds at high concentrations enable hybridoma growth in a protein-free medium. Biotechnol. Lett. **9**, 259-264

Köves, K., Arimura, A. (1989): Solid-phase adsorption method for removing undesired antibodies from polyclonal antiserum. J. Histochem. Cytochem. **37**, 903-908

Kozel, T.R., Hermerath, C.A. (1988): Benzoquinone activation of Cryptococcus neoformans capsular polysaccharides for construction of an immunoaffinity column. J. Immunol. Meth. **107**, 53-58

Kranz, D.M., Billing, P.A., Herron, J.N., Voss, E.W., Jr. (1980): Modified hybridoma methodology: Antigen-directed chemically mediated cell fusion. Immunol. Commun. **9**, 639-651

Kricka, L.J., Stott, R.A.W., Thorpe, G.H.G. (1988): Enhanced chemiluminiscence enzyme immunoassays.

In: Collins, W.P (ed.) Complementary Immunoassays, pp. 169-179, J. Wiley & Sons, Chichester

Kristiansen, T. (1978): Matrix-bound antigens and antibodies. In: Hoffmann-Ostenhof, O., Breitenbach, M., Koller, F., Kraft, D., Scheiner, O. (eds.), Affinity Chromatography, pp. 191-206

Kristiansen, T., Sparrman, M., Moreno-Lopez, J. (1979): Immobilized lectins for isolation of virus and virus glycoproteins. In: Egly, J.M. (ed.): Affinity Chromatography and Molecular Interactions, Editions INSERM, Paris, pp. 217-230

Kronvall, G., Williams, R.C. (1969): Differences in antiprotein A activity among IgG subgroups. J. Immunol. **103**, 828-833

Kubo, R.T., Born, W., Kappler, J.W., Marrack, P., Pigeon, M. (1989): Characterization of a monoclonal antibody which detects all murine αß T-cell receptors. J. Immunol. **142**, 2736-2742

Kvalheim, G., Fodstad, O., Pihl, A., Nustad, K., Pharo, A., Ugelstad, J., Funderud, S. (1987): Elimination of B-lymphoma cells from human bone marrow: Model experiments using monodisperse magnetic particles coated with primary monoclonal antibodies, Cancer Res. **47**, 846-851

Kyhse-Andersen, J. (1984): Electroblotting of multiple gels: a simple apparatus without buffer tank for rapid transfer of proteins from polyacrylamide to nitrocellulose. J. Biochem. Biophys. Meth. **10**, 203-209

Laemmli, U.K. (1970): Cleavage of structural proteins during the assembly of the head of bacteriophage T4, Nature **227**, 680-684

Lambert, K.J., Boraston, R., Thompson, P.W., Birch, J.R. (1987): Production of monoclonal antibodies using large-scale cell culture. Developments in Industrial Microbiol. **27**, 101-106

Larrick, J.W., Buck, D.W. (1984): Practical aspects of human monoclonal antibody production. BioTechniques **2**, 6-14

Larsson, P.-O., Glad, M., Hansson, L., Mansson, M.O., Ohlson, S., Mosbach, K. (1983) High-performance liquid chromatography. In: Giddings, J.C. et al. (eds.) Advances in Chromatography, Vol. 21, Marcel Dekker Inc., New York, pp. 41-85

Lasch, J., Irwig, M., Koelsch, R., David, H., Marx, I. (1975): Studies of the distribution of proteins bound to CNBr-activated Sepharose 4B at the electron-microscopic level. Eur. J. Biochem. **60**, 163-167

Lasch, J., Janowski, F. (1988): Leakage stability of ligand-support conjugates under operational conditions. Enzyme Microb. Technol. **10**, 312-314

Lasch, J., Koelsch, R. (1978): Enzyme leakage, multipoint attachment of agarose-bound enzyme preparations. Eur. J. Biochem. **82**, 181-186

Lasch, J., Koelsch, R., Kühnau, R. (1985): Homogeneity, stability of enzyme-support-conjugates. Proc. 16th FEBS Congress, Pt. C, pp. 243-249

Lasch, J., Koelsch, R., Weigel, S., Blaha, K., Turkova, J. (1982): Final affinity support characterization: (in)homogeneity, stability of ligand-matrix linkage. In: Gribnau, T.C.J., Visser, J., Nivard, R.J.F. (eds.) Affinity Chromatography and Related Techniques. Elsevier Sci. Publ., Amsterdam, pp. 245-254

Le, M.S., Robertston, J.P., Gollan, K.L. (1988): Novel approach to biological material preparation by membrane chromatography. Data Sheet Dr. H. Knauer Wissenschaftliche Geräte KG, Bad Homburg

Lea, T., Smeland, E. Funderud, S., Vartdal, F., Davies, C., Beiske, K., Ugelstad, J. (1986): Characterization of human mononuclear cells after positive selection with immunomagnetic particles. J. Immunol. **23**, 509-519

Lee, C.-Y. G., Huang, Y.-S., Hu, P.-C., Gomel, V., Menge, A.C. (1982): Analysis of sperm antigens by sodium dodecyl sulphate gel/protein blot radioimmunobinding method. Anal. Biochem. **123**, 14-22

Lee, I.H., Meyerhoff, M.E. (1988): Enzyme-linked flowinjection immunoassay using immobilized secondary antibodies, Microchim. Acta **111**, 207-221

Lee, K.N., Birckbichler, P.J., Fesus, L. (1986): Purification of human erythrocyte transglutaminase by immunoaffinity chromatography, Prep. Biochem. **16**, 321-335

Lee, S.-M., Gustafson, M.E., Pickle, D.J., Flickinger, M.C., Muschik, G.M., Morgan, A.D., Jr. (1986): Large scale purification of murine anti-melanoma monoclonal antibodies. J. Biotechnol. **4**, 189-204

Leivestad, T., Gaudernack, G., Ugelstad, J., Thorsby, E. (1986): Positive selection of activated T cells of the T8 (CD8) sub-type by immunomagnetic separation, Tissue Antigens **28**, 46-52

Leivestad, T., Gaudernack, G., Ugelstad, J., Vartdal, F., Thorsby, E. (1987): Isolation of pure and functionally active T4 and T8 cells by positive selection with antibody-coated monosized magnetic microspheres, Transplant. Proc. Vol.XIX, 265-267

Lemoli, R.M., Gobbi, M., Tazzari, L., Tassi, C., Dinota, A., Visani, G., Grassi, G., Mazza, P., Cavo, M., Tura, S. (1989): Bone marrow purging for multiple myeloma by avidin-biotin immunoadsorption, Transplantation **47**, 385-387

Lemoli, R.M., Gobbi, M., Tazzari, P.L., Grassi, G., Dinota, A. Gherlinzoni, F., Mazza, P., Tura, S. (1988): Avidin-biotin immunoadsorption for ex vivo bone marrow purging: effect of percentage of target cells and flow rate, Haematologica **73**, 183-185

LeNoble, W.J., Kelm, J. (1980): Chemie in komprimierten Lösungen. Angew. Chem. **92**, 887-902

Leong, M.M.L., Milstein, C., Pannel, R. (1986): Luminiscent detection for immunodot, Western, and Southern blots. J. Histochem. Cytochem. **34**, 1645-1650

LESSER, G.J., LEE, R.H., ZEHFUS, M.H., ROSE, G.D. (1987): Hydrophobic interactions in proteins. In: Protein Engineering. A.R. Liss Inc., New York, pp. 175-179

LEUTE, R., ULLMANN, E., GOLDSTEIN, A., HERZENBERG, L.(1972): Spin immunoassay technique for determination of morphine, Nature, New Biol. **236**, 93-94

LEUTE, R.K., ORTH, H.D.(1978): Prinzip und Anwendung des homogenen Enzymimmunoassays (EMIT^{TM}). In: VOGT, W. (ed.) Enzymimmunoassay, Grundlagen und praktische Anwendung, Georg Thieme Verlag Stuttgart, pp.. 10-19,

LEUVERING, J.H.W., THAL, P.J.H.M., VAN DER WAART, M., SCHUURS, A.H.W.M. (1980): Sol particle agglutination immunoassay for human chorionic gonadotropin, Fresenius Z. Anal. Chem. **301**, 132

LEVY, H.B., SOBER, H.A. (1960): A simple chromatographic method for preparation of gamma-globulin. Proc. Soc. Exp. Biol. Med. **103**, 250-256

LEVY, J.A., LEE. H.M., KAWAHATA, R.T., SPITLER, L.E. (1984): Purification of monoclonal antibodies from mouse ascites eliminates contaminating infectious mouse type C viruses and nucleic acids. Clin. Exp. Immunol. **56**, 114-120

LI, J.K., BARKER, B., KOWALIK, T. (1987): Rapid alkaline blottransfer of viral dsRNAs. Anal. Biochem. **163**, 210-218

LIAPIS, A.I., ANSPACH, B., FINDLEY, M.E., DAVIES, J., HEARN, M.T.W., UNGER, K.K. (1989): Biospecific adsorption of lysozyme onto monoclonal antibody ligand immobilized on nonporous silica particles. Biotechnol. Bioengng. **34**, 467-477

LIM, P.L. (1987): Isolation of specific IgM monoclonal antibodies by affinity chromatography using alkaline buffers. Mol. Immunol. **24**, 11-15

LIMIT, J.M., MOUSSEBOIS, C.H., CAMBIASO, C,L., VAERMAN, J.P., MASSON, P.L. (1979): Particle counting immunoassay. IV. The use of $F(ab')_2$ fragments and N_ε-chloroacetyl lysine N-carboxyanhydride for their coupling to polystyrene latex particles. J. Immunol. Meth. **28**, 25-34

LIN, W., KASAMATSU, H. (1983): On electrotransfer of polypeptides from gels to nitrocellulose membranes. Anal. Biochem. **128**, 302-311

LINDMARK, R., THOREN-TOLLING, K., SJÖQUIST, J. (1983): Binding of immunoglobulins to protein A and immunoglobulin levels in mammalian sera. J. Immunol. Meth. **62**, 1-13

LIVINGSTON, D.M. (1975): Immunoaffinity chromatography of proteins. Meth. Enzymol. **34**, 723-731

LOCASIO-BROWN, L., PLANT, A.L., HORVATH, V. and DURST, R.A. (1990): Liposome flow injection immunoassay: Implications for sensitivity, dynamic range, and antibody regeneration. Anal. Chem. **62**, 2587-2593

LÖFÅS, S., JOHNSSON, B. (1990): A novel hydrogel matrix on gold surfaces in surface plasmon resonance sensors for fast and efficient covalent immobilization of ligands. J. Chem. Soc., Chem. Commun. **1990**, 1526-1528

LOONY, C.(1984): High sensitive light scattering immunoassays. J. Clin. Immunoassay **7**, 90-95

LOW, D. (1988): Purification by process chromatography. Pharm. Manuf. Int. **1988**, 273-279

LOWRY, O.H., ROSEBROUGH, N.J., RANDALL, R.J. (1951): Protein measurement with the Folin phenol reagent. J. Biol. Chem. **193**, 265-275

LUNDBLAD, A., SCHROER, K., ZOPF, D. (1984): Affinity purification of glucose-containing oligosaccharides using a monoclonal antibody. J. Immunol. Meth. **68**, 227-234,

LUNDIN, K.E.A., OVIGSTAD, E., SOLLID, L.M., GJERTSN, H.A., GAUDERNACK, G., THORSBY, E. (1989): Positive selection of Tac (CD25) positive cells following T-cell activation. J. Immunogenet. **16**, 185-191

LUONG, H.T., NGUYEN, A.-L., MALE, K.B. (1987): Affinity cross-filtration for purifying biomolecules. Bio/Technology **5**, 564-566

LUZIO, J.P., NEWBY, A.C., HALES, C.N. (1974): Immunological isolation of rat fat-cell plasma membranes. Biochem. Soc. Trans. **2**, 1385-1386

LUZIO, J.P., NEWBY, A.C., HALES, C.N. (1976): A rapid immunological procedure for the isolation of hormonally sensitive rat fat-cell plasma membrane. Biochem. J. **154**, 11-21

LUZIO, J.P., STANLEY, K.K. (1983): The isolation of endosome-derived vesicles from rat hepatocytes. Biochem. J. **216**, 27-36

MADARA, P.J., BANGHART, L.R., JACK, L.J.W., NEIRA, L.M., MATHER, I.H. (1990): Affinity purification of polyclonal antibodies from antigen immobilized in situ in sodium dodecyl sulfate-polyacrylamide gels. Anal. Biochem. **187**, 246-250

MAJORS, R. E. (1989): New columns for chromatography, a review. LC-GC International **2**, 10-18

MALAN BOREL, I., GENTILE, T., ANGELUCI, J., MARGNI, R.A., BINAGHI, R.A. (1990): Assymmetric Fab glycosylation in guinea-pig IgG1 and IgG2. Immunol. **70**, 281-283

MALM, B. (1987): A method for the isolation of monoclonal antibodies from large volumes of serum-containing hybridoma cell culture supernatants. J. Immunol. Meth. **104**, 103-109

MANCINI, G., CARBONARA, A.O., HEREMANS, J.F. (1965): Immunochemical quantitation of antigens by single radial immunodiffusion. Immunochemistry **2**, 235-254

MANIL, L., MOTTE, P., PERNAS, P., TROALEN, F., BOHUON, C., BELLET, D. (1986): Evaluation of protocols for purification of mouse monoclonal antibodies. J. Immunol. Meth.. **90**, 25-37

Marburg, S., Flagagan, M.E., Tolman, R.L. (1989): Chemistry on solid supports: Defining events and titers by use of cleavable, assayable linking molecules. Anal. Biochem. **181**, 242-249

Matson, R.S., Little, M.C. (1988): Strategy for the immobilization of monoclonal antibodies on solid-phase supports. J. Chromatogr. **458**, 67-77

Mattew, W.D., Tsavaler, L., Reinhardt, L.P. (1981): Identification of a synaptic vesicle-specific membrane protein with a wide distribution in neuronal and neurosecretory tissue. J. Cell. Biol. **91**, 257-269

Mattiasson, B., Nilsson, H. (1977): An enzyme immunoelectrode. Assay of human serum albumin and insulin. FEBS Lett. **78**, 251-254

McCue, J.P., Sasagawa, P.K., Hein, R.H. (1988): Changes induced in antibodies by isolation methods. Biotechnol. Appl. Biochem. **10**, 63-71

McGregor, J.L., Borchier, J., Wild, F., Follea, G., Trzeciak, M.C., James, E., Dechavanne, M., McGregor, L., Clementson, K.J. (1983): Monoclonal antibodies against platelet membrane glycoproteins. Eur. J. Biochem. **131**, 427-436

McKinney, M.M., Parkinson, A. (1987): A simple non-chromatographic procedure to purify immunoglobulins from serum and ascites fluid. J. Immunol. Meth. **96**, 271-278

Melamed, M.D., Green, N.M. (1963): Avidin. Purification and composition. Biochem. J. **89**, 591-599

Mencke, M.W., Weicker, H., Wolf, G.A., Fiehn, W., Feraudi, M. (1986): Reliability of immunoglobulin determination by two methods. Clin. Chim. Acta **155**, 89-94

Menozzi, F.D., Vanderpoorten, P., Dejaffe, P., Miller, A.O.A. (1987): One-step purification of mouse monoclonal antibodies by mass ion exchange chromatography on Zetaprep. J. Immunol. Meth. **99**, 229-233

Merisko, E.M., Farquhar, M.G., Palade, G.E. (1982): Coated vesicle isolation by immunoadsorption on *Staphylococcus aureus* cells. J. Cell. Biol. **92**, 846-857

Messner, D.J., Griffith, G., Kornfeld, S. (1989): Isolation and characterization of membranes from bovine liver which are highly enriched in mannose-6-phosphate receptors. J. Cell. Biol. **108**, 2149-2162

Meyerhoff, M.E., Rechnitz, G.A. (1979): Electrode-based enzyme immunoassays using urease conjugates. Anal. Biochem. **95**, 483-493

Micheel, B., Karsten, U., Fiebach, H., Porstmann, T., Denner, J. (1984): The detection of distinct epitopes of human alpha-fetoprotein (AFP) by solid phase radioimmunoassay using hybridoma culture fluid. Biomed. Biochim. Acta **11**, 1317-1323

Milios, J., Leong, A. S.-Y. (1987): The application of the avidin-biotin technique to previously stained histological sections, Stain Technol. **62**, 411-416

Milstein, C., Cuello, A.C. (1983): Hybrid hybridomas and their use in immunochemistry. Nature **305**, 537-540

Mirande, M., Kellermann, O., Wallen, J.-P. (1982): Macromolecular complexes from sheep and rabbit containing seven aminoacyl-tRNA synthetases. II. Structural characerization of the polypeptide components and immunological identification of the methionyl-tRNA synthetase subunit. J. Biol. Chem. **257**, 11049-11050

Mizra, I.H., Wilkin, T.J., Cantarini, M., Moore, K. (1987): A comparison of spleen and lymph node cells as fusion partners for the raising of monoclonal antibodies after different routes of immunization. J. Immunol. Meth. **105**, 235-243

Mohr, P., Pommerening, K. (1985): Affinity Chromatography - Practical and Theoretical Aspects. Marcel Dekker Inc., New York

Monestier, M., Debbas, M.E., Zhou, S. (1989): Rat monoclonal antibodies to murine IgM determinants: Application to antibody purification. Hybridoma **8**, 631-637

Moreaux, T., Leydecker, M.-T., Meyer, C. (1989): Purification of nitrate reductase from *Nicotiana plumbaginifolia* by affinity chromatography using 5-AMP-Sepharose and monoclonal antibodies. Eur. J. Biochem. **179**, 617-620

Mozhaev, V.V., Sergeeva, M.V., Belova, A.B., Khmelnitsky, Y.L. (1990): Multipoint attachment to a support protects enzyme from inactivation by organic solvents: α-chymotrypsin in aqueous solutions of alcohols and diols. Biotechnol. Bioengng. **35**, 653-659

Müller, R. (1980): Calculation of average antibody affinity in anti-hapten sera from data obtained by competetive radioimmunoassay. J. Immunol. Meth. **34**, 345-352

Murakami, H. (1984): Serum-free cultivation of plasmacytomas and hybridomas. In: Barnes, D.W. (ed.) Methods for Serum-free Culture of Neuronal and Lymphoid Cells, Alan R. Liss Inc., New York, pp. 197-205

Murakami, H. (1989): Serum-free media used for cultivation of hybridomas. In: Mizraki, A. (ed.) Monoclonal Antibodies: Production and Application, Alan R. Liss Inc., New York, pp. 107-141

Muramatsu, H., Dicks, J.M., Tamiya, E., Karube, I. (1987): Piezoelectric crystal biosensor modified with protein A for determination of immunoglobulins. Anal. Chem. **59**, 2760-2763

Muramatsu, H., Kajiwara, K., Tamiya, E., Karube, I. (1986): Piezoelectric immunosensor for the detection of *Candida albicans* microbes. Anal. Chim. Acta **188**, 257-261

Murphy, R.F., Imam, A., Hugehes, A.E., Mcguckern, M.J., Buchanan, K.D., Conlon, J.M., Elmore, D.T. (1976): Avoidance of strongly chaotropic eluents for immunoaffinity chromatography by chemical modification of immobilized ligand. Biochim. Biophys. Acta **420**, 87-96

Myhre, E.B., Kronvall, G. (1981): Immunoglobulin specificities of defined types of Streptococcal Ig receptors. In: Holm, S.E., Christensen, P. (eds.) Basic Concepts of Streptococci and Streptococcal Diseases, Redbook Ltd., Chertsey, Surrey, pp. 209-210

Nakamura, K. Tanaka, T., Kuwahara, A., Takeo, K. (1985): Microassay for proteins on nitrocellulose filter using protein dye-staining procedure. Anal. Biochem. **148**, 311-319

Nakamura, K., Hashimoto, T., Kato, Y., Shimura, K., Kasai, K.-I. (1990): Tresyl-acitvated support for high-performance affinity chromatography. J. Chromatogr. **510**, 101-113

Nau, D.R. (1986): A unique chromatographic matrix for rapid antibody purification. BioChromatography **1**, 82-94

Nau, D.R. (1990): Design of chromatographic matrices for the purification and analysis of antibodies. In: Hancock, W. (ed.) High Performance Liquid Chromatography in Biotechnology, John Wiley & Sons, New York, Chapter **13**, pp. 399-530

Nau, D.R. (1988 a): Chromatographic analysis and characterization of antibodies and antibody preparations. In: Nau, D.R. (ed.) Characterization and Analysis of Antibodies and Antibody Preparations, VHC Publishers, New York (cited in: Nau, 1989a)

Nau, D.R. (1988 b): Die Reinigung von Antikörpern mit BAKERBOND ABx - Application Note J.T. BAKER, 1st. ed.

Nau, D.R. (1988): The role of hydrophobic interaction chromatography in antibody purification - mobile phase optimization. Information Bulletin J.T. Baker B.V.

Nau, D.R. (1989 a): Chromatographic methods for antibody purification and analysis. BioChromatography **4**, 4-18

Nau, D.R. (1989 b): Chromatographic analysis and purification of antibodies. In: Swaminathan, B., Prakash, G. (eds.) Nucleic Acid and Monoclonal Antibody Probes, Marcel Dekker, Inc., New York-Basel, pp. 383-430

Nau, D.R. (1989 c): Optimization of mobile phase conditions for antibody purification on a mixed-mode chromatographic matrix. BioChromatography **4**, 131-143

Neoh, S.H., Gordon, C., Potter, A., Zola, H. (1986): The purification of mouse monoclonal antibodies from ascitic fluid. J. Immunol. Meth. **91**, 231-236

Neurath, A.R., Brunner, R. (1969): Fractionation of proteins with different isoelectric points by Rivanol. Experientia **25**, 668-671

Ngo, T.T., Khatter, N. (1990): Chemistry and preparation of affinity ligands useful in immunoglobulin isolation and serum protein separation. J. Chromatogr. **510**, 281-291

Nielsen, R.G., Wilson, G.S. (1987): Characterization of adsorption on the stationary phase using high-performance immunoaffinity chromatography. J. Chromatogr. **423**, 41-50

Nilsson, I.M., Jonsson, S., Sundquist, S.B., Ahlberg, A., Bergentz, S.E. (1981): A procedure for removing high titer antibodies by extracorporeal protein A-Sepharose adsorption in hemophilia: Substitution therapy and surgery in patients with hemophilia B and antibodies, Blood **58**, 38-44

Nisonoff, A., Palmer, J.L. (1964): Hybridization of half molecules of rabbit gamma globulin. Science **143**, 376-379

Nisonoff, A., Rivers, M.M. (1961): Recombination of a mixture of univalent antibody fragments of different specificity. Arch. Biochem. Biophys. **93**, 460-462

Nollstadt, K.H., Karhanis, Y.D., Gnozzio, M.J., Crane, M.St.J., Gurnett, A.M., Schmatz, D.M., Turner, M.J. (1989): Potential of the sulfobetaine detergent Zwittergent 3-12 as a desorbing agent in biospecific and bioselective affinity chromatography. J. Chromatogr. **497**, 87-100

Nopper, B., Kohen, F., Wilchek, M. (1989): A thiophilic adsorbent for the one-step high performance liquid chromatography purification of monoclonal antibodies. Anal. Biochem. **180**, 66-71

Norwood, T.H. (1976): Dimethylsulfoxide enhances polyethylene glycol mediated somatic cell fusion. Somat. Cell. Genet. **2**, 263-270

Nygren, H., Stenberg, M. (1989): Immunochemistry at interfaces. Immunology **66**, 321-327

O'Shannessy, D.J. (1990): Hydrazino-derivatized supports in affinity chromatography. J. Chromatogr. **510**, 13-21

O'Shannessy, D.J., Wilchek, M. (1990): Immobilization of glycoconjugates by their oligosaccharides: use of hydrazino-derivatized matrices. Anal. Biochem. **191**, 1-8

Oellerich, M. (1979): Anwendung der EMIT-Technik beim Drogen-screening. In: VOGT, W. (ed.) Praktische Anwendung des Enzymimmunasays in klinischer Chemie und Serologie, Georg Thieme Verlag Stuttgart, pp. 66-75

Ogden, J.R., Leung, K. (1988): Purification of murine monoclonal antibodies by caprylic acid. J. Immunol. Meth. **111**, 283-284

Ohlson, S., Gustafsson, S. (1988 a): Protein G - a new tool for the analysis and purification of antibodies. BioMedia **1**, 6-11

Ohlson, S., Nilsson, R., Niss, U., Kjellberg, B.-M., Freiburghaus, C. (1988 b): A novel approach to monoclonal antibody separation using high performance liquid affinity chromatography (HPLAC) with SelectiSpher-10 Protein G. J. Immunol. Meth. **114**, 175-180

OI, V.T., JONES, P.P., HERZENBERG, L.A. (1978): Properties of monoclonal antibodies to mouse Ig allotypes, H-2 and Ia antigens. Current Topics Microbiol. Immunol. **81**, 115-129

OKAMURA, H., RAGUET, S., BELL, A., GAGNON, J., KELLY, P.A. (1989): Purification and sequence analysis of rat liver prolactin receptor. J. Biol. Chem. **244**, 5904-5910

OKUMURA, K., TAKEMORI, T., TOKUHISA, T., TADA, T. (1977): Specific enrichment of the suppressor T cell bearing I-J determinants. Parallel functional, serological characterizations. J. Exptl. Med. **146**, 1234-1245

OLIVER, R.W.A. (ed.): (1989) HPLC of Macromolecules - a Practical Approach. IRL Press, Oxford

OLMSTED, J.B. (1988): Affinity purification of antibodies from blots. In: BJERRUM, O.J., HEEGAARD, N.H.H. (eds.): CRC Handbook of Immunoblotting of Proteins, Vol. 2, CRC Press, London, pp. 94-97

OLSON, W.C., LEUNG, S.K., YARMUSH, M.L. (1989): Recovery of antigens from immunoadsorbents using high pressure. Bio/Technoloy **7**, 369-373

ONO, T., TUAN, R.S. (1990): Double staining of immunoblot using enzyme histochemistry and india ink. Anal. Biochem. **187**, 324-327

OSTERHAUS, A., UYTDEHAAG, F. (1985): Lymphocyte hybridomas: Production and use of monoclonal antibodies. In: Animal Cell Biotechnology, Academic Press Inc., London, Vol. 2, pp. 49-69

ÖSTLUND, C. (1986): Large-scale purification of monoclonal antibodies. TIBTECH **4**, 288-293

ÖSTLUND, C., BORWELL, P., MALM, B. (1987): Process-scale purification from cell culture supernatants. Monoclonal antibodies. Dev. Biol. Stand. **66**, 367-375

OUCHTERLONY, Ö. (1962): In-gel methods for immunological analysis. II. In: Progr. Allergy **6**, S. Karger, Basel, pp. 30-154

PALFREYMAN, J.W., VIGROW, A., BUTTON, D., GLANCY, H. (1988): Simple method for scanning immunoblots. J. Immunol. Meth. **109**, 199-201

PARHAM, P. (1983): Monoclonal antibodies against HLA products and their use in immunoaffinity purification. Meth. Enzymol., **92**, 110-138

PARKER, C.W.(1990): Immunoassays, Meth. Enzymol. **182**, 700-718

PARKER, T.S., STUDEBAKER, J.F. (1988): Low density lipoprotein pheresis: selective immunoadsorption of plasma lipoproteins from patients with premature atherosclerosis. Meth. Enzymol. **137**, 466-478

PARRY, R.P., LOVE, C.A., ROBINSON, G.A. (1990): Detection of Rubella antibody using an optical immunosensor. J. Virol. Meth. **27**, 39-48

PATURLE, L., WEHLAND, J., MARGOLIS, R.L., JOB, D. (1989): Complete separation of tyrosinated and nontyrosinable brain tubulin subpopulation using affinity chromatography. Biochem. **28**, 2698-2704

PAVLU, B., JOHANSSON, U., NYHLEN, C., WICHMAN, A. (1986): Rapid purification of monoclonal antibodies by high-performance liquid chromatography. J. Chromatogr. **359**, 449-460

PB Scientific Posters 1990: Thin Dry Film Multilayer Immunoassay and Self-Contained Fluorogenic ELISA for the Clinical Laboratory: 7 Scientific Posters published by **PB Diagnostics Systems, Inc., Westwood, MA, U.S.A.**; presented at the International Congress of Clinical Chemistry, San Francisco, California U.S.A., July, 1990

PENG, L., CALTON, G.J., BURNETT, J.W. (1987): Evaluation of activation methods with cellulose beads for immunosorbent purification of immunoglobulins. J. Biotechnol. **5**, 255-265

PERRY, G.A., JACKSON, J.D., McDONALD, T.L., CROUSE, D.A., SHARP, J.G. (1985): Purification of monoclonal antibodies using HPLC. Prep. Biochem. **14**, 431-447

PETKOV, L., SAJDOK, J., RAE, K., SUCHOVA, M., KAS, J., TURKOVA, J. (1990): Activation of galactose-containing glycoprotein and solid supports by galactose oxidase in presence of catalase for immobilization purposes. Biotechnology Techniques **4**, 25-30

PFEFFER, S.R., KELLY, R.B. (1985): The subpopulation of brain-coated vesicles that carries synaptic vesicle proteins contains two unique polypeptides, Cell **40**, 949-957

PFEIFFER, N., WYLIE, D.E., SCHUSTER, S.M. (1987): Immunoaffinity chromatography utilizing monoclonal antibodies. J. Immunol. Meth. **97**, 1-9

PFÜLLER, U. (1986) Mizellen, Vesikel, Mikroemulsionen. VEB Verl. Volk u. Gesundheit, Berlin, p. 15

PHILIPS, A.V., ROBBINS, D.J., COLEMAN, M.S., BARKLEY, M.D. (1987): Immunoaffinity purification and fluorescence studies of human adenosine deaminase. Biochem. **26**, 2893-2903

PHILLIPS, A.P., MARTIN, K.L., HORTON, W.H. (1984): The choice of methods for immunoglobulin IgG purification: Yield and purity of antibody activity. J. Immunol. Meth. **74**, 385-393

PHILLIPS, T.M., MORE, N.S., QUEEN, W.D., HOLOHAN, T.V., KRAMER, N.C., THOMPSON, A.M. (1984a): High-performance affinity chromatography: a rapid technique for the isolation and quantitation of IgG from cerebral spinal fluid. J. Chromatogr. **317**, 173-179

PHILLIPS, T.M., QUEEN, W.D., MORE, N.S., THOMPSON, A.M. (1985): Protein A-coated glass beads. Universal support medium for high-performance immunoaffinity chromatography. J. Chromatogr. **327**, 213-219

PIERCE (1990): Catalog & Handbook, Vol. **1**, Pierce Europe B.V., 3260 Out Beijerland, The Netherlands, Chapter D, p. 2

PLACE, J.F., SUTHERLAND, R.M., DÄHNE, C. (1985): Optoelectronic immunosensors: A review of optical immunoassay at continuous surfaces. Biosensors **1**, 321-354

PODUST, V.N., LAVRIK, O.I., NASHEUER, H.-P., GROSSE, F. (1989): DNA-polymerase α-DNA primase from human placenta: Immunoaffinity purification and preliminary characterization, FEBS Lett. **245**, 14-16

PORATH, J. (1974): General methods and coupling procedures. Meth. Enzymol. **34**, 13-30

PORATH, J. (1987): Thiophilic interaction and the selective adsorption of proteins. Trends in Biotechnol. **15**, 225-229

PORATH, J., MAISANO, F., BELEW, M. (1985): Thiophilic adsorption - a new method for protein fractionation. FEBS Lett. **185**, 306-310

PORSTMANN, B., PORSTMANN, T., NUGEL, E. (1981): Comparison of chromogens for the determination of horseradish peroxidase as a marker in enzyme immunoassay. J. Clin. Chem. Biochem. **19**, 435-439

POSSILICO, E.G., KALLELIS, M.S., GEORGE, J.M. (1987): Large-scale production and purification of monoclonal antibodies using cellular microencapsulation. In: SEAVER, S.S. (ed.) The Commercial Production of Monoclonal Antibodies, Marcel Dekker Inc., New York-Basel, pp 139-157

POWELL, M.J., HANSEN, D.E. (1989): Catalytic antibodies - a new direction in enzyme design. BioEngng. **3**, 69-75

PRICE, C., TRULL, A., BERRY, D., GORMAN, E. (1987): Development and validation of particle-enhanced turbidimetric immunoassay for C-reactive protein. J. Immunol. Meth. **99**, 205-211

PRICKETT, K.S., AMBERG, D.C., HOPP, T.P. (1989): A calcium- dependent antibody for identification and purification of recombinant protein. BioTechniques **7**, 580-589

PROGRAIS, L.J., Jr., HAMMER, C.H., KATHUSHA, K., FRANK, M.M. (1987): Purification of C1 inhibitor: A new approach for the isolation of this biologically important plasma protease inhibitor. J. Immunol. Meth. **99**, 113-122

PRUSIK, Z., KASICKA, V. (1985): Micropreparative isotachophoretic electrodesorption of monoclonal antibodies from an affinity adsorbent. J. Chromatogr. **320**, 81-88

PUTNAM, J.E. (1987): Monoclonal antibody production in a ceramic matrix. In: SEAVER, S.S. (ed.) The Commercial Production of Monoclonal Antibodies, Marcel Dekker Inc., New York, pp. 119-138

RAO, L.V.M. (1988): Characterization of anti-tissue factor antibody and its use in immunoaffinity purification of human tissue factor. Thromb. Res. **51**, 373-384

RAYMOND, Y., SUH, M. (1986): Lymph node primary immunization of mice for the production of polyclonal and monoclonal antibodies. J. Immunol. Meth. **93**, 103-106

Réactifs IBF (1983): Ultrogel R, Magnogel R and Trisacryl R. Practical guide for use in affinity chromatography and related techniques. Villeneuve-la-Garenne

READING, C.L. (1982): Theory and methods for immunization in culture and monoclonal antibody production. J. Immunol. Meth. **53**, 261-291

REDEUILH, G., SECCO, C., BAULIEU, E.-E. (1985): The use of biotinyl estradiol-avidin system for the purification of "non-transformed" estrogen receptor by biohormonal affinity chromatography. J. Biol. Chem. **260**, 3996-4002

REED, K.C., MANN, D.A. (1985): Rapid transfer of DNA from agarose gels to nylon membranes. Nucleic Acids Res. **13**, 7207-7221

REIK, L.M., MAINES, S.L., RYAN, D.E., LEVIN, W., BANDIERA, S., THOMAS, P.E. (1987): A simple, non-chromatographic purification procedure for monoclonal antibodies. J. Immunol. Meth. **100**, 123-130

REINHART, M.P., MALAMUD, D. (1982): Protein transfer from isoelectric focousing gels: The native blot. Anal. Biochem. **123**, 229-235

REISER, J., WARDALE, J. (1981): Immunological detection of specific proteins in total cell extracts by fractionation in gels and transfer to diazophenylthioether paper. Eur. J. Biochem. **114**, 569-575

RENNEBERG, R., SCHÖBLER, W., SCHELLER, F. (1983): Amperometric enzyme sensor based immunoassay for factor VIII related antigen. Anal. Lett. **16**, 1279-1289

REUVENY, S., VELEZ, D., MILLER, L., MACMILLAN, J.D. (1986): Comparison of cell propagation methods for their effect on monoclonal antibody yield in fermentors. J. Immunol. Meth. **86**, 61-69

RHODES, M., BIRCH, J. (1988): Large-scale production of proteins from mammalian cells. Biotechnology **6**, 518-523

RICHARDSON, J.P., LUZIO, J.P. (1986): Immunoaffinity purification of subcellular particles and organelles. Appl. Biochem. Biotechnol. **13**, 133-145

RICHARDSON, J.P., SIDDLE, K., LUZIO, J.P. (1984): Immunoaffinity purification of intact, metabolically active, cholinergic nerve terminals from mammalian brain. Biochem. J. **219**, 647-654

RIMMELZWAAN, G.F., GROEN, J., JUNTTI, N., TAPPEMA, J.S. UYTDEHAAG, F.G.C., OSTERHAUS, A.D.M.E (1987): Purification of infectious canine Parvovirus from cell culture by affinity chromatography with monoclonal antibodies. J. Virol. Meth. **15**, 313-322

RITZ, J., SCHLOSSMAN, S.E. (1982): Utilization of monoclonal antibodies in treatment of leukemia and lymphoma. Blood **59**, 1-11

ROBINS, R.A., EMBLETON, M.J., PIMM, M.V., BETES, D.S., CHARLESTON, A., MARKHAM, A.J., BALDWIN, R.W. (1990): Bispecific antibody that binds carcinoembryonic antigen and Ricin toxin A chain cytotoxic for gastrointestinal tract tumor cells. J. Natl. Canc. Inst. **82**, 1295-1296

Robinson, G.A. (1990): Abstr. 1st World Congress on Biosensors, May 2nd-4th, Singapore, p. 37-39

Roederer, J.E., Bastiaans G.J. (1983): Microgravimetric immunoassays with piezoelectric crystals. Anal. Chem. **55**, 2333-2336

Rohringer, R., Holden, D.W. (1985): Protein blotting: Detection of proteins with colloidal gold, and of glycoproteins and lectins with biotin-conjugated and enzyme probes. Anal. Biochem. **144**, 118-127

Roitt, I.M., Brostoff, J., Male, D.K. (1989): Immunology, Gower Medical Publ. Ltd., London, 2nd edition

Roman, L.M., Hubbard, A.L. (1984): A domain-specific marker for the hepatocyte plasma membrane: III. Isolation of canalicular membrane by immunoadsorption. J. Cell. Biol. **98**, 1497-1504

Rordorf, C., Gambke, C., Gordon, J. (1983): A multidot immunobinding assay for autoimmunity and the demonstration of novel antibodies against retroviral antigens in the sera of MRL mice. J. Immunol. Meth. **59**, 105-112

Rosebrough, S.F., Grossman, Z.D., McAfee, J.G. (1986): Purification of fibrin-specific monoclonal antibodies from ascites fluid by preparative isoelectric focusing. Immunol. Lett. **12**, 147-151

Ross, A.H., Herlyn, D., Koprowski, H. (1987): Purification of monoclonal antibodies from ascites using ABx liquid chromatography column. J. Immunol. Meth. **102**, 227- 231

Rousseaux, J., Picque, M.T., Bazin, H., Biserte, G. (1981): Rat IgG subclasses: Differences in affinity to protein A-Sepharose. Mol. Immunol. **18**, 639-645

Rubinstein, K.E., Schneider, R.S., Ullman, E.F. (1972): "Homogeneous" enzyme immunoassay. A new immunochemical technique. Biochem. Biophys. Res. Commun. **47**, 846-851

Russo, C., Callegaro, L., Lanza, E., Ferrone, S. (1983): Purification of IgG monoclonal antibodies by caprylic acid precipitation. J. Immunol. Meth. **65**, 269-271

Saal, S.D., Parker, T.S., Gordon, B.R., Studebaker, J., Hudgins, L., Ahrens, E.H., Rubin, A.L. (1986): Removal of low-density lipoproteins in patients by extracorporeal immunoadsorption, Amer. J. Med. **80**, 583-589

Sada, E., Katoh, S., Kondo, A., Kiyokawa, A. (1986): Effects of coupling method and ligand concentration on adsorption equilibrium in immunoaffinity chromatography. J. Chem. Engng. Japan **19**, 502-506

Sada, E., Katoh, S., Yamanaka, K., Sohma, Y. (1989): Effects of antigen molecular weight on immunoadsorption equilibrium in immunoaffinity chromatography. J. Ferment. Bioengng. **68**, 37-39

Saint-Blancard, J., Kirzin, J.M., Riberon, P., Petit, F., Foucart, J., Girot, P., Boschetti, E. (1982): A simple and rapid procedure for large scale preparation of IgGs and albumin from human plasma by ion exchange and affinity chromatography. In: Gribnau, T.C.J., Visser, J., Nivard, R.J.F. (eds.): Affinity Chromatography and Related Techniques. Elsevier Sci. Publ., Amsterdam, pp. 305-312

Sairam, M.R., Porath, J. (1976): Isolation of antibodies to protein hormones by bioaffinity chromatography on divinyl-sulfonyl Sepharose. Biochem. Biophys. Res. Commun. **69**, 190-196

Samuel, D., Abuknesha, R.A. (1990): Single-step method for the purification of anti-FITC antibodies by use of a coumarin immunoadsorbent. J. Immunol. Meth. **133**, 133-139

Sandgren, M.E., DeLuca, H.F.(1989): An immunoradiometric assay for 1,25-dihydroxyvitamin D3 receptor. Anal. Biochem. **183**, 57-63

Santucci, A., Soldani, P., Lozzi, L., Rustici, M., Bracci, L., Petreni, S., Neri, P. (1988): High performance liquid chromatography immunoaffinity purification of antibodies and antibody fragments. J. Immunol. Meth. **114**, 181-185

Sarvas, H.O., Seppälä, I.J.T., Tähtinen, T., Peterfy, P., Mäkelä, O. (1983): Mouse IgG antibodies have subclass associated affinity differences. Mol. Immunol. **20**, 239-246

Sato, H., Kidaka, T., Hori, M. (1987): Leakage of immobilized IgG from therapeutic immunoadsorbents. Appl. Biochem. Biotechnol. **15**, 145-158

Sato, H., Watanabe, K., Azuma, J., Kidaka, T., Hori, M. (1989): Specific removal of IgE by therapeutic immunosorption system. J. Immunol. Meth. **118**, 161-168

Saunders, G.C. (1979): The art of solid-phase enzyme immunoassay including selected protocols. In: Immunoassays in Clinical Laboratory, Alan R. Liss Inc., New York, pp. 99-118

Scatchard, G. (1949): The attractions of proteins for small proteins and ions. Ann. N.Y. Acad. Sci. **51**, 660-672

Scheller, F., Schubert, F. (1989): Biosensoren. Akademie Verlag Berlin, pp. 255-281,

Schibeci, A., Wade, A.W., Depew, W.T., Szewczuk, M.R. (1986): Analysis of serum antibody repertoires by isoelectric focusing and capillary blotting onto nitrocellulose paper. J. Immunol. Meth. **89**, 201-205

Schierenburg, E. (1987): Laser-induced cell fusion. In: Sowers, A.E. (ed.) Cell Fusion, Plenum Publ. Corp., New York, pp. 409-418

Schlom, J. (1988): Monoclonal antibodies in cancer therapy: The present and the future. BioPharm Sept. 1988, 44-48

Schlossman, S.F., Hudson, L. (1973): Purification of lymphocyte populations on digestible immunosorbent. J. Immunol. **110**, 313-315

Schmidt, C. (1989): The purification of large amounts of monoclonal antibodies. J. Biotechnol. **11**, 235-252

SCHMITZ, G., BOETTCHER, A., KAHL, H.G., BRÜNING, T. (1988): Purification of monoclonal antibodies against the low-density lipoprotein receptor by preparative isotachophoresis. J. Chromatogr. Biomed. Appl. **431**, 327-342

SCHULTZE, H.E., HAUPT, H., HEIDE, K., HEIMBERGER, N., SCHWICK, H.G. (1965): Comparative investigations of purified Diphtheria and Tetanus T-components and their fragments. Immunochemistry **2**, 273-284

SCHULZE-OSTHOFF, K., MICHELS, E., OVERWIEN, B., SORG, C. (1989): Electroelution of antigens immobilized on antibody-linked affinity matrices. Anal. Biochem. **177**, 314-317

SCHUURS, A.H.W.M., GRIBNAU, T.C.J., LEUVERING, J.H.W. (1982): Use of immobilized reagents in immunoassay. In: GRIBNAU, T.C.J., VISSER, J., NIVARD, R.J.F. (eds.) Affinity Chromatography and Related Techniques, Elsevier Sci. Publ., Amsterdam, pp. 343-356

SCHWARTZ, W.E., CLARK, F.M., SABRAN, I.B. (1986): Process- scale isolation and purification of immunoglobulin G. LC-GC Magazine **4**, 442-448

SCHWENZER, B., NEEF, B., BUBLITZ, R., EHLE, H., HORN, A. (1987): Large-scale purification intraluminal alkaline phosphatase from calf intestine by immunosorbent affinity chromatography. Biomed. Biochim. Acta **46**, 15-21

SCOTT, D.W. (1976): Antifluorescein affinity columns: Isolation and immunocompetence of lymphocytes that bind fluoresceinated antigen in vivo or in vitro. J. Exp. Med. **144**, 69-78

SCOTT, R.W., DUFFY, S.A., MOELLERING, B.J., PRIOR, C.(1987): Purification of monoclonal antibodies from large scale mammalian cell culture perfusion systems. Biotechnol. Progr. **3**, 49-56

SCOUTEN, W.H. (1987): A survey of enzyme coupling techniques. Meth. Enzymol. **135**, 30-65. cf. also NGO, T.T. (1986): Methods of activating hydroxyl groups of a polymer carrier using 3-fluoro-1-methyl pyridinium toluene-4-sulfonate. U.S. patent 4,582,875

SEAVER, S.S. (1987): The Commercial Production of Monoclonal Antibodies, Marcel Dekker Inc., New York-Basel

SECHER, D.S., BURKE, D.C. (1980): A monoclonal antibody for large-scale purification of human leukocyte interferon, Nature **285**, 446-450

SELF, C.H.(1985): Enzyme amplification - A general method applied to provide an immunoassisted assay for placental alkaline phosphatase. J. Immunol. Meth. **76**, 389-393

SEPPÄLÄ, I., SARVAS, H., PETERFY, F., MÄKELÄ, O. (1981): The four subclasses of IgG can be isolated from mouse serum using protein A-Sepharose. Scand J. Immunol. **14**, 335-342

SHARON, N. (1979): Application of lectins to cell fractionation: In: EGLY, J.M. (ed.): Affinity Chromatography and Molecular Interactions, Edition INSERM, Paris, pp. 197-205,

SHEPPARD, A.J., HUGHES, M., STEPHEN, J. (1987): Affinity purification of tetanus toxin using polyclonal and monoclonal antibody immunoadsorbents. J. Appl. Bacteriol. **62**, 335-348

SINGER, K.H., JOHNSTON, C., AMOS, D.B., SCOTT, D.W. (1978): Selective depletion and enrichment of alloreactive cytolytic effector lymphocytes using antifluorescein affinity columns, Cell. Immunol. **36**, 75-85

SIPS, R. (1948): On the structure of catalyst surface. J. Chem. Phys. **16**, 490-495

SISSON, T.H., CASTOR, C.W. (1990): An improved method for immobilizing IgG antibodies on protein A-agarose. J. Immunol. Meth. **127**, 215-220

SJÖGREN-JANSSON, E., JEANSSON, S. (1985): Large-scale production of monoclonal antibodies in dialysis tubing. J. Immunol. Meth. **84**, 359-364

SMITH, G.E., SUMMERS, M.D. (1980): The bidirectional transfer of DNA and RNA to nitrocellulose or diazobenzyloxymethyl-paper. Anal. Biochem. **109**, 123-129

SMITH, G.J., MCFARLAND, R.D., REISNER, H.M., HUDSON, J.S. (1984): Lymphoblastoid cell-produced immunoglobulins: Preparative purification from culture medium by hydroxylapatite chromatography. Anal. Biochem. **141**, 432-436

SOLSKY, R.L., RECHNITZ, G.A. (1979): Preparation and properties of an antibody-selective membrane electrode. Anal. Chim. Acta **123**, 135-141

SOMNIER, F.E., LANGVAD, E. (1989): Plasma exchange with selective immunoadsorption of anti-acetylcholinereceptor antibodies. J. Neuroimmunol. **22**, 123-127

SOUTHERN, E.M. (1975): Detection of specific sequences among DNA fragments separated by gel electrophoresis. J. Mol. Biol. **98**, 503-517

SPITZ, M., SPITZ, L., THORPE, R., EUGUI, E. (1984): Intraspleenic primary immunization for the production of monoclonal antibodies. J. Immunol. Meth. **70**, 39-43

SRINIVASAN, R., RUCKENSTEIN, E. (1980): Role of physical forces in hydrophobic interaction chromatography. Separat. Purificat. Meth. **9**, 267-370

STAERZ, U.D., BEVAN, M.J. (1986): Hybrid hybridoma producing a bispecific monoclonal antibody that can focus effector T-cell activity. Proc. Natl. Acad. Sci. U.S.A.. **83**, 1453-1457

STÄHLI, C., STAEHELIN, T., MIGGIANO, V., SCHMIDT, J., HARING, P. (1980): High frequencies of antigen specific hybridomas: Dependence on immunization parameters and prediction. J. Immunol. Meth. **32**, 297-304

STANISLAWSKI, M., COEUR-JOLY, G. (1972): Biogel-adsorbed insoluble protein derivatives for the isolation of antibodies. Biochimie **54**, 203-208

Stanker, L.H., Branscomb, E., Vanderlaan, M., Jensen, R.H. (1986): Monoclonal antibodies recognizing single amino acid substitutions in hemoglobin. J. Immunol. **136**, 4174-4180

Stanker, L.H., Vanderlaan, M., Juarez-Salinas, H. (1985): One-step purification of mouse monoclonal antibodies from ascites fluid by hydroxylapatite chromatography. J. Immunol. Meth. **76**, 157-169

Stanley, C.J., Cox, R.B., Carosi, M.F., Turner, A.F.P. (1988): Amperometric enzyme-amplified immunoassay. J. Immunol. Meth. **112**, 153-161

Stanley, C.J., Johannsson, A., Self, C.H. (1985): Enzyme amplification can enhance both the speed and the sensitivity of immunoassays. J. Immunol. Meth. **83**, 89-95

Steinbuch, M., Audran, R.R (1969): The isolation of IgG from mammalian sera with the aid of caprylic acid. Arch. Biochim. Biophys. **134**, 279-284

Steindl, F., Jungbauer, A., Wenisch, E., Himmler, G., Katinger, H. (1987): Isoelectric precipitation and gel chromatography for purification of monoclonal IgM. Enzyme Microb. Technol. **9**, 361-364

Stenberg, E., Persson, B., Roos, H., Urbaniczky, C. (1991): Quantitative determination of surface concentration of protein with surface plasmon resonance by using radiolabeled proteins. J. Colloid Interface Sci., in press

Stenberg, M., Nygren, H.N. (1982): A receptor ligand reaction studied by a novel analytical tool - the elipsometer isoscope. Anal. Biochem. **127**, 183-192

Stephen, J., Gallop, R.G.C., Smith, H. (1966): Separation of antigens by immunological specifity. Use of disulphide-linked antibodies as immunosorbents. Biochem. J. **101**, 717-720

Stephenson, J.R., Lee. J.M., Wilton-Smith, P.D. (1984): Production and purification of murine monoclonal antibodies: Aberrant elution from protein A-Sepharose 4B. Anal. Biochem. **142**, 189-195

Stevens, F.J. (1987): Modification of an ELISA-based procedure for affinity determination: Correction necessary for use with bivalent antibody. Mol. Immunol. **24**, 1055-1060

Stevens, F.J., Carperos, W.E., Monafo, W.J., Greenspan, N.S. (1988): Size-exclusion HPLC analysis of epitopes. J. Immunol. Meth. **108**, 271-278

Steward, M.W., Petty, R.E. (1972): The use of ammonium sulfate globulin precipitation for determination of affinity of anti-protein antibodies in mouse serum. Immunology **22**, 747-756

Stocks, S.J., Brooks, D.E. (1989): Production and isolation of large quantities of monoclonal antibody using serum-free medium and fast protein liquid chromatography. Hybridoma **8**, 241-247

Stoffel, W., Borberg, H,, Grewe, W. (1981): Application of specific extracorporal removal of low density lipoprotein in familial hypercholesterolaemie, Lancet **2**, 1005-1007

Stoffel. W., Demant, T. (1981): Selective removal of apolipoprotein B-containing serum lipoproteins from blood plasma, Proc. Natl. Acad. Sci. U.S.A. **78**, 611-615

Stone, M.J., Metzger, H.J. (1968): Study of macromolecular interactions by equilibrium molecular sieving. J. Biol. Chem. **243**, 5049-5055

Stott, D.I. (1989): Immunoblotting and dot blotting. J. Immunol. Meth. **119**, 153-187

Stott, D.I., McLearie, J., Marsden, H.S. (1985): A gel transfer-tank for immunoblotting and its application for analysis of nuclear proteins. Anal. Biochem. **149**, 454-460

Sturgeon, C.M., Kennedy, J.F. (1980) A quick-reference summary of recent literature on molecular immobilization and bioaffinity phenomena. Enzyme Microb. Technol. 1 and following volumes

Surek, B., Latzko, E. (1984): Visualization of antigenic proteins blotted onto nitrocellulose using the immuno-gold staining (IGS) method. Biochem. Biophys. Res. Comm. **121**, 284-289

Suzuki, T., Liu, P., Wang, J.H. (1987): Rapid purification of phospholamban by monoclonal antibody immunoaffinity chromatography. Biochem. Cell. Biol. **65**, 302-309

Swaab, D.F., Pool, C.W. (1975): Specificity of oxytocin and vasopressin immunoflurescence. J. Endocrinol. **66**, 263-272

Sweet, C., Stephen, J., Smith, H. (1974): Purification of influenca viruses by disulfide-linked immunosorbents derived from rabbit antibody. Immunochemistry **11**, 295-304

Swingle, M., Tiselius, A. (1951): Tricalcium phosphate as an adsorbent in the chromatography of proteins. Biochem. J. **48**, 171-174

Takamiya, O., Funahashi, S., Yoshioka, K. (1986): Preparation of factor VII-depleted plasma by immunoaffinity chromatography of insolubilized anti-factor VII, Med. Lab. Sci. **43**, 215-219

Tanimori, H., Yoshida, K., Motomura, H., Kitada, K., Yagisawa, S., Kitagawa, S. (1987): Purification of two specific antibodies against drug and carrier protein molecules. Chim. Pharm. Bull. (Tokyo) **35**, 2062-2070

Tanswell, P. Albert, W., Glatz, C., Treffert, C., Linke, R., Staehler, F.(1979): Bestimmung des menschlichen Thyrotropins (hTSH) mittels Enzymimmunoassay. In: Vogt, W. (ed.) Praktische Anwendung des Enzymimmunoassays in klinischer Chemie und Serologie, Georg Thieme Verlag Stuttgart, pp. 91-97,

Tarditi, L., Mariani, M. (1990): Purification of bispecific monoclonal antibodies secreted by tetradomas. Bio-Radiations **74**, 1-3

Taylor, R.F. (1985): A comparison of various commercially available liquid chromatographic supports for immobilization of enzymes and immunoglobulins. Anal. Chim. Acta **174**, 241-248

TEMPONI, M., KAGESHITA, T., PEROSA, F., ONO, R., OKADA, H., FERRONE, S.(1989): Purification of murine IgG monoclonal antibodies by precipitation with caprylic acid: Comparison with other methods of purification. Hybridoma **8**, 85-95

TEMPONI, M., KEKISH, U., FERRONE, S. (1988): Immunoreactivity and affinity of murine IgG monoclonal antibodies purified by caprylic acid precipitation. J. Immunol. Meth. **115**, 151-152

TERASAKI, P.I., MCCLELLAND, J.D. (1964): Microdroplet assay of human serum toxins. Nature **204**, 998-1000

TERMAN, D.S., BUFFALOE, G., MATTIOLI, C., COOK, G., TILLQUIST, R., SULLIVAN, M., AYNS, J.C. (1979): Extracorporeal immunoadsorption: initial experience in human systemic lupus erythematosus. Lancet **2**, 824-827

TERMAN, D.S., YOUNG, J.B., SHEARER, W.T., AYNS, C., LEHANE, D., MATTIOLI, C., ESPADA, R., HOWELL, J.F., YAMAMOTO, T., ZALESKI, H.I., MILLER, L., FROMMER, P., FELDMAN, L., HENRY, J.F., TILLQUIST, R., COOK, G., DASKAL, Y. (1981): Preliminary observations of the effects of brea. New Engl. J. Med. **305**, 1195-1200

TESSER, G.I., FISCH, H.-U., SCHWYZER, R. (1974): Limitations of affinity chromatography: solvolytic detachment of ligands from polymeric supports. Helv. Chim. Acta **57**, 1718-1730

THELU, J., CHUMPITAZI, B., AMBROSE-THOMAS, P. (1989): Purification of *plasmodium falciparum* exoantigens by spuncolumn and chromatography, Ann. Trop. Med. Parasitol. **83**, 11-18

THOMAS, D.E., LANSDORP, P.M. (1988): Immunoadsorption of T cells onto glass beads using tetramolecular complexes of monoclonals antibodies. J. Immunol. **112**, 219-226

THOMAS, D.E., SUTHERLAND, H.J., LANSDORP, P.M. (1989): Specific binding and release of cells from beads using cleavable tetrameric antibody complexes. J. Immunol. Meth. **120**, 221-231

THORPE, R., PERRY, M.J., CALLUS, M., GAFFNEY, P.J., SPITZ, M. (1984): Single shot intraspleenic immunization: An advantageous procedure for the production of monoclonal antibodies specific for human fibrin fragments. Hybridoma **3**, 381-386

TIJSSEN, P. (1985): Practice and Theory of Enzyme Immunoassay (Laboratory Techniques in Biochemistry and Molecular Biology, Vol. 15), Elsevier Sci. Publ., Amsterdam

TIMASHEFF, S.N., ARAKAWA, T. (1989): Stabilization of protein structure by solvents. In: CREIGHTON, T.E. (ed.) Protein Structure - a Practial Approach, CRL Press, Oxford, pp. 331-345

TISELIUS, A., HJERTEN, S., LEVIN, Ö. (1956): Protein chromatography on calcium phosphate columns. Arch. Biochem. Biophys. **65**, 132-155

TONEGAWA, S. (1983): Somatic generation of antibody diversity. Nature **302**, 575-581

TOWBIN, H., GORDON, J. (1984): Immunoblotting and dot immunobinding - current status and outlook. J. Immunol. Meth. **72**, 313-340

TOWBIN, H., STAEHELIN, T., GORDON, J. (1979): Electrophoretic transfer of proteins from polyacrylamide gels to nitrocellulose sheets: Procedure and some applications, Proc. Natl. Acad. Sci. U.S.A.. **76**, 4350-4356

TRELEAVEN, J.G., GIBSON, F.M., UGELSTAD, J., REMBAUM, A., PHILIP, T., KEMSHEAD, J.T. (1984): Removal of neuroblastoma cells from bone marrow with monoclonal antibodies conjugated to magnetic microspheres, Lancet **I**, 70-73,

TRUCCO, M., DE PETRIS, S. (1981): Stabilization of protein structure by solvents. In: LEFKOVITS, I., PERNIS, B. (eds.) Immunological Methods, Vol. 2, Academic Press, New York, pp. 1-26

TRUCCO, M.M., STOCKER, J.W., CEPPELLINI, R. (1978): Monoclonal antibodies against human lymphocyte antigens. Nature **273**, 666-668

TRUFFA-BACHI, P., WOFSY, L. (1970): Specific separation of cells by affinity columns, Proc. Natl. Acad. Sci. U.S.A. **66**, 685-692

TU, Y.Y., PRIMUS, F.J., GOLDENBERG, D.M. (1988): Temperature affects binding of murine monoclonal IgG antibodies to protein A. J. Immunol. Meth. **109**, 43-47

TURESKY, R.J., FORSTER, C.M., AESCHBACHER, H.U., WURZENER, H.P., SKIPPER, P.L., TRUDEL, L.J., TANNENBAUM, S.R. (1989): Purification of the food-born carcinogens 2-amino-3-methylimidazo[4.5-f] quinoline and 2-amino-3,8-dimethyl imidazo[4.5-f] quinoxaline in heated meat products by immunoaffinity chromatography. Carcinogenesis **10**, 151-156

TURKOVA, J. (1978): Affinity Chromatography. J. Chromatogr. Library Vol. 12. Elsevier Sci. Publ., Amsterdam etc., pp. 13-87.

TURKOVA, J., PETKOV, L., SAJDOK, J., KAS, J., BENES, M.J. (1990): Carbohydrates as a tool for oriented immobilization of antigens and antibodies. J. Chromatogr. **500**, 585-593

URIOS, P., CITTANOVA, N.(1990): Adaption of fluorescence polarization immunoassay to the assay of macromolecules. Anal. Biochem. **185**, 308-312

VAESSEN, E.T.M.J., KREIKE, J., GROOT, G.S.P. (1981): Simple method for quantitation of single proteins in complex mixtures, FEBS Lett. **124**, 193-196

VARTDAL, F., GAUDERNACK, G., FUNDERUD, S. BRATLIE, A. LEA, T., UGELSTAD, J., THORSBY, E. (1986): HLA class I and II typing using cells positively selected from blood by immunomagnetic isolation - a fast and reliable technique. Tissue Antigens **28**, 301-312

VARTDAL, F., KVALHEIM, G., LEA, T., BOSNES, V., GAUDERNACK, G., UGELSTAD, J., ALBRECHTSEN, D.

(1987): Depletion of T lymphocytes from human bone marrow: Use of magnetic monosized polymer microspheres coated with lymphocyte-specific monoclonal antibodies, Transplantation **43**, 366-371

Vedeler, C.A., Matre, R., Kristoffersen, E.K. (1989): Solubilization of human peripheral nerve Fc receptors and purification of a functional 40 kDa receptor, Immunol. Lett. **22**, 281-286

Verwey, W.F. (1940): A type-specific antigenic protein derived from the Staphylococcus. J. Exp. Med. **71**, 635-644

Vockley, J., Bednarz, K., Harris, H. (1984): Purification of monoclonal antibodies to human alkaline phosphatase by antigen immunoaffinity chromatography: Comparison of their molar binding values. J. Immunol. Meth. **74**, 23-30

Vu Hai, M.T., Jolivet, A., Ravet, V. Lorenzo, F., Pierrot-Applanat, M., Citerne, M., Milgrom, E. (1989): Novel monoclonal antibodies against human uterine progesterone receptor. Mapping of receptor immunogenic domains. Biochem. J. **260**, 371-376

Wagener, C., Clark, B.R., Rickard, K.J., Shively, J.E. (1983): Monoclonal antibodies for carcinoembryonic antigen and related antigens as a model system: Determination of affinities and specificities of monoclonal antibodies by using biotin-labeled antibodies and avidin as precipitating agent in a solution phase immunoassay. J. Immunol. **130**, 2302-2307

Walker, D. (1988): Selection of a Western blotting detection system, Internat. Biotechnol. Lab. Dec. **88**, 8-11

Walzel, H., Brock, J., Franz, H., Ziska, P. (1989): Detection and quantitation of ligand leakage from lectin affinity columns. Biomed. Biochim. Acta **48**, 221-226

Ward, M.D., Buttry, D.A. (1990): In situ interfacial mass detection with piezoelectric transducers. Science **249**, 1000-1007

Weber, G., Dirckamer, H.G. (1983): The effect of pressure on proteins and other biomolecules. Quart. Rev. Biophys. **16**, 89-112

Wedel, von R.J. (1987): Mass culture of mouse and human hybridoma cells in hollow-fiber culture. In: Seaver, S.S. (ed.) The Commercial Production of Monoclonal Antibodies, Marcel Dekker Inc., New York, pp. 159-173

Weetall, H.H., Lee, M.J. (1989). Antibodies immobilized on inorganic supports. Appl. Biochem. Biotechnol. **22**, 311-330

Weihing, R.R. (1983): Purification of HeLa cell high molecular weight actin binding protein and its identification in HeLa cell plasma membrane ghosts and intact HeLa cells. Biochem. **22**, 1839-1847

Weile, Y., Renbin, Z. (1989): HPLC of biopolymers, pharmaceuticals, and natural products. J. Chromatogr. Sci. **27**, 626-652

Weir, D.M. (ed.) (1978): Handbook of Experimental Immunology, Blackwell Sci. Publ., London, Vol. 1

Weiss, M., Eisenstein, Z. (1987): A simple method to optimize elution from affinity chromatography. J. Liquid Chromatogr. **10**, 2815-2824

Westwood, S.A., Luzio, J.P., Flockhard, D.A., Siddle, K. (1979): Investigation of subcellular distribution of cyclic AMP phosphodiesterase in rat hepatocytes, using rapid immunological procedure for the isolation of plasma membrane. Biochim. Biophys. Acta **583**, 454-466

Whittle, N., Adair, J., Schlom, J., Raubitschek, A., Colcher, D., Bodmer, M. (1987): Expression in COS cells of mouse-human chimaeric B 72.3 antibody. Prot. Engng. **1**, 499-505

Wholtjen, H., Dessy, R. (1979): Surface acoustic wave probe for chemical analysis. I. Introduction and instrument description. Anal. Chem. **51**, 1458-1464

Wide, L., Porath, J.(1966): Radioimmunoassay of protein with the use of Sephadex-Coupled antibodies. Biochim. Biophys. Acta **130**, 257-260

Wigzell, H., Andersson, R. (1969): Cell separation on antigen-coated columns: Elimination of high rate antibody forming cells and immunological memory cells. J. Exp. Med. **129**, 23-26

Wilchek, M., Miron, T., Kohn, J. (1984): Affinity chromatography. Meth. Enzymol. **104**, 3-55

Wilton-Smith, P. (1987): Automating the production of monoclonal antibodies. Internat. Lab., April 1987, 62-66

Winkler, M. E., Bringman, T., Marks, B. J. (1986): The purification of fully active recombinant transforming growth factor produced in *Escherichia coli*. J. Biol. Chem. **261**, 13838-13843

Wormmeester, J. F., Stiekema, F., De Grott, K. (1984): A simple method for immunoselective cell separation with the avidin-biotin system. J. Immunol. Meth. **67**, 389-394

Worthington, J., Chan, C.-T. J., Byfield, P. G. H. (1986): Novel separation method for serum immunoglobulins. FEBS Lett. **211**, 123-128

Yalow, R.S., Berson, S.A.(1959): Assay of plasma insulin in human subjects by immunological methods. Nature **184**, 1648-1649

Yamakawa, Y., Chiba, J. (1988): High performance liquid chromatography of mouse monoclonal antibodies on spherical hydroxyapatite beads. J. Liquid Chromatogr. **11**, 665-681

Yang, Y.-C., Ciarleatta, A.B., Temple, P.A., Chung, M.P., Kovacic, S., Witek-Gianotti, J.S., Leary, A.C., Kriz, R., Donahue, R.E., Wong, G.G., Clark, S.C. (1986): Human IL-3 (multi-CSF): Identification by expression cloning a novel hematopoietic growth factor related to murine IL-3, Cell **47**, 3-10

Yarmush, M., Olson, W.C. (1988): Electrophoretic elution from biospecific adsorbents: Principles, methodology, and applications. Electrophoresis **9**, 111-120

Yokoyama, C., Shinjo, F., Yoshimota, T., Yamamoto, S., Oates, J.A., Brash, A.R. (1986): Aracchidonate 12-lipoxigenase purified from porcine leukocytes by immunoaffinity chromatography and its reactivity with hydroperoxyeicosatetraenoic acids. J. Biol. Chem. **261**, 16714-16721

Yoshida, T., Takamura, S., Suzuki, S. (1989): A simplified method for purification of an antitumor acidic glycoprotein from *Streptomyces pyogenes*. J. Antibiot. **42**, 448-453

Young, W.W., Jr., Tamura, Y., Wolock, D.M., Fox, J.W. (1984): Staphylococcal protein A binding to the Fab fragments of mouse monoclonal antibodies. J. Immunol. **133**, 3163-3166

Zara, J.J., Wood, R.D., Boon, P., Kim, C.-H., Pomato, N., Bredehorst, R., Vogel, C.-W. (1991): A carbohydrate-directed heterobifunctional cross-linking reagent for the synthesis of immunoconjugates. Anal. Biochem. **194**, 156-162

Zeng, C., Suzuki, Y., Alpert, E. (1990): Polyethylene glycol significantly enhances the transfer of membrane immunoblotting. Anal. Biochem. **189**, 197-201

Zhao, Y.-J., Belew, M. (1986): The effect of various coupling methods on the adsorption of serum proteins by immobilized concanavalin A. Biotechnol. Appl. Biochem. **8**, 75-82

Zimmermann, U., Scheurich, P. (1981): High frequency fusion of plant protoplasts by electric fields. Planta **151**, 26-32

References added in proof

Chapter 1

Jones, P. T. (1992): Antibody engineering. Biochem. Soc. Transact. **20**, 203-207

Zola, H. (1990): Laboratory Methods in Immunology, Vol. I and II. CRC Press, Inc., London

Chapter 2; Chapter 3

Domen, P.L., Nevens, J.R., Malla, A.K., Hermanson, G.T., Klenk, D.C. (1990): Site-directed immobilization of proteins. J. Chromatogr. **510**, 293-302

Gorchakov, V.D., Sakodynskii, K.I., Lebedin, Yu.S., Chuchalin, A.G. (1991): Immunoadsorbents for clinical use: ex vivo immunoglobulin D removal in allergy. J. Chromatogr. **563**, 166-171

Langlotz, P., Kroner, K. H. (1992): Surface-modified membranes as a matrix for protein purification. J. Chromatogr. **591**, 107-113

Morehead, H.W., Talmadge, K.W., O'Shannessy, D.J., Siebert, C.J. (1991): Optimization of oxidation of glycoproteins – an assay for predicting coupling to hydrazide chromatographic supports. J. Chromatogr. **587**, 171-176

Pflüger, E., Müller, E.A., Anderer, F.A. (1990): Preservation of cytotoxic function during multi-cycle immunomagnetic cell separations of human NK cells using a new type of magnetic bead. J. Immunol. Meth. **129**, 163-173

van Ginkel, L.A. (1991): Immunoaffinity chromatography, its application and limitations in multi-residue analysis of anabolizing and doping agents. J. Chromatogr. **564**, 363-384

Wimalasena, R., Wilson, G.S. (1992): Factors affecting the specific activity of immobilized antibodies and their biologically active fragments. J. Chromatogr. **572**, 85-102

Zara, J.J., Wood, R.D., Boon, P., Kim, C.-H., Pomato, N., Bredehorst, R., Vogel, C.-W. (1991): A carbohydrate-directed heterobifunctional cross-linking reagent for the synthesis of immunoconjugates. Anal. Biochem. **194**, 156-162

Chapter 3; Chapter 4

Butler, J. E. (1991): Immunochemistry of Solid-Phase Immunoassay. CRC Press Inc., London

Chaiken, I., Rosè, S., Karlsson, R. (1992): Analysis of macromolecular interactions using immobilized ligands. Anal. Biochem. **201**, 197-210

Deldado, C., Anderson, R. J., Francis, G. E., Fisher, D. (1991): Separation of cell mixtures by immunoaffinity cell partitioning: strategies for low abundance cells. Analyt. Biochem. **192**, 322-328

Dyer, P. A. (1992): Immuno-mediated cell separation methods. Biochem. Soc. Transact. **20**, 230-233

Hansel, T. T., De Vries, I. J. M., Iff, T. Rihs, S., Wandzilak, M., Betz, S., Blaser, K., Walker, C. (1991: An improved immunomagnetic procedure for the isolation of highly purified human blood eosinophils. J. Immunol. Methods **145**, 105-110

Highsmith, F., Regan, T., Clark, D., Drohan, W., Tharakan, J. (1992): Evaluation of CNBr, FMP and hydrazide resins for immunoaffinity purification of Factor IX. BioTechniques **12**, 418-423

Tsay, Y. G., Lin, C. I. Lee, J. Gustafson, E. K., Appelqvist, R., Magginetti, P., Norton, R., Teng, N., Charlton, D. (1991): Optical biosensor assay (OBA). Clin. Chem. **37**, 1502-1505

Turksen, K., Aubin, J. E. (1991): Positive and negative immunoselection for enrichment of two classes of osteoprogenitor cells. J. Cell Biol. **114**, 373-384

van Emon, J., Lopez-Avila, V. (1992): Immunochemical methods for environmental analysis. Anal. Chem. **64**, 78A-88A

Werner, R. G., Berthold, W., Hoffmann, H., Walter, J., Werz, W. (1992): Immunological techniques in biotechnology research. Biochem. Soc. Transact. **20**, 221-226

Subject Index

- M.R. Waterman, E.R. Simpson: Mechanisms of Regulation of Steroid Hydroxylase Gene Expression
- M. Okamoto, Y. Nonaka: Structure and Function of Adrenal Mitochondrial Cytochrome P-450 $_{11\beta}$
- S. Takemori, S. Kominami: Adrenal Microsomal Cytochrome P-450 Dependent Reactions in Steroidogenesis and Biochemical Properties of the Enzymes Involved therein
- R. Megges, M. Müller-Frohne, D. Pfeil, K. Ruckpaul: Microbial Steroid Hydroxylating Enzymes in Glucocorticoid Production

Volume 4

Microbial and Plant Cytochchromes P-450: Biochemical Characteristics Geneting Engineering and Practical Implications

Edited by Klaus Ruckpaul / Horst Rein

1991. IX, 240 pages – 71 figures
46 tables – 150 mm x 230 mm
Hardcover DM 98,–
ISBN 3-05-500460-4

From the Contents:
- H. Rein, K. Ruckpaul: Introduction
- O. Asperger, H.P. Kleber: Distribution and Diversity of Bacterial Cytochromes P-450
- S.A. Martinis, J.D. Ropp, S.G. Sligar, I.C. Gunsalus: Molecular Recognition by Cytochrome P-450cam Substrate Specifity, Catalysis and Electron Transfer
- H.-G. Müller, W.-H. Schunck, E. Kärgel: Cytochromes P-450 in Alkane-Assimilating-Yeasts
- Y. Yoshida, Y. Aoyama: Cytochromes P-450 in the Ergosterol Biosynthesis
- T. Hudnik-Plevnik, K. Breskvar: Cytochrome P-450 from Rhizopus nigricans
- Y. Yabusaki, H. Ohkawa: Genetic Engineering on Cytochrome P-450 Monooxygenases
- F. Durst: Biochemistry and Physiology of Plant Cytochrome P-450

Volume 5

Membrane Organization and Phospholipid Interaction of Cytochrome P-450

Edited by Klaus Ruckpaul / Horst Rein

1991. VIII, 210 pages – 61 figures
10 tables – 150 mm x 230 mm
Hardcover DM 210,–
ISBN 3-05-500461-2

From the Contents:
- K. Ruckpaul, H. Rein: Introduction
- P. Nuhn: Physicochemical Basis and Biological Properties of Membranes
- S.A.E. Finch, A. Stier: Rotational Diffusion of Homo- and Heterooligomers of Cytochrome P-450, the Functional Significance of Cooperativity and the Membrane Structure
- C.Richter, E.E. Dilorio: Analysis of the Membrane-Bound Cytochrome P-450 System by the Flash Photolysis Technique
- D.Schwarz: Rotational Motion and Membrane Topology of the Microsomal Cytochrome P-450 System as Analysed by Saturation Transfer EPR
- A.G. Krainev, L.M. Weiner: Localization of Active Centres of Endoplasmic Proteins in Membranes
- H. de Groot, I. Anundi, H. Sies: Cytochrome P-450 and Lipid Peroxidation

Volume 6

Cytochrome P-450 Dependent Biotransformation of Endogenous Substrates

Edited by Klaus Ruckpaul / Horst Rein

1991. VIII, 206 pages – 30 figures
14 tables – 150 mm x 230 mm
Hardcover DM 210,–
ISBN 3-05-501284-4

Bei Fragen zur Produktsicherheit wenden Sie sich bitte an:
If you have any questions regarding product safety,
please contact:

Walter de Gruyter GmbH
Genthiner Straße 13
10785 Berlin
productsafety@degruyterbrill.com